Controversies in Assisted Reproduction

To Dr. Ayten Murat, a very distinguished obstetrician and gynecologist,

for her incredible support during the production of this book

(BR)

I dedicate this to Professor Botros Rizk who transformed a friendly professional

conversation into this book, which does not aim to provide the ultimate answers

to all controversies in reproductive medicine but aims to encourage critical

thinking, open-mindedness, and acceptance that some clinical interventions we

practice now may or may not be corroborated by robust evidence in the future

(YK)

Controversies in Assisted Reproduction

Edited by

**Botros Rizk, MD, MA, FRCOG,
FRCS, HCLD, FACOG, FACS**
Medical Director, California Elite Fertility
Pasadena, California, USA and Shanghai, China
President, Middle East Fertility Society
and formerly Professor and Head, Reproductive Endocrinology & Infertility
Department of Obstetrics & Gynecology
University of South Alabama
Mobile, Alabama, USA

Yakoub Khalaf, MB BCh, MSc, MD, FRCOG, MFFP
Professor of Reproductive Medicine and Surgery
Guy's and St Thomas' Hospital *and* King's College London,
and Head, Fertility Service
Director, Assisted Conception Unit and Centre
for Pre-Implantation Genetic Diagnosis
Guy's and St Thomas' Hospital
London, UK

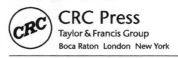
CRC Press
Taylor & Francis Group
Boca Raton London New York

CRC Press is an imprint of the
Taylor & Francis Group, an **Informa** business

CRC Press
Taylor & Francis Group
6000 Broken Sound Parkway NW, Suite 300
Boca Raton, FL 33487-2742

© 2020 by Taylor & Francis Group, LLC
CRC Press is an imprint of Taylor & Francis Group, an Informa business

No claim to original U.S. Government works

Printed on acid-free paper

International Standard Book Number-13: 978-0-8153-7458-9 (Paperback)
978-0-8153-7463-3 (Hardback)
978-1-351-24169-4 (eBook)

Library of Congress Control Number: 2020930158

Visit the Taylor & Francis Web site at
http://www.taylorandfrancis.com

and the CRC Press Web site at
http://www.crcpress.com

Contents

Contributors

Mohamed A. Aboulghar
Department of Obstetrics and Gynecology
Faculty of Medicine
Cairo University
and
The Egyptian IVF Center, Maadi
Cairo, Egypt

Mona M. Aboulghar
Department of Obstetrics and Gynecology
Faculty of Medicine
Cairo University
and
The Egyptian IVF Center, Maadi
Cairo, Egypt

Shima Elbakhit Albasha
Department of Obstetrics and Gynecology
Hamad Medical Corporation
Doha, Qatar

Jad Farid Assaf
AUBMC Haifa Idriss Fertility Center
and
Department of Obstetrics and Gynecology
American University of Beirut Medical Center
Beirut, Lebanon

Johnny Awwad
AUBMC Haifa Idriss Fertility Center
and
Department of Obstetrics and Gynecology
American University of Beirut Medical Center
Beirut, Lebanon

M. Yusuf Beebeejaun
King's Fertility
King's College Hospital
London, United Kindom

Siladitya Bhattacharya
School of Medicine
Cardiff University
Wales, United Kingdom

Christophe Blockeel
Centre for Reproductive Medicine
Universitair Ziekenhuis Brussel
Brussels, Belgium

David Bolumar
Igenomix Foundation
and
Department of Obstetrics and Gynecology
University of Valencia/INCLIVA
Valencia, Spain

Fadi Choucair
AUBMC Haifa Idriss Fertility Center
and
Department of Obstetrics and Gynecology
American University of Beirut Medical Center
Beirut, Lebanon

Panagiotis Drakopoulos
Centre for Reproductive Medicine
Universitair Ziekenhuis Brussel
Brussels, Belgium

Chantal Farra
Department of Pathology and Laboratory
    Medicine
American University of Beirut Medical Center
Beirut, Lebanon

Human Fatemi
Medical Department
IVI Middle East
Abu Dhabi and Dubai, United Arab Emirates

and

Medical Department
IVI Middle East
Muscat, Oman

Andy Greenfield
Mammalian Genetics Unit
Medical Research Council Harwell Institute
Oxfordshire, United Kingdom

Dalia Khalife
Department of Obstetrics and Gynecology
American University of Beirut Medical Center
Beirut, Lebanon

Efstratios Kolibianakis
Unit for Human Reproduction
First Department of Obstetrics and Gynaecology
    Medical School
Aristotle University of Thessaloniki
Thessaloniki, Greece

Barbara Lawrenz
Medical Department
IVI Middle East
Abu Dhabi, United Arab Emirates

and

Obstetrical Department
Women's University Hospital Tuebingen
Tuebingen, Germany

Shari Mackens
Centre for Reproductive Medicine
Universitair Ziekenhuis Brussel
Brussels, Belgium

Abha Maheshwari
Department of Aberdeen Fertility Centre
NHS Grampian
Aberdeen, United Kingdom

Neena Malhotra
Department of Obstetrics and Gynecology
All India Institute of Medical Sciences
New Delhi, India

Laura Melado
Medical Department
IVI Middle East
Abu Dhabi and Dubai, United Arab Emirates

Nicole C. Michel
Department of Reproductive Endocrinology
University of South Alabama
Mobile, Alabama

Pavlidi Olga
Unit for Human Reproduction
First Department of Obstetrics and Gynecology
    Medical School
Aristotle University of Thessaloniki
Thessaloniki, Greece

Biljana Popovic-Todorovic
Centre for Reproductive Medicine
Universitair Ziekenhuis Brussel
Brussels, Belgium

Annalisa Racca
Centre for Reproductive Medicine
Universitair Ziekenhuis Brussel
Brussels, Belgium

Abdel-Maguid Ramzy
Department of Obstetrics and
    Gynecology
Cairo University
and
Kasr Al-Aini IVF Center
Cairo, Egypt

Samuel Santos-Ribeiro
IVI-RMA Lisboa
Lisbon, Portugal

Alejandro Rincón
Igenomix SL
Valencia, Spain

Natalie Shammas
Medical Student
Georgetown University School of
    Medicine
Washington, DC

Carlos Simón
Igenomix SL
and
Igenomix Foundation
and
Department of Obstetrics and
    Gynecology
University of Valencia/INCLIVA
Valencia, Spain

and

Department of Obstetrics and
    Gynecology
Stanford University
Stanford, California

and

Department of Obstetrics and Gynecology
Baylor College of Medicine
Houston, Texas

Elsie Sowah
St. George's University of London
MBBS Programme at University of Nicosia
     Medical School
Nicosia, Cyprus

Hans-Peter Steiner
Inst. f. IVF
IVF Future
IVFETFLEX.COM
Graz, Austria

Sesh K. Sunkara
Division of Women's Health
Faculty of Life Sciences and Medicine
King's College London
London, United Kindom

Vasilios Tanos
University of Nicosia Medical School
and
Aretaeio Hospital
Nicosia, Cyprus

Diana Valbuena
Igenomix SL
Valencia, Spain

Christos A. Venetis
School of Women's and Children's Health
and
Centre for Big Data Research in Health
Faculty of Medicine
University of New South Wales
New South Wales, Australia

1

The Use of Ovarian Markers

Neena Malhotra and Siladitya Bhattacharya

Introduction

Ovarian reserve is a term used to describe a woman's reproductive potential and is a reflection of her pool of primordial follicles or, more specifically, the number and quality of oocytes in her ovaries (1). Each woman is born with approximately 2 million primordial follicles, but this number drops to 400,000 around menarche as a consequence of follicular atresia (2). Follicle numbers fall further with age, and the rate of decline is faster when women are in their mid-30s. This decline in fertility potential is specific for an individual woman and is influenced by race as well as genetic and environmental factors.

The ideal ovarian reserve test should be convenient, reproducible, display little if any intracycle and intercycle variability, and demonstrate high specificity to minimize the risk of false diagnoses. At the same time, the test should be able to identify women with an abundance of ovarian reserve and those who are likely to respond vigorously to ovarian stimulation in the context of fertility treatment. A number of biomarkers have been used over the last few decades to predict ovarian response and pregnancy outcomes, including live birth in women undergoing *in vitro* fertilization (IVF). These include hormonal assessments and ultrasound parameters.

Hormonal biomarkers include serum early follicular (basal) levels of follicle-stimulating hormone (FSH), estradiol (E2), inhibin B, and anti-Müllerian hormone (AMH), as well as dynamic tests that measure gonadotropins and estradiol levels in response to stimulation, like the clomiphene citrate challenge test (CCCT), GnRH-agonist stimulation test (GAST), or exogenous FSH ovarian reserve test (EFORT).

Ultrasonographic assessments include antral follicle count (AFC) and ovarian volume. The number of antral follicles reflects the size of the remaining follicular pool and correlates with the number of oocytes retrieved following stimulation. Ovarian volume declines with advancing age and is a potential indicator of ovarian reserve.

This chapter considers the basic principles governing the use of diagnostic tests and reviews common tests of ovarian reserve including their role in predicting fertility with and without assisted reproduction treatment.

Understanding Diagnostic Tests

As diagnostic tests are seldom 100% accurate, tests need to be validated by comparing them with an ideal test or a gold standard in a suitable population of patients. A valid test is able to identify most people with a particular condition and exclude most people without that condition such that a positive test result means that the disorder in question is present (3). Conventionally, four terms are used to qualify the validity of a test—sensitivity, specificity, positive predictive value, and negative predictive value (Figure 1.1). Sensitivity is the true positive rate that expresses how good the test is for correctly identifying those with the condition. In contrast, specificity is the true negative rate that tells us how good a test is for correctly excluding people without the condition.

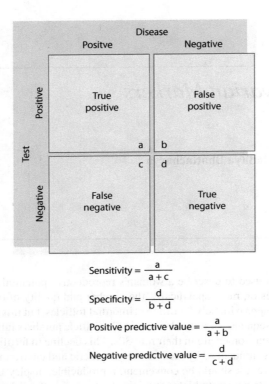

FIGURE 1.1   Calculation of test validity. (With permission from Grimes D, Schulz K. *Lancet*. 2002;359[9309]:881–4.)

As both sensitivity and specificity represent a retrospective analysis of results that have already been collected, their clinical use is limited. In real life, clinicians need to know the predictive value of the test, i.e., whether a patient who tests positive actually has the disease or condition in question. Positive predictive value is the posttest probability of a positive test. It tells the clinician what the probability of having that condition is if the patient tests positive. Negative predictive value tells the clinician the probability of a patient not having a condition if the patient tests negative. It is customary to express the validity of the test by plotting sensitivity against one minus specificity and measure the area under the curve (AUC). AUC is an effective way to summarize the overall diagnostic accuracy of the test by plotting values between 0 and 1 (Figure 1.2), where a value of 0 indicates a totally inaccurate test and a value of 1 a perfectly accurate test. An AUC of 0.5 indicates an inability to diagnose patients with and without a particular condition, while 0.8–1.0 is considered excellent (6).

The prevalence of disease in a population affects the performance of screening tests. Even excellent tests have poor predictive value positives in low-prevalence settings. For example, a valid test of ovarian reserve will have a better positive predictive value in women attending a fertility clinic than in a general population of asymptomatic women. Hence, knowledge of the approximate prevalence of disease is a prerequisite to interpreting screening test results. Inappropriate application or interpretation of screening tests can rob people of their perceived health, initiate harmful diagnostic testing, and squander health-care resources. From a clinical perspective, key questions about tests include the following: Is it relevant, i.e., can the test be used in the relevant patient group? Is it affordable, acceptable, and better than the test normally used? And crucially, Will it inform the choice of treatment?

Early Follicular Follicle-Stimulating Hormone

Levels of basal FSH in the early follicular phase have been used as a biomarker for the prediction of response to ovarian stimulation during *in vitro* fertilization (IVF) (7,8). The test is based on the feedback inhibition of FSH pituitary secretion by ovarian hormones. Women with normal ovarian activity should produce sufficient

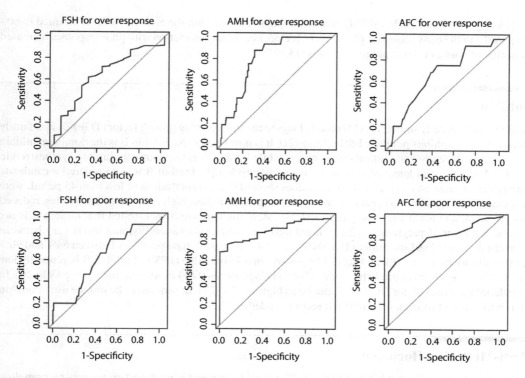

FIGURE 1.2 Receiver operating characteristic curves and area under the curve for a number of common ovarian reserve tests. (With permission from Nardo L et al. *Fertil Steril.* 2009;92[5]:1586–93.)

levels of ovarian hormones at this early stage of the menstrual cycle to suppress FSH levels within a normal range. Elevated serum FSH levels suggest poor production of ovarian estrogen by a smaller follicular pool consistent with diminished ovarian reserve (DOR). However, basal FSH testing has several major limitations, including significant intercycle and intracycle variability (9,10) and limited sensitivity when used in isolation. Measurement of both FSH and estradiol on cycle day 3 may therefore help decrease the incidence of false-negative testing. Despite its limitations, FSH is commonly used as an ovarian reserve test, and high values have been associated with both poor ovarian response and failure to achieve pregnancy (11). FSH has relatively high specificity (45%–100%) for poor response to ovarian stimulation (usually defined as less than four retrieved oocytes) using cutoff points beyond 10 IU/L (10–20 IU/L), but its sensitivity is generally poor (11%–86%) (11,12). In terms of predicting lack of conception, FSH testing is still specific (50%–100%) but much less sensitive (3%–65%) using similar cutoffs (11,12). This test is still clinically useful since an abnormally elevated FSH result implies DOR (high positive predictive value); however, normal levels do not rule out DOR, as the majority of these women will have a normal FSH test result (low negative predictive value). Moreover, a single abnormal FSH value in a woman younger than 40 years of age may not predict a poor response to stimulation or failure to achieve pregnancy (13) and should prompt repeat testing.

Estradiol

Basal estradiol between days 2 and 5 of the menstrual cycle has poor inter- and intracycle reliability as a test of ovarian reserve (14). In isolation, basal estradiol does not discriminate between women with or without DOR, when used to interpret response to ovarian stimulation or pregnancy outcome (15–17). Basal estradiol alone should therefore not be used to screen for DOR. The test has some value as an additional test in the interpretation of a "normal" basal serum FSH value, as an early rise in serum estradiol concentrations is a characteristic of reproductive aging that can result in a spuriously low basal

FSH level (18). When the basal FSH concentration is "normal" but the estradiol level is elevated (>60–80 pg/mL) in the early follicular phase, there is evidence for an association with poor response, increased cancellation rates, or lower pregnancy rates (15,19,20).

Inhibin B

Inhibin is structurally similar to AMH and belongs to the transforming growth factor (TGF)-β superfamily that selectively inhibits pituitary FSH release (21). It is now known that inhibin B is the dominant inhibin produced in the early and midfollicular phases, while inhibin A is the dominant inhibin synthesized in the late follicular and luteal phases of the menstrual cycle (21). Inhibin B was considered a candidate biomarker for ovarian reserve, and initial studies showed that concentrations of less than 45 pg/mL were associated with age above 35 years, poor response to gonadotropins, high cycle cancellation rates, reduced oocyte yield, and lower pregnancy rates (22,23). Most studies have demonstrated that inhibin B is not a good predictor of pregnancy (12,24). It exhibits high intracycle variability, and levels vary between menstrual cycles (25). Low inhibin B in the range of 40–45 pg/mL has specificity between 64% and 90% and sensitivity between 40% and 80%. The positive predictive value (PPV) of inhibin B is generally low (19%–22%) and negative predictive value (NPV) is high (95%–97%) in women undergoing IVF (26). In populations at high risk for DOR, PPV can be as high as 83% (27). In summary, the routine use of inhibin B as a measure of ovarian reserve is not recommended (1,12,24).

Anti-Müllerian Hormone

AMH is a glycoprotein that belongs to the TGF-β superfamily and is produced exclusively by granulosa cells of small and large preantral and small antral follicles (28). AMH production begins *in utero* at around 36 weeks by the fetal ovary and is measurable in infants; however, its levels rise in young women, beginning in adolescence and peaking at about 25 years of age (29). There is a gradual decline in AMH levels until it is undetectable a few years prior to menopause. AMH has a negative effect on early folliculogenesis by inhibiting recruitment of primary follicles from the primordial pool, preventing selection of follicles by FSH, and diminishing aromatase production (30,31). As AMH is secreted by follicles up to 6 mm mainly during normal early folliculogenesis, it is relatively independent of gonadotropin control—a feature that allows testing anytime throughout the cycle. Initial studies suggested that AMH levels were relatively stable throughout the menstrual cycle in normo-ovulatory women (32–34); however, later studies suggest fluctuations within a menstrual cycle (35–37). While this issue remains highly debated, evidence suggests that these fluctuations are limited to younger women (38) and those with high AMH levels (36) but are of little relevance in patients with low ovarian reserve (36,38).

AMH is considered the most sensitive of all the ovarian reserve tests and the first to be altered in aging ovaries (39). In a systematic review of studies in women undergoing controlled ovarian stimulation with gonadotropins, low AMH cutoff points (0.1–1.66 ng/mL) had sensitivities ranging between 44% and 97% and specificities ranging between 41% and 100% for prediction of poor ovarian response (28). A meta-analysis including 28 studies showed that AMH had good predictive ability for poor ovarian response, with an AUC of 0.78 (40). The ability of AMH in predicting ovarian hyperstimulation during gonadotropin stimulation displayed sensitivities ranging from 53% to 90.5% and specificities ranging from 70% to 94.9%, with cutoff values of 3.36–5.0 ng/mL (28). However, despite its strong correlation with ovarian response to stimulation in assisted reproductive technology (ART), AMH is a poor predictor of nonpregnancy with sensitivities between 19% and 66%, and specificities between 55% and 89% when using cutoffs ranging from less than 0.1 to 1.66 ng/mL (41).

Recent data from the Society for Assisted Reproductive Technology (SART) showed that women with extremely low AMH (<0.16 ng/mL) had an average cycle cancellation rate of 54% and an overall live birth rate per cycle starting at 9.5% (42), highlighting the view that denying infertility treatment solely on the basis of AMH levels is not advisable. In a recent systematic review and meta-analysis on the predictive ability of AMH for implantation and clinical pregnancy in women undergoing ART, it was suggested that AMH has some association with implantation and clinical pregnancy but that its predictive ability is weak (43). A recent analysis of the SART database on the association of AMH with live birth analyzed over 85,000 non-preimplantation genetic diagnosis fresh and frozen embryo transfer and concluded that AMH was a poor predictor of live birth when used independently (44). However, similar analysis from the database could give meaningful conclusions on the potential of AMH on predicting live birth. A major limitation of testing AMH for ovarian reserves relates to assay variability and lack of standardized international assay. There were two different assays used—Immunotech Beckman Coulter (IBC, Marseille, France) assay and Diagnostic Systems Laboratories Inc. (DSL, Webster, Texas) assay—which were developed independently with different antibodies and reported very different results, using different units. This problem was overcome by manufacturing both enzyme-linked immunosorbent assays (ELISAs) and the development of a new assay by the same company (Gen II, Beckman Coulter Inc., Brea, California), which combines the best features of both (45). However, several studies have demonstrated intra-assay/interassay differences, between-laboratory differences, and sample stability and storage issues related to the Gen II assay as well (46). To overcome some of these issues, automated AMH assay platforms are available that offer greater precision (fourfold), faster turnaround time (18 minutes versus 6 hours), and greater sensitivity (10-fold) compared to current ELISA-based assays (47,48). This should resolve the confusion over interpretation of the AMH results.

Considering a wide inter-/intra-assay difference, fertility clinics are relying on age-specific AMH as provided by several studies in prognosticating and decisions in regard to treatment (49–51). These reference values are age appropriate and not referenced to a general population of women independent of age. As a general rule, the lower limits of age-appropriate serum AMH values in 5-year age intervals are given approximately as follows: 0.5 ng/mL for 45 years, 1 ng/mL for 40 years, 1.5 ng/mL for 35 years, 2.5 ng/mL for 30 years, and 3.0 ng/mL for 25 years. These are conservative estimates, as the most widely used AMH assay, Gen II, reports about 30%–40% higher mean values compared to these guidelines (52).

Besides biological age, possible factors influencing interpretation of AMH include reproductive and lifestyle patterns. Elevated AMH levels are associated with polycystic ovary syndrome (PCOS) (53,54), while decreased AMH levels can be found with ovarian suppression with oral contraceptive pills or GnRH agonist administration, which return to baseline within 3–4 months of oral contraceptive discontinuation (55). AMH levels cannot be reliably used to express the ovarian reserves, as these would be inaccurate in these women. Lifestyle modifications including smoking, low vitamin D levels, and obesity have also been linked with low serum AMH levels (56).

Dynamic Ovarian Reserve Tests

Clomiphene Citrate Challenge Test

The clomiphene citrate challenge test (CCCT) involves measurements of serum FSH before (cycle day 3) and after (cycle day 10) treatment with clomiphene citrate (100 mg daily, cycle days 5–9). The test is based on the fact that rising inhibin B and estradiol levels from a growing cohort of ovarian follicles will suppress FSH in women with responsive ovaries. In women with DOR, the follicular cohorts will generate less inhibin B and estradiol, resulting in decreased negative feedback inhibition of FSH secretion and higher stimulated FSH concentrations. An elevated FSH concentration after clomiphene stimulation is suggestive of DOR. Studies of CCCT results have observed significant intercycle variability in stimulated FSH levels and in the difference between basal and stimulated estradiol and inhibin B concentrations, which limits the reliability of the CCCT (57,58).

Exogenous FSH Ovarian Reserve Test

This ovarian reserve screening method involved baseline measurement of FSH and E2, followed by administration of a standard intramuscular (IM) dose (300 IU) of purified FSH on day 3. E2 levels were rechecked 24 hours later. IVF with GnRH-a and human menopausal gonadotropin (hMG) was undertaken two menstrual cycles later, and the post-FSH E2 increment (Δ E2) and the baseline FSH values (b FSH) were evaluated and compared with the subsequent quality of the ovarian response in IVF and pregnancy outcome. This test consumes considerable time and therefore is rarely used, besides producing a high false-positive rate (12) as mentioned in a systematic review. The test is not recommended in clinical settings.

GnRH-Agonist Stimulation Test

The physiologic response to gonadotropin-releasing hormone agonists (GnRH-a), with an initial E2 rise followed by profound suppression in E2 levels, is well accepted. Subsequently, it was hypothesized that latent impairments in ovarian reserve might be uncovered by recording differences in endogenous gonadotropin and E2 levels after GnRH-a administration (59). In contrast to the CCCT, both pituitary gonadotropin output and the ovarian response can be assessed by this technique. This approach was later formalized as a screening tool known as the GnRH-a stimulation test (60). When used in regularly cycling women, GAST appears to demonstrate high accuracy in prediction of poor response and was considered a candidate for more extensive confirmatory research (12).

The overall diagnostic accuracy of the previously mentioned dynamic ovarian reserves was assessed in a systematic review (61) that concluded that the diagnostic odds of abnormal CCCT for nonpregnancy were 2.11 (95% confidence interval [CI], 1.04–4.29) at FSH greater than 10 IU/L (day 3 or 10). The diagnostic accuracy of GAST and EFORT could not be quantified in this systematic review due to inconsistencies in the test methodology across available studies. The suggestion from this review was to abandon the use of dynamic tests for ovarian reserve assessments (61).

Ovarian Response to Gonadotropin Stimulation

Response to gonadotropin is one of the best dynamic tests, as it is a testimony to the primordial pool or reserves that ovary bears. Poor ovarian response to ovarian stimulation is identified by a reduced follicular response with reduced number of oocytes retrieved to maximal stimulation during IVF. In defining the poor ovarian response, the European Society of Human Reproduction and Embryology (ESHRE) working group proposed the Bologna criteria that two of the following criteria be present to accept a given low response to stimulation as a poor ovarian response: (a) advanced maternal age or any other risk factor for poor ovarian response, (b) a previous poor ovarian response, and (c) an abnormal ovarian reserve test. Two episodes of poor ovarian response after maximal stimulation are sufficient to define a patient as a poor responder in the absence of advanced maternal age or an abnormal ovarian reserve test (62). Besides the number of oocytes retrieved, embryology data including fertilization rate, cleavage patterns, embryo granularity, fragmentation, day of embryo transfer, and cell number at transfer are more meaningful than the hormonal, sonographic, and other dynamic assessments prior to the IVF cycle. In the setting with recently demonstrated good or poor ovarian response, the ovarian reserve tests are sufficient, and it is unnecessary to repeat testing with hormone and ultrasound processes (1).

Antral Follicular Count

AFC is defined as the sum of follicles measuring 2–10 mm in both ovaries visualized by ultrasound during the early follicular phase (day 2–4) of the menstrual cycle. It is important to emphasize that these measurements are done in a two- or three-dimensional mode using a transvaginal probe between 8 and 12 MHz. The advantages of AFC include the ease and opportunistic nature of the procedure, the ability to generate an immediate result, and good intercycle and interobserver reliability if done by experienced health professionals (12). Technical challenges in obese patients can reduce the precision of AFC (41), while intracycle and interobserver variations can be caused by differences in operator training, criteria for measuring antral follicles, and differences in ultrasound technology. Intercycle and intracycle variability due to operator-related factors have been noted.

In a meta-analysis, a low AFC has been shown to be strongly associated with poor ovarian response to ovarian stimulation during IVF but less predictive for pregnancy. In women undergoing IVF, an AFC of three to four follicles (both ovaries combined) has high specificity (73%–97%) for poor ovarian response but low sensitivity (9%–73%) for poor ovarian response (12). In another meta-analysis, the AUC for AFC in predicting poor ovarian response was 0.76 (40). In predicting nonpregnancy, AFC is still specific

(64%–98%) but much less sensitive (7%–34%) (12). However, both AFC and AMH have been shown to be valid tests for identifying women at risk for ovarian hyper stimulation syndrome (OHSS).

Previous work has shown that the two tests are comparable in terms of accuracy (41), but secondary analysis of data from a randomized trial (63) has suggested that AMH may be a better predictor of number of oocytes retrieved.

Ovarian Volume

Calculation of ovarian volume is based on the formula of an ellipsoid measuring each ovary in three planes (D1 × D2 × D3 × 0.52 = volume) and using the mean ovarian volume, which is the average volume of both ovaries in the same individual. However, this may not be reliable in situations when there is ovarian pathology including PCOS, endometriomas, and large cysts (1). Some studies report significant intercycle variability, but this observation is not consistent (64). When ovarian volume is acquired and stored by three-dimensional ultrasound, intra- and interobserver variability are minimized, but this may require specialized equipment (65). Overall, ovarian volume correlates with number of follicles and retrieved oocytes but not as well with pregnancy (66). Low ovarian volume, typically less than 3 mL, or low mean diameter, less than 2 cm, predicts poor response to ovarian stimulation with high specificity (80%–90%) and a wide range of sensitivity (11%–80%) (25), but overall, it is fair to conclude that ovarian volume has a poor predictability as a biomarker.

Clinical Utility of Ovarian Reserve Tests

In *In Vitro* Fertilization

Historically, ovarian reserve tests were developed for women undergoing ART procedures in order to identify those that are likely to have a diminished or exaggerated ovarian response to hormonal stimulation. AMH and AFC predict ovarian response, such as the number of follicles, the number of oocytes retrieved, the number of embryos, and cancellation rate, with reasonable efficiency (67). Although both tests are comparable in terms of test accuracy for ovarian response and nonconception, AMH is considered by some to have an edge due to the subjective elements associated with AFC assessment.

AMH less than 0.5 ng/mL predicts poor ovarian response in IVF (defined as less than four oocytes) (68). These women need careful counseling and protocols that optimize oocyte yield. Women with AMH levels greater than 1.0 ng/mL and <3.5 ngm/mL are expected to have a normal response to ovarian stimulation with standard agonist or antagonist stimulation protocols (52). Levels of AMH greater than 3.5 ngm/mL are associated with a risk of OHSS and should prompt caution when planning stimulation protocols (69). While ongoing live birth is the most clinically relevant indicator of success, most tests of ovarian reserve are poor predictors of this key outcome. An individual patient data (IPD) meta-analysis based on 1008 patients undergoing fertility treatment demonstrated a weak association of AMH with ongoing pregnancy (40). Although AMH is associated with live birth after assisted conception, its predictive accuracy is poor (44).

Results from a recent randomized trial indicate that in women undergoing IVF/intracytoplasmic sperm injection (ICSI), individualized FSH dosing based on ovarian reserve testing by AFC does not improve live birth rates or reduce costs as compared to a standard FSH dose (70). In women with predicted poor response, a personalized approach to ovarian stimulation based on AFC is unable to enhance live birth rates but does increase costs (71). However, in women with a predicted hyperresponse (based on AFC of greater than 15), a reduced dose of gonadotropins for ovarian stimulation results in comparable cumulative life birth rates in comparison with a standard dose but reduces the overall risk of ovarian hyperstimulation (72).

Use of Ovarian Biomarkers beyond Assisted Reproduction

Beyond IVF, ovarian reserve tests have found limited utility in the management of women with fertility problems. They have not been found to be more useful than age alone in the prediction of pregnancy in women presenting with unexplained infertility or mild male infertility (73).

A number of studies suggest that AMH levels along with age are useful in predicting age at menopause with accuracy in women at advanced ages (74,75). However, in a recent individual participant data meta-analysis, the additional predictive value of AMH (compared to age alone) was minimal (age alone C-statistic 84%; age + AMH HR 0.66 95% CI 0.61–0.71, C-statistic 86%), although the accuracy of AMH as a predictive test increased with decreasing age of menopause (76).

With advances in cancer detection and therapy, more young women are surviving cancers; however, the major concerns among survivors is the loss of ovarian function and fertility. With the availability of AMH, it has been possible to detect the iatrogenic loss in ovarian reserves by measuring this biomarker pre- and posttreatment with chemotherapy or radiotherapy (77). Further, AMH levels are useful in planning fertility-preserving options and counseling accordingly.

There is sufficient evidence to suggest that AMH is involved in the pathogenesis of PCOS, and levels correlate with the severity of the condition. A cutoff of AMH greater than 5.0 ng/mL has been shown to be highly diagnostic of PCOS (AUC 0.973, sensitivity 92%, specificity 97%), and it has been suggested that this should be incorporated as a diagnostic criterion (54).

Use in the General Population

Whether ovarian reserve tests should be offered to women without immediate fertility concerns is a contentious subject. In the last few decades, there has been an increase in the age of first planned pregnancy as women continue to delay childbearing in their pursuit of higher education and careers. This has created a space for ovarian reserve testing to inform reproductive decisions such as cryopreservation of oocytes in order to preserve future fertility. Proponents of ovarian reserve testing suggest that many women might modify their plans for childbearing on the basis of their ovarian reserve test results. However, the opponents of such testing feel that it adds to anxiety and negative psychological impact that may have a bearing on their decisions on career and marital relationship. There is no consensus on the routine testing of ovarian reserves in the general population. From a methodological perspective, ovarian reserve tests, like AMH, are some distance away from fulfilling the criteria for an ideal screening test. The positive predictive value is likely to be poor in an unselected population of younger women in whom the prevalence of diminished ovarian reserve is low. It is also unclear how often screening should be performed, what the potential physical and psychological impacts of screening might be, and what interventions are available for those who test positive.

Conclusion

Age-related decline in oocyte quality and quantity undermines the success rate of IVF. There is a need for an ovarian reserve test that can predict live birth. AMH and AFC are able to estimate ovarian response but not live birth with any degree of accuracy. AMH has the advantage of being a more objective measure as well as slightly superior in identifying any chance of pregnancy.

REFERENCES

1. Practice Committee of the American Society for Reproductive Medicine. Testing and interpreting measures of ovarian reserve: A committee opinion. *Fertil Steril.* 2015;103(3):e9–e17.
2. Tal R, Seifer D. Ovarian reserve testing: A user's guide. *Am J Obstet Gynecol.* 2017;217(2):129–40.
3. Greenhalgh T. How to read a paper: Papers that report diagnostic or screening tests. *Br Med J.* 1997;315(7107):540–3.
4. Grimes D, Schulz K. Uses and abuses of screening tests. *Lancet.* 2002;359(9309):881–4.
5. Nardo L, Gelbaya T, Wilkinson H et al. Circulating basal anti-Müllerian hormone levels as predictor of ovarian response in women undergoing ovarian stimulation for in vitro fertilization. *Fertil Steril.* 2009;92(5):1586–93.
6. Hosmer D, Lemeshow S. *Applied Logistic Regression.* 2nd ed. New York, NY: Wiley; 2000.

7. Scott R, Toner J, Muasher S et al. Follicle-stimulating hormone levels on cycle day 3 are predictive of *in vitro* fertilization outcome. *Fertil Steril.* 1989;51(4):651–4.
8. Toner J, Philput C, Jones G, Muasher S. Basal follicle-stimulating hormone level is a better predictor of in vitro fertilization performance than age. *Fertil Steril.* 1991;55(4):784–91.
9. Scott R, Hofmann G, Oehninger S, Muasher S. Intercycle variability of day 3 follicle-stimulating hormone levels and its effect on stimulation quality in *in vitro* fertilization. *Fertil Steril.* 1990;54(2):297–302.
10. Kwee J, Schats R, McDonnell J et al. Intercycle variability of ovarian reserve tests: Results of a prospective randomized study. *Hum Reprod.* 2004;19(3):590–5.
11. Esposito M, Coutifaris C, Barnhart K. A moderately elevated day 3 FSH concentration has limited predictive value, especially in younger women. *Hum Reprod.* 2002;17(1):118–23.
12. Broekmans F, Kwee J, Hendriks D et al. A systematic review of tests predicting ovarian reserve and IVF outcome. *Hum Reprod Update.* 2006;12(6):685–718.
13. Roberts J, Spandorfer S, Fasouliotis S et al. Taking a basal follicle-stimulating hormone history is essential before initiating *in vitro* fertilization. *Fertil Steril.* 2005;83(1):37–41.
14. Fanchin R, Taieb J, Lozano D et al. High reproducibility of serum anti-Müllerian hormone measurements suggests a multi-staged follicular secretion and strengthens its role in the assessment of ovarian follicular status. *Hum Reprod.* 2005;20(4):923–7.
15. Evers J, Slaats P, Land J et al. Elevated levels of basal estradiol-17β predict poor response in patients with normal basal levels of follicle-stimulating hormone undergoing *in vitro* fertilization. *Fertil Steril.* 1998;69(6):1010–4.
16. Phophong P, Ranieri D, Khadum I et al. Basal 17β-estradiol did not correlate with ovarian response and in vitro fertilization treatment outcome. *Fertil Steril.* 2000;74(6):1133–6.
17. Bancsi L, Broekmans F, Eijkemans M et al. Predictors of poor ovarian response in in vitro fertilization: A prospective study comparing basal markers of ovarian reserve. *Fertil Steril.* 2002;77(2):328–36.
18. Ranieri D, Quinn F, Makhlouf A et al. Simultaneous evaluation of basal follicle-stimulating hormone and 17β-estradiol response to gonadotropin-releasing hormone analogue stimulation: An improved predictor of ovarian reserve. *Fertil Steril.* 1998;70(2):227–33.
19. Licciardi F, Liu H, Rosenwaks Z. Day 3 estradiol serum concentrations as prognosticators of ovarian stimulation response and pregnancy outcome in patients undergoing *in vitro* fertilization. *Fertil Steril.*;64(5):991–4.
20. Smotrich D, Widra E, Gindoff P et al. Prognostic value of day 3 estradiol on *in vitro* fertilization outcome. *Obstet Gynecol Surv.* 1996;51(4):235–7.
21. Soules M, Battaglia D, Klein N. Inhibin and reproductive aging in women. *Maturitas.* 1998;30(2):193–204.
22. Klein N, Illingworth P, Groome N et al. Decreased inhibin B secretion is associated with the monotropic FSH rise in older, ovulatory women: A study of serum and follicular fluid levels of dimeric inhibin A and B in spontaneous menstrual cycles. *J Clin Endocrinol Metab.* 1996;81(7):2742–5.
23. Seifer D, Lambert-Messerlian G, Hogan J et al. Day 3 serum inhibin-B is predictive of assisted reproductive technologies outcome. *Fertil Steril.* 1997;67(1):110–4.
24. Creus M, Penarrubia J, Fabregues F et al. Day 3 serum inhibin B and FSH and age as predictors of assisted reproduction treatment outcome. *Hum Reprod.* 2000;15(11):2341–6.
25. McIlveen M, Skull J, Ledger W. Evaluation of the utility of multiple endocrine and ultrasound measures of ovarian reserve in the prediction of cycle cancellation in a high-risk IVF population. *Hum Reprod.* 2007;22(3):778–85.
26. Muttukrishna S, McGarrigle H, Wakim R et al. Antral follicle count, anti-Müllerian hormone and inhibin B: Predictors of ovarian response in assisted reproductive technology? *BJOG.* 2005;112(10):1384–90.
27. Muttukrishna S, Suharjono H, McGarrigle H, Sathanandan M. Inhibin B and anti-Müllerian hormone: Markers of ovarian response in IVF/ICSI patients? *BJOG.* 2004;111(11):1248–53.
28. La Marca A, Sighinolfi G, Radi D et al. Anti-Müllerian hormone (AMH) as a predictive marker in assisted reproductive technology (ART). *Hum Reprod Update.* 2010;16(2):113–30.
29. Rajpert-De Meyts E, Jørgensen N, Græm N et al. Expression of anti-Müllerian hormone during normal and pathological gonadal development: Association with differentiation of Sertoli and granulosa cells. *J Clin Endocrinol Metab.* 1999;84(10):3836–44.
30. Durlinger A, Gruijters M, Kramer P et al. Anti-Müllerian hormone attenuates the effects of FSH on follicle development in the mouse ovary. *Endocrinology.* 2001;142(11):4891–9.
31. Grossman M, Nakajima S, Fallat M, Siow Y. Müllerian-inhibiting substance inhibits cytochrome P450 aromatase activity in human granulosa lutein cell culture. *Fertil Steril.* 2008;89(5):1364–70.

32. Hehenkamp W, Looman C, Themmen A et al. Anti-Müllerian hormone levels in the spontaneous menstrual cycle do not show substantial fluctuation. *J Clin Endocrinol Metab.* 2006;91(10):4057–63.

33. La Marca A, Stabile G, Artenisio A and Volpe A. Serum anti-Müllerian hormone throughout the human menstrual cycle. *Hum Reprod.*;21(12):3103–7.

34. Tsepelidis S, Devreker F, Demeestere I et al. Stable serum levels of anti-Müllerian hormone during the menstrual cycle: A prospective study in normo-ovulatory women. *Hum Reprod.* 2007;22(7):1837–40.

35. Wunder D, Bersinger N, Yared M, et al. Statistically significant changes of anti-Müllerian hormone and inhibin levels during the physiologic menstrual cycle in reproductive age women. *Fertil Steril.* 2008;89(4):927–33.

36. Sowers M, McConnell D, Gast K et al. Anti-Müllerian hormone and inhibin B variability during normal menstrual cycles. *Fertil Steril.* 2010;94(4):1482–6.

37. Hadlow N, Longhurst K, McClements A et al. Variation in antimüllerian hormone concentration during the menstrual cycle may change the clinical classification of the ovarian response. *Fertil Steril.* 2013;99(6):1791–7.

38. Overbeek A, Broekmans F, Hehenkamp W et al. Intra-cycle fluctuations of anti-Müllerian hormone in normal women with a regular cycle: A re-analysis. *Reprod Biomed Online.* 2012;24(6):664–9.

39. Kelsey T, Anderson R, Wright P et al. Data-driven assessment of the human ovarian reserve. *Mol Hum Reprod.* 2012;18(2):79–87.

40. Broer S, van Disseldorp J, Broeze K et al. Added value of ovarian reserve testing on patient characteristics in the prediction of ovarian response and ongoing pregnancy: An individual patient data approach. *Hum Reprod Update.* 2013;19(1):26–36.

41. Broer S, Mol B, Hendriks D, Broekmans F. The role of anti-Müllerian hormone in prediction of outcome after IVF: Comparison with the antral follicle count. *Fertil Steril.* 2009;91(3):705–14.

42. Seifer D, Tal O, Wantman E et al. Prognostic indicators of assisted reproduction technology outcomes of cycles with ultralow serum antimüllerian hormone: A multivariate analysis of over 5,000 autologous cycles from the society for assisted reproductive technology clinic outcome reporting system database for 2012–2013. *Fertil Steril.* 2016;105(2):385–93.e3.

43. Iliodromiti S, Kelsey T, Wu O et al. The predictive accuracy of anti-Müllerian hormone for live birth after assisted conception: A systematic review and meta-analysis of the literature. *Hum Reprod Update.* 2014;20(4):560–70.

44. Tal R, Seifer D, Wantman E et al. Antimüllerian hormone as a predictor of live birth following assisted reproduction: An analysis of 85,062 fresh and thawed cycles from the society for assisted reproductive technology clinic outcome reporting system database for 2012–2013. *Fertil Steril.* 2018;109(2):258–65.

45. Nelson S, La Marca A. The journey from the old to the new AMH assay: How to avoid getting lost in the values. *Reprod Biomed Online.* 2011;23(4):411–20.

46. Broer S, Broekmans F, Laven J, Fauser B. Anti-Müllerian hormone: Ovarian reserve testing and its potential clinical implications. *Hum Reprod Update.* 2014;20(5):688–701.

47. Nelson S, Pastuszek E, Kloss G et al. Two new automated, compared with two enzyme-linked immunosorbent, anti-Müllerian hormone assays. *Fertil Steril.* 2015b;104(4):1016–1021.e6.

48. van Helden J, Weiskirchen R. Performance of the two new fully automated anti-Müllerian hormone immunoassays compared with the clinical standard assay. *Hum Reprod.* 2015;30(8):1918–26.

49. Almog B, Shehata F, Suissa S et al. Age-related normograms of serum antimüllerian hormone levels in a population of infertile women: A multicenter study. *Fertil Steril.* 2011;95(7):2359–63.e1.

50. Barad D, Weghofer A, Gleicher N. Utility of age-specific serum anti-Müllerian hormone concentrations. *Reprod Biomed Online.* 2011;22(3):284–91.

51. Seifer D, Baker V, Leader B. Age-specific serum anti-Müllerian hormone values for 17,120 women presenting to fertility centers within the United States. *Fertil Steril.* 2011;95(2):747–50.

52. La Marca A, Papaleo E, Grisendi V et al. Development of a nomogram based on markers of ovarian reserve for the individualisation of the follicle-stimulating hormone starting dose in in vitro fertilisation cycles. *BJOG.* 2012;119(10):1171–9.

53. Pigny P, Jonard S, Robert Y, Dewailly D. Serum Anti-Müllerian hormone as a surrogate for antral follicle count for definition of the polycystic ovary syndrome. *J Clin Endocrinol Metab.* 2006;91(3):941–5.

54. Dewailly D, Gronier H, Poncelet E et al. Diagnosis of polycystic ovary syndrome (PCOS): Revisiting the threshold values of follicle count on ultrasound and of the serum AMH level for the definition of polycystic ovaries. *Hum Reprod.* 2011;26(11):3123–9.

55. Bentzen J, Forman J, Pinborg A et al. Ovarian reserve parameters: A comparison between users and non-users of hormonal contraception. *Reprod Biomed Online.* 2012;25(6):612–9.

56. Dólleman M, Verschuren W, Eijkemans M et al. Reproductive and lifestyle determinants of Anti-Müllerian hormone in a large population-based study. *J Clin Endocrinol Metab.* 2013;98(5):2106–15.

57. Hannoun A, Abu Musa A, Awwad J et al. Clomiphene citrate challenge test: Cycle to cycle variability of cycle day 10 follicle stimulating hormone level. *Clin Exp Obstet Gynecol.* 1998;25(4):155–6.

58. Hendriks D, Broekmans F, Bancsi L et al. Repeated clomiphene citrate challenge testing in the prediction of outcome in IVF: A comparison with basal markers for ovarian reserve. *Hum Reprod.* 2005;20(1):163–9.

59. Garcia J. Gonadotropin-releasing hormone and its analogues: Applications in gynecology. *Clin Obstet Gynecol.* 1993;36(3):719–26.

60. Winslow K, Toner J, Brzyski R, et al. The gonadotropin-releasing hormone agonist stimulation test—A sensitive predictor of performance in the flare-up *in vitro* fertilization cycle. *Fertil Steril.* 1991;56(4):711–7.

61. Maheshwari A, Gibreel A, Bhattacharya S, Johnson N. Dynamic tests of ovarian reserve: A systematic review of diagnostic accuracy. *Reprod Biomed Online.* 2009;18(5):717–34.

62. Ferraretti A, La Marca A, Fauser B et al. ESHRE consensus on the definition of "poor response" to ovarian stimulation for *in vitro* fertilization: The Bologna criteria. *Hum Reprod.* 2011;26(7):1616–24.

63. Nelson S, Klein B, Arce J. Comparison of antimüllerian hormone levels and antral follicle count as predictor of ovarian response to controlled ovarian stimulation in good-prognosis patients at individual fertility clinics in two multicenter trials. *Fertil Steril.* 2015a;103(4):923–30.e1.

64. Elter K, Si'smanoglu A, Durmusoglu F. Intercycle variabilities of basal antral follicle count and ovarian volume in subfertile women and their relationship to reproductive aging: A prospective study. *Gynecol Endocrinol.* 2005;20(3):137–43.

65. Mercé L, Gómez B, Engels V et al. Intraobserver and interobserver reproducibility of ovarian volume, antral follicle count, and vascularity indices obtained with transvaginal 3-dimensional ultrasonography, power Doppler angiography, and the virtual organ computer-aided analysis imaging Pr. *J Ultrasound Med.* 2005;24(9):1279–87.

66. Frattarelli J, Lauria-Costab D, Miller B et al. Basal antral follicle number and mean ovarian diameter predict cycle cancellation and ovarian responsiveness in assisted reproductive technology cycles. *Fertil Steril.* 2000;74(3):512–7.

67. Arce J, Nyboe Andersen A, Fernández-Sánchez M et al. Ovarian response to recombinant human follicle-stimulating hormone: A randomized, anti-Müllerian hormone–stratified, dose–response trial in women undergoing *in vitro* fertilization/intracytoplasmic sperm injection. *Fertil Steril.* 2014;102(6):1633–40.e5.

68. Gnoth C, Schuring A, Friol K et al. Relevance of anti-Müllerian hormone measurement in a routine IVF program. *Hum Reprod.* 2008;23(6):1359–65.

69. Huang X, Wang P, Tal R et al. A systematic review and meta-analysis of metformin among patients with polycystic ovary syndrome undergoing assisted reproductive technology procedures. *Int J Gynaecol Obstet.* 2015;131(2):111–6.

70. van Tilborg T, Oudshoorn S, Eijkemans M et al. Individualized FSH dosing based on ovarian reserve testing in women starting IVF/ICSI: A multicentre trial and cost-effectiveness analysis. *Hum Reprod.* 2017a;32(12):2485–95.

71. van Tilborg T, Torrance H, Oudshoorn S, et al. Individualized versus standard FSH dosing in women starting IVF/ICSI: An RCT. Part 1: The predicted poor responder. *Hum Reprod.* 2017b;32(12):2496–505.

72. Oudshoorn S, van Tilborg T, Eijkemans M et al. Individualized versus standard FSH dosing in women starting IVF/ICSI: An RCT. Part 2: The predicted hyper responder. *Hum Reprod.* 2017;32(12):2506–14.

73. van Rooij I, Broekmans F, Hunault C et al. Use of ovarian reserve tests for the prediction of ongoing pregnancy in couples with unexplained or mild male infertility. *Reprod Biomed Online.*2006;12(2):182–90.

74. Freeman E, Sammel M, Lin H et al. Contribution of the rate of change of antimüllerian hormone in estimating time to menopause for late reproductive-age women. *Fertil Steril.* 2012;98(5):1254–9.e2.

75. Broer S, Eijkemans M, Scheffer G et al. Anti-Müllerian hormone predicts menopause: A long-term follow-up study in normoovulatory women. *J Clin Endocrinol Metab.* 2011;96(8):2532–9.

76. Depmann M, Eijkemans M, Broer S et al. Does AMH relate to timing of menopause? Results of an individual patient data meta-analysis. *J Clin Endocrinol Metab.* 2018;103(10):3593–600.

77. Anderson R, Rosendahl M, Kelsey T, Cameron D. Pretreatment anti-Müllerian hormone predicts for loss of ovarian function after chemotherapy for early breast cancer. *Eur J Cancer.* 2013;49(16):3404–11.

2

Use of Molecular Markers of Endometrial Receptivity

Alejandro Rincón, David Bolumar, Diana Valbuena, and Carlos Simón

Introduction

Humans are an inefficient species from a reproductive point of view. Compared to other mammals, our success rates of conception and live births are on average one-third and one-half, respectively (1). Successful implantation and subsequent embryonic invasion and endometrial decidualization result from a complex synergetic process that entails coordination of a euploid embryo obtained by careful embryonic selection, endometrial status, and the dialogue established between the embryo and endometrium (2).

On the maternal side, this synchronic phenomenon occurs during a short self-limited and hormone-dependent period of time called the *window of implantation* (WOI). This occurs when the endometrium—a highly dynamic tissue that covers the womb and undertakes a complex remodeling process during the menstrual cycle—undergoes a morphofunctional transition to a receptive phenotype, in which the blastocyst can efficiently implant onto the luminal epithelium to subsequently invade the decidualized stromal compartment. The existence of the WOI has been largely acknowledged, with the first reports published in the 1950s. At that point in time, investigators identified 34 embryos from hysterectomy samples in the luteal phase and observed that only those from tissue after day 20 had successfully implanted (3). Later, the Wilcox hypothesis placed the WOI at days 8–10 after ovulation in natural cycles (4). However, this indication is not used in current clinical practice. Today, the WOI is generally accepted to open during the mid-secretory phase, specifically on the fifth day after progesterone exposure, and remains open for about 2–3 days. This period is canonically described as days 5.5–9.5 after ovulation, which corresponds to days 20–24 in a canonical menstrual cycle (5).

The modulation of the progress of the endometrial phases has been largely studied to identify patterns of change or single molecules that can be measured simply and precisely, giving rise to reliable markers of endometrial receptivity. In addition, modifications that affect different endometrial tissue strata, namely, luminal epithelium, glandular epithelium, and stromal and vascular compartments, have also been studied in depth.

The luminal epithelium undergoes a series of modifications, including progressive loss of cell polarity, flattening of the apical surface, and appearance of microvilli, also known as pinopods. These cellular structures have been one of the best markers of endometrial receptivity since the 1950s. Additionally, study of the endometrial luminal surface has discovered molecules that display modulation during different stages of the menstrual cycle. Consequently, special emphasis has been placed on those that vary during the secretory phase, offering possible candidates for biomarkers of endometrial receptivity, such as mucins, integrins, cytokines, chemokines, and growth factors.

Further, conformational change of the secretory glands in the glandular epithelia stratum facilitates dissemination of uterine secretions. These endometrial exudates, along with serum transudates, residual products of womb cell apoptosis, and, in the case of effective fertilization, substances released by the embryo (6), compose a viscous liquid that is secreted into the endometrial cavity and is known as endometrial fluid (EF). EF has various functions, such as immunologic defense, blastocyst microenvironment preparation, adhesion and early implantation, and placentation processes. Consequently, it has been proposed as a source of putative receptivity biomarkers.

Decidualization takes place in the stromal compartment, which involves dramatic morphologic and functional differentiation of endometrial stromal cells (ESCs) into decidual cells guided by a progesterone-dependent and complex interactive process (7). Subsequently, decidualized ESCs trigger the production of prolactin (PRL), which is considered a decidualization biomarker. Further, accumulation of glycogen and lipids builds up inside these cells, which now evolve into a bigger and more rounded shape. Eventually, vascularization increases around the implantation area.

In 1950, Noyes et al. described an objective method for endometrial evaluation (8). This was a milestone in gynecological diagnosis and anatomical medicine, adding importance for the first time to the endometrial factor. However, after more than 60 years of experience, the histological timeline of the endometrium as a predictive method of receptivity does not play a relevant role in current clinical practice. New molecular and -omic technologies are more accurate and replicable alternatives that have displaced classical techniques, which have been questioned in numerous retrospective (9,10), prospective (11,12), and randomized studies (13,14).

These new techniques have uncovered specific genetic, transcriptomic, and proteomic profiles from patients' biological samples that can be used as biomarkers. Overall, due to advanced scientific knowledge and emerging new technologies based on next-generation sequencing (NGS), evaluation of the endometrial state has become reality. Moreover, new trends for the characterization and search for molecular markers in biological fluids such as EF constitute an alternative to traditional, invasive sampling methods. Further, EF and peripheral blood can be painlessly obtained by aspiration during the same cycle in which the embryo transfer is performed without affecting implantation rates (15).

Endometrial Receptivity Biomarkers

For many decades, the first system for endometrial dating developed by Noyes and collaborators was accepted as the gold standard to evaluate the human endometrium under both normal and pathologic conditions (8). The method was originally based on histological analysis of menstrual cycle components that change rapidly but consistently throughout the cycle. The approximate variation of eight morphologic factors from endometrial biopsies was used to determine the day of the menstrual cycle: gland mitosis, pseudostratification of nuclei, basal vacuolation, glandular secretion, stromal edema, pseudodecidual reaction, stromal mitosis, and leukocytic infiltration.

However, the authors warned about the limitations of the method: variation in these eight factors was unable to determine the exact day during the proliferative stage and could at most discern between early, middle, and late stages. Nonetheless, the dating was accurate for the secretory phase, mainly based on changes in glandular cells (mitosis, pseudostratification, basal vacuolization, and secretion) during the first week and guided by changes in the stromal compartment (edema, pre-decidual reaction, mitosis, and leukocyte infiltration) during the second week of the secretory phase. The study also indicated that given natural variation in menstrual cycle length, the timeline could indicate progression of sequential phases characterized by their histological appearance rather than actual days of the menstrual cycle. Many later studies demonstrated such limitations in Noyes' criteria.

A 2004 study demonstrated high prevalence of a time lag in endometrial biopsies from fertile women, making it possible to observe discrepancies of up to 3–4 days compared to a timeline based on the day of ovulation. Moreover, histological analysis was unable to differentiate between infertile women and fertile controls independently of the criterion used to define the time lag in biopsies. The study even showed a trend toward higher phases length variation in fertile compared to infertile women. Results were confirmed both for mid-luteal phase, where the WOI is located, and late luteal phase biopsies (14).

Reproducibility of the endometrial dating system based on histological criteria has also been criticized regarding a series of flaws in the original methodology. First and foremost, biopsies from infertile women were used to develop a normal endometrial histological model. Second, the day of the menstrual cycle correlating with histology in tissue specimens was determined by counting back from the next menses, assuming a canonical secretory phase of 14 days. Finally, the study did not consider intra- and interobserver bias to interpret the histology (13). Considering these flaws, reevaluation of the definite accuracy and clinical usefulness of Noyes, criteria for endometrial dating of the secretory phase in healthy, regularly cycling, fertile women showed that changes in the eight Noyes' factors are much less variable than originally described, preventing discrimination of the specific luteal day. Further, variability of interpretation between observers fluctuates around one day, histological time lag between patients increases toward the end of the secretory phase, and variability in histological maturation is quite common among women (13).

These limitations highlighted an increasing necessity for new markers of endometrial receptivity to improve implantation ratios after euploid embryo transfer, in an effort to avoid transfer of multiple embryos and associated risk of multiple pregnancies and derived obstetric problems (16). Additionally, it is important to consider that the retrieval of an endometrial biopsy during the WOI damages the functional layer of the endometrium, preventing the progression of pregnancy when conducted during the transfer cycle and thus delaying transfer until the following cycle. A promising alternative to biopsies is the analysis of markers in the EF, whose retrieval does not disturb implantation in the transfer cycle (15). The need to delay the transfer cycle reinforces the concern of intercycle WOI variability in naturally cycling patients. This situation can be controlled by cycles of hormonal replacement therapy (HRT) or controlled ovarian stimulation (COS), which allow the WOI to be established in days P+5 and hCG+7, respectively.

The first attempts to obtain new markers of endometrial receptivity were based on immunohistochemistry techniques to identify endometrial proteins with specific expression patterns around the WOI. Based on this principle, HSP 24 kDa (HSP 27) was observed to be more present in the luminal epithelium, where it reached maximum expression by day 21 in the cycle and thus coincides with the WOI. In the glandular epithelium, HSP 24 kDa expression peaked by the middle of the cycle (17). Calcitonin was also proposed as a WOI marker because its mRNA expression in human endometrium reached a maximum at days 19–21 in the menstrual cycle, while this hormone was not significantly expressed previous to ovulation or in the late secretory phase (18).

Combined expression profiles of cadherins 6 and 11, both for mRNA and protein, have also been proposed as possible WOI markers. In the stromal compartment, cadherin 6 was found highly expressed during the follicular phase and then markedly decreased as cells entered decidualisation. Reduction in cadherin 6 expression coincides with an increase in cadherin 11 expression in the same cell compartment, at the point when the endometrium is preparing for implantation. Thus, the inverse expression patterns of cadherins 6 and 11 in stromal cells could serve as a marker of endometrial maturity (19) (Figure 2.1).

During the same year, antiadhesion molecules were being studied, specifically mucin 1 (MUC-1). The associated cell surface is a highly glycosylated high molecular weight protein glycocalyx that covers luminal epithelium cells, forming a gel-like secretion. For this reason, mucins indirectly protect cells from pathogen infection, avoiding cell surface–pathogen contact and later putative adhesion. *MUC-1* is overexpressed around 36 hours following the luteinizing hormone (LH) peak (20), and its deposition avoids cell areas covered by pinopods, favoring blastocyst implantation.

FIGURE 2.1 First after Noyes proposed molecular markers for endometrial dating. (a) The 24-kDa HSP (HSP-27) expression throughout the menstrual cycle in both the luminal and glandular epithelium. Degree of change was measured using an arbitrary 4-point scale. (b) Densitometric quantitation of Northern blots for cadherins 11 and 6 mRNAs, normalized to the absorbance values obtained for the 18S rRNA. Samples were obtained from human endometrial stroma during late follicular (A), mid-luteal (B), and late luteal (C) phases of the menstrual cycle. Results are standardized relative to the cadherin mRNA levels and are represented (mean ± standard error; $n = 3$) in the bar graphs (*$P < 0.05$). (c) Expression levels for calcitonin mRNA from human endometrial biopsies obtained in different days of the menstrual cycle. (c1) Calcitonin and GAPDH mRNA RT-PCR amplification and Southern blot. (c2) Densitometric quantitation of the previously obtained calcitonin mRNA signals, normalized versus the GAPDH internal control (c1). Results are expressed relative to GAPDH and are plotted as the mean ± standard error for at least three separate experiments. (d) Percentage of endometria showing pinopods and αvβ3 integrin in epithelial cells for different postovulatory days. (e) Correlations between the endometrial tissue dating (postovulatory days) and LIF ($r = 0.105$, $P = 0.594$) or GdA ($r = 0.376$, $P = 0.048$) in endometrial secretions. ([a] Adapted from Ciocca D et al. *J Clin Endocrinol Metab.* 1983;57(3):496–9. [b] Adapted from Getsios S et al. *Dev Dyn.* 1998;211(3):238–47. [c] Adapted from Kumar S et al. *J Clin Endocrinol Metab.* 1998;83(12):4443–50. [d] Adapted from Creus M et al. *Hum Reprod.* 2002;17(9):2279–86. [e] Adapted from Van der Gaast M et al. *BJOG.* 2008;116(2):304–12.)

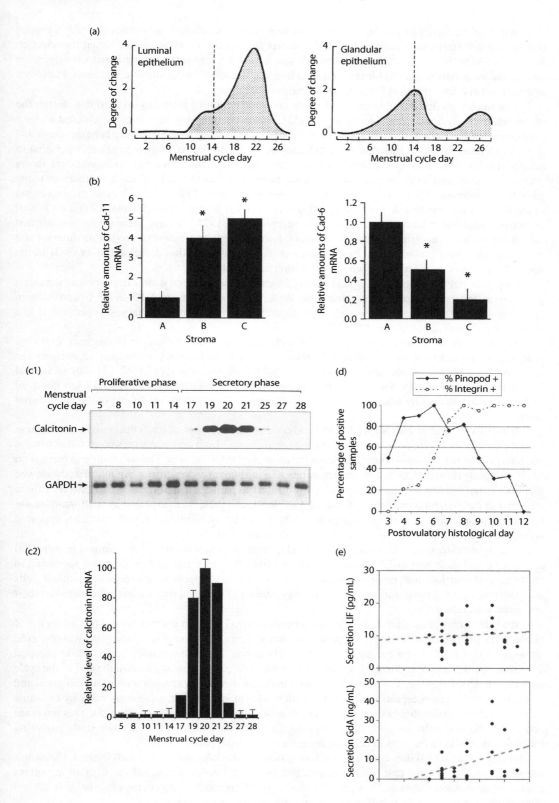

Endometrial receptivity markers

Contrary to the family of mucins, integrins are largely known adhesion molecules that play a crucial role in cell–cell interactions, cell–extracellular matrix (ECM) communication, and signal transduction from the ECM to the cell. Some integrins are transmembrane heterodimers that increase their expression and modulation during the mid-luteal stage, aiding implantation (endometrial epithelium–blastocyst interactions) and later invasion throughout the endometrial lining.

The presence, plasma membrane distribution, and modulation of integrins are variable during the menstrual cycle, so molecules such as $\alpha 1\beta 1$, $\alpha 4\beta 1$, and $\alpha v\beta 3$ integrins have been considered under a predictive endometrial status. The expression levels of $\beta 1$ and $\beta 3$ integrin families have been demonstrated to be modulated by blood estrogen (E2) and progesterone (P4) levels, showing different patterns in epithelial cells. The $\beta 1$ family is constitutively expressed during the menstrual cycle, while $\beta 3$ shows greater variation, and its decreased expression has been linked to reduced uterine receptivity in many pathologic conditions. Nevertheless, E2 and P4 were shown to have differential effects on the expression of the different integrin families, thus suggesting the combined interpretation of blood E2 and P4 as well as integrin expression levels for predicting the receptive status (21). Several groups have investigated the role of the integrin family to find a correlation between gene expression or protein modulation and endometrium timing and/or status. Peyghambari et al. demonstrated that decreased $\beta 1$ or $\alpha 4\beta 1$ in the stromal compartment is correlated with implantation failure (IF) (22).

Osteopontin (OPN), the classical ligand of the $\beta 3$ subunit, also has been widely described in numerous publications for its high expression during the WOI. For this reason, the OPN-$\alpha v\beta 3$ ligand-integrin complex, which is generated in the envelope of the luminal epithelium cell surface, was postulated as a marker of endometrial receptivity (23).

Currently, there are commercial tests that measure the level of these possible biomarkers. *E-Tegrity* analyzes the presence of the $\beta 3$ subunit by using immunohistochemistry techniques to evaluate the endometrial state. Another example is *ReceptivaDx* (BCL6 Test), which needs a LH+7–LH+10 endometrial biopsy, buffered in formalin, for the immunostaining process. In addition to evaluating $\beta 3$, it is designed to predict endometriosis by assessing *BCL6* levels to detect inflammatory conditions of the endometrial lining (24).

However, in agreement with Noyes' histological criteria (8), expression of $\alpha v\beta 3$ integrins in combination with the formation of pinopods in the endometrial epithelium—both dependent on sex steroid hormones and analyzed from biopsies—constitute two of the most cited WOI markers. The $\alpha v\beta 3$ integrin expression has been closely related to the histological maturation of the human endometrium. An initial study showed that almost half of the endometrial samples from infertile patients had abrogated expression of these integrins in the glandular epithelial cells during the WOI, and these were also absent in all out-of-phase biopsies corresponding to the mid-luteal phase of the cycle (25). In addition, integrins suddenly appeared on day 20 of the menstrual cycle, coinciding with the start of the WOI.

Pinopods are cytoplasmic protrusions that develop from the apical surface of the luminal endometrial epithelium, and their role in EF absorption and in lifting the epithelial surface has been suggested to facilitate endometrium and embryo interactions (26). Pinopods appear when epithelial luminal cells start the process of depolarization to promote implantation (27), prompting a correlation between their appearance and the WOI.

A study by Creus et al. analyzed the relation between $\alpha v\beta 3$ integrin expression and the formation of pinopods (11) but detected no direct temporal correlation. The expression of $\alpha v\beta 3$ integrins was observed between days LH+7–8 and increased progressively during the postovulatory stage, while pinopod formation seemed to occur during days LH+4–8, with subsequent reduction toward the end of the cycle (see Figure 2.1). Likewise, the study found no correlation between expression of $\alpha v\beta 3$ integrins and progesterone/estrogen receptors or serum levels of the hormones. In fact, a previous study by the same group found no relationship between the expression of $\alpha v\beta 3$ integrins and fertility (25). This temporal and spatial variability in mentioned markers expression was confirmed in a subsequent study analyzing the expression of both markers in consecutive cycles of infertile patients (12).

Cytokines and chemokines constitute another group of molecules that draw much interest. Cytokines are small soluble proteins that rule autocrine, paracrine, and endocrine signaling, with an important impact for immunomodulation. They act by joining a specific receptor to trigger the modulation of several physiologic processes, such as cell proliferation, differentiation, and maturation.

The most studied cytokine family is interleukin-6 (IL-6), which is related to blastocyst implantation. Its main purpose is immunoglobulin production inside activated B cells. IL-6 mRNA increases during the mid-secretory phase and subsequently decreases in the late-secretory phase, so it has been postulated as a putative endometrial receptivity biomarker during the WOI (28). Complementary to IL-6, which is mostly present in the luminal and glandular epithelial layer (28), IL-11 and IL-15 are overrepresented in the stromal compartment during decidualization (29). Therefore, these interleukins may represent another possible biomarker.

The main reported chemokines are secreted by macrophages during the first implantation stage, including monocyte chemotactic protein 1 (MCP-1), IL-8, and RANTES, which have receptors CXCR1, CCR5, and CCR2B, respectively, in the stromal compartment (30).

Meanwhile, studies of different growth factors have highlighted the heparin-binding epidermal growth factor (EGF)-like growth factor (HB-EGF). HB-EGF is a glycoprotein from the EGF family secreted by macrophages and monocytes, which play a crucial role in epidermal injury healing, epithelialization, cell proliferation modulation, and decidualization. HB-EGF appears in the luminal epithelial layer, and its expression is modulated during the menstrual cycle, progressing from basal expression during the proliferative stage to maximum expression during the mid-secretory phase (31). Considering its ease of determination together with its modulation during the cycle and possible functions related to adhesion and implantation, HB-EGF is considered an endometrial biomarker candidate.

Different groups have described the expression of cyclin E in endometrium in relation to endometrial hyperplasia and cancer (32,33). However, from a reproductive point of view, this molecule could be an effective biomarker for endometrial receptivity. Cyclin E is expressed in the cytoplasm of glandular epithelial cells during the proliferative phase up to day 18 of the menstrual cycle, at which time its localization moves to the nuclear compartment.

Therefore, Kliman's group created the Endometrial Function Test (EFT), which can identify the presence of cyclin E and p27 in endometrial biopsies through an immunohistochemical approach (34). Considering the publication indicates that fertile women only express cyclin E up until roughly day 19 of the cycle, as opposed to infertile patients who only show cyclin E after this point, patients with an abnormal EFT profile could have a defect in stroma and glands communication. Consequently, a normal profile does not guarantee successful implantation, and an abnormal EFT result only appears to be associated with pregnancy failure (35).

More recently, glycodelin A (GdA) and leukemia inhibitory factor (LIF) were proposed as putative indicators of endometrial receptivity that could be identified in endometrial secretions. Investigators tried to establish a correlation between their expression and endometrial maturity measured by different biopsy-based criteria, such as Noyes' criteria and progesterone receptor/Ki-67 immunohistochemical labeling. They found that LIF, an inflammatory cytokine derived from the IL-6 family, is overexpressed in the human endometrium around the time of implantation, but no correlation was found between LIF levels and degree of endometrial maturity. In contrast, GdA expression significantly increased during the WOI and correlated to increased endometrial histological maturity. Moreover, higher levels of GdA were observed in endometrial secretions of fertile compared to infertile patients (36) (see Figure 2.1).

Endometrial Receptivity Biomarkers: Transcriptomic Biomarkers

In order to globally study the different phases of the endometrium and its receptivity state, new -omic techniques are needed. Trying to find a single mechanism or molecule that regulates the complexity of the whole process turns into a simplistic view. Transcriptomics instead offers a massive approach in which all mRNAs and subsequent proteins can be directly and indirectly determined, measured, and evaluated. This could provide a general understanding of the endometrial environment during each phase of the cycle, including the mid-secretory phase and the WOI.

During 2003–2006, the combined work of pioneering groups (37–39) set the ball rolling to demonstrate that the analysis and subsequent evaluation of endometrial transcriptomic profiles during the different phases of the menstrual cycle could be used not only as a biomarker of receptivity but also as a procedure for continuous dating of the endometrium. These works revealed novel and valuable information, highlighting the complex but high potential of the methodology (40).

In 2003, Simon's group used microarrays to compare the transcriptomic profiles of fertile *in vitro* fertilization (IVF) patients during the same natural cycle in days LH+2 versus LH+7, obtaining 211 significantly regulated genes (fold-change >3) (37). In 2004, Rogers and collaborators published an endometrial transcriptome profile during the menstrual cycle. This microarray study of natural cycle samples reported the differences between pre-receptive stages and receptivity using endometrial biopsies (38).

Moreover, this work postulated the possibility of studying gene expression in the different endometrium layers. One of the first transcriptomic works thus appeared one year later, which used microarrays to evaluate the differential expression between epithelial and stromal cells. In addition, this group hypothesized that WFDC2 and MMP7 in the luminal epithelia layer and decorin and TIMP1 in the stromal compartment could be used as markers during the natural cycle (LH+7) (41). This work started a race to search for transcriptomic biomarkers.

During the same year, Mirkin compared the transcriptomic modulation during two states of the cycle (LH+2 versus LH+8) and reported a differential expression of *ANXA4*, *FOXO1A*, and *SPP1* (42). In 2006, Giudice's group and Lessey's group together used microarray technology to analyze 28 specimens through whole-genome phenotyping (39). The authors identified four endometrial phenotypes—proliferative, early secretory, mid-secretory, and late secretory—highlighting the potential of this approach.

In 2008, Franchi et al. compared the differences between stroma and epithelium during days 16, 21, and 24 in the cycle and identified some differentially expressed mRNA, including IL-15, IL-15Ra, OPN, DAF, and αvβ3 integrin (43). One year later, Gaide et al. added to the list *IL-8* and *adrenomedullin* in the glandular epithelium and MMP1, MMP3, MMP9, MMP12, TIMP1, TIMP3, PLAU, and PLAT in the stromal compartment (44).

Endometrial Receptivity Analysis Revolution

In 2009, the Endometrial Receptivity Analysis (ERA) test was developed and patented, and subsequently launched in 2011, taking advantage of all the scientific evidence accumulated over the previous 10 years of research on endometrial biomarkers, transcriptomics, and genes involved in the menstrual cycle (45). This new state-of-the-art diagnostic method was microarray based and coupled to an in-home machine-learning predictive algorithm to evaluate and diagnose a woman's endometrial receptivity status, categorizing each endometrial transcriptome between different cycle stages mainly as non-receptive or receptive.

The high values of specificity (0.88) and sensitivity (0.99) of this method, in addition to its efficacy and consistency, have been widely demonstrated in a comparative study between the ERA molecular approach and the classic Noyes' histological method for endometrial dating. Moreover, consistency analysis in which different samples taken from the same woman on the same cycle day but during different cycles over 2–3 years demonstrated high similarity profiles and a consistent endometrial pattern (46,47).

As previously mentioned, the lack of synchronization between the carefully selected embryo and the receptive endometrium is one of the most relevant causes of recurring implantation failure. Therefore, to determine the optimal moment for embryo transfer, an accurate molecular diagnostic technique is mandatory. The ERA test compares each patient's transcriptomic profile, consisting of the differential expression of 236 selected genes, to all previously categorized samples. The method requires an endometrial biopsy that should be carried out on day P+5, after 120 hours of exogenous progesterone administration during a HRT cycle, or on day LH+7, taken 7 complete days after the LH peak during the natural cycle (Figure 2.2).

The ERA test currently uses NGS technology, which is a step forward in terms of speed, multiplexing, security, traceability, and cost efficiency—further benefiting not only patients who have undergone recurring implantation failure, but also patients who wish to know their endometrial status before performing an embryo transfer during IVF treatment. The improved algorithm is capable of segregating the endometrial status into seven different phases: proliferative, 2 days pre-receptive, 1 day pre-receptive,

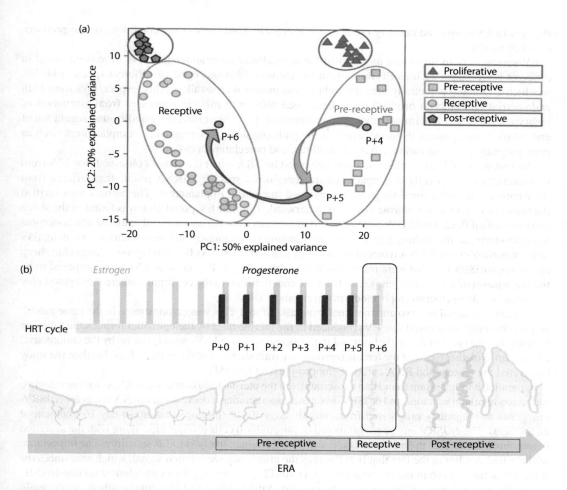

FIGURE 2.2 Endometrial Receptivity Analysis predictor principal component analysis (PCA) and endometrial development during a hormonal replacement therapy (HRT) cycle. (a) PCA plot obtained from three endometrium specimens of the same patient taken at different HRT cycles. First and second results were taken after 4 and 5 full days with exogenous progesterone administration, P+4 and P+5, respectively, showing a pre-receptive state. The third specimen, taken at P+6, shows a receptive endometrial profile. (b) The endometrial evolution during the HRT cycle. P+4 and P+5 biopsies were pre-receptive, while the P+6 biopsy was centered in the receptive stage, coinciding with the personalized time to perform the embryo transfer (pET).

early receptive, receptive, late receptive, and post-receptive. This precisely limits the WOI and subsequently allows personalized embryo transfer (PET), thus increasing the chance of pregnancy.

Today, after 10 years of clinical experience and more than 60,000 patients, ERA is the only molecular diagnostic test with widely demonstrated reproducibility and clinical applicability. Moreover, the ERA testing laboratory and its personnel are fully licensed by Clinical Laboratory Improvement Amendments (CLIA).

Extracellular Vesicles: Endometrial Receptivity Markers for the Future?

The term *extracellular vesicles* (EVs) was coined to broadly describe the different membrane-enclosed structures that are released by cells under different conditions. Although many specialized EVs groups have been described, they are generally classified into three main classes according to their biogenetic origin: apoptotic bodies, microvesicles, and exosomes. EVs are released by cells in response to different stimuli, both under physiologically normal and pathologic conditions. Different stimuli further trigger changes in EV cargo and delivery rates, which eventually could reflect the conditions of the producer cells/organs (54).

EV secretion is an important mechanism for intercellular communication. EVs have been found in different body fluids, such as EF throughout the menstrual/estrous cycle of different species (48–53), in which EVs could potentially mediate embryo and maternal crosstalk. In this respect, EVs from both endometrial and embryo origins/targets have been attributed roles in processes from promotion of embryo development and implantation, enhancement of trophoblast migratory ability, and regulation of endometrial angiogenesis to participation in the pathophysiology of pregnancy complications, such as early pregnancy loss, gestational diabetes mellitus, and preeclampsia (54).

The first work addressing this issue was published in 2013, when the authors observed that EVs from endometrial epithelial cells in primary culture contained a specific miRNA profile that differed from their parent cells, with some target genes involved in embryo implantation. The authors also verified the presence of EVs in the uterine fluid (53). Afterward, a similar EV population was found in the sheep uterine luminal fluid. These EVs were enriched in proteins from the endometrial epithelia and conceptus trophectoderm, distinguishing a specific cargo signature for pregnancy and non-pregnancy. Of note, EVs were conveyors of small RNA molecules, including gag and env RNAs from endogenous Jaagsiekte sheep retrovirus (enJSRV), which were transmissible to surrounding cells. As such, EVs were proposed to be the mechanism of transport of env genes from the endometrium to the conceptus, where these genes play an essential role in embryo trophectoderm development (50).

Later, bidirectional embryo and maternal crosstalk through EVs was demonstrated in the same model. *In vivo* observations showed that EVs produced in the uterine fluid by the epithelial lining were taken up by both the embryo and the epithelium and that conceptus-derived EVs were taken up by the endometrial epithelium. No other tissue of the female reproductive tract showed uptake of these EVs. Further, the study uncovered the protein and RNA cargo of embryo-derived EVs (51).

In parallel, another group found that exosomes from the uterine fluid contained mRNAs for interleukins, interferon regulatory factors, and enJSRV-env genes, appreciating a decrease in mRNA levels for enJSRV-env genes as pregnancy progressed from roughly days 10–12 (preimplantation) to day 16 (moment of attachment). The enJSRV-env genes promoted trophectoderm cells proliferation along with the secretion of interferon tau (IFNT) in an exosome dose-dependent manner, likely via TLR signaling. The importance of these findings lies in the fact that IFNT acts as the pregnancy recognition signal, which announces the presence of the embryo to the uterus around days 10–12 of pregnancy for its attachment on day 16 (52).

Finally, a recent work in the same model reasserted the luminal and glandular epithelia as the main producers of EVs and demonstrated a cyclic variation in uterine lumen EVs levels. More importantly, this study established a hormonal regulation of EVs secretion, where progesterone was shown to regulate EV production and enrichment in a specific subset of miRNAs (55).

Communication between the mother and the peri-implantation embryo through EVs has also been demonstrated in humans. An initial study showed exosomes containing hsa-miR-30d being transferred from endometrial epithelial cells to the murine embryo trophoblast, where the miRNA was internalized. It is important to note that the effect of miR-30d modified embryo expression pattern, increasing expression of genes coding for embryo adhesion molecules (48). Posteriorly, a second group demonstrated *in vitro* that the proteome of EVs produced by human endometrial epithelial cells is regulated by steroid hormones, thus varying with the progression of the menstrual cycle. Importantly, the proteome of exosomes under receptive phase hormonal conditions showed potential implications in embryo implantation. In fact, those exosomes were internalized by human trophoblastic cells, enhancing their adhesive capacity (56).

EVs are also produced by the embryo and participate both in crosstalk with the endometrium (51) and in self-paracrine regulation (57). In the final case, murine embryonic stem cells from the inner cell mass were shown to generate microvesicles that contacted the trophoblast layer and enhanced migration ability of trophoblast cells in culture, either as isolated cells or in the whole embryo. Further, injection of these microvesicles inside the blastocoel of E3.5 blastocysts increased their implantation efficiency (57). Another group working with a pig model observed that EVs from a trophectoderm cell line were able to stimulate proliferation of endothelial cells *in vitro*, thus becoming potential regulators of maternal endometrial angiogenesis. In fact, the authors demonstrated bidirectional EV communication. These vesicles contained miRNA and protein cargo including species with annotated functions in angiogenesis.

TABLE 2.1

Main Functions of Extracellular Vesicles (EVs) in Embryo–Maternal Crosstalk for Embryo Implantation Promotion Classified by Their Origin and Targets

EV Main Features	Origin	Target	Functions	References
Wide variety of origins: serum transudates, residues from womb cell apoptosis, endometrial epithelial cells, and conceptus. Variations throughout the menstrual cycle.	Endometrium	Endometrium	Promotion of embryo implantation (specific miRNA cargo).	Ng et al. (53)
		Embryo	Embryo development (enJSRV *env* gene RNA) and subsequent priming of the endometrium for embryo harboring.	Burns et al. (50,51); Ruiz-González et al. (52)
			Promotion of embryo implantation (miR-30d, specific protein cargo, influenced by uterine hormones—functional with trophectoderm).	Vilella et al. (48); Greening et al. (56)
			Progesterone cyclic regulation of endometrial epithelial EV levels and cargo.	Burns et al. (55)
	Embryo	Endometrium	Regulation of endometrial angiogenesis (specific miRNA and protein cargo) and uterine spiral arteries remodeling.	Bidarimath et al. (58); Salomon et al. (59)
		Embryo	Enhancing of trophoblast cells' migratory ability and implantation efficiency (laminin, fibronectin).	Desrochers et al. (57)

Source: Adapted from Simon C et al. *Endocr Rev.* 2018;39(3):292–332.

Nonetheless, care should be taken with these results, because they were obtained from *in vitro* cell cultures, and pigs are a species with epitheliochorial placentation—therefore, important differences are likely to be present in human physiology (58).

In line with these results, a previous study showed that extravillous trophoblast cells (HTR-8/SVneo and Jeg3)-derived exosomes promote vascular smooth muscle cells migration, a process involved in human uterine spiral arteries remodeling in successful pregnancies (59). However, different trophoblast cell lines produced different migration results, raising the possibility that cell origin, content, and bioactivity of the exosomes may importantly affect their pro-migratory activity. Thus, these results cannot be directly extrapolated *in vivo*.

This information (Table 2.1) postulates that EVs are still underexploited mediators of embryo implantation promotion, where not only the mother regulates the endometrium to harbor an embryo and enhance embryo invasive properties, but also the embryo announces its presence to the mother while modifying the endometrial lining for its imminent encounter. These facts, alongside EVs mid-secretory endometrial functions and cyclically regulated content, reinforce the interest in the EVs from the EF as potential markers of endometrial receptivity (54,60,61).

Future Directions

Evolution of diagnostic methodologies, advancement of bioinformatics, development of social models, and colonization of new market niches continue to drive the search for improved endometrial receptivity biomarkers. However, some new conditions have been proposed to develop such biomarker tests, including noninvasive techniques, painless sampling methods, or those that can be used during the same cycle (active conception cycle) without assuming additional cost or delay to a process that is awkward for many patients.

An optimistic approach would involve obtaining samples from liquid tissues or fluids, such as peripheral blood, urine, or EF. In addition to the emerging interest in EF EVs, this uterine secretion also provides other perspectives. For instance, Chan et al. obtained an expression profile of the differentially expressed genes between isolated cells from uterine aspirates, taken in a minimally invasive way, during days LH+2 and LH+7 of the cycle (62). Moreover, a study of molecules of interest present during the WOI revealed the existence of two new possible biomarkers—PGE2 and PGF2α, prostaglandins that could predict the optimal moment of implantation in the previous 24 hours and thus constitute possible non-invasive biomarkers of endometrial receptivity (63). Although these markers have not yet obtained clinical translation, they constitute a basis for future research.

In addition, contributions of the microbiome to the endometrial factor must not be overlooked. Despite not yet being considered a proper biomarker of receptivity, the prevalence of a microbiologically favorable uterine microenvironment can be a factor for good prognosis for implantation, reducing its efficiency in negative conditions (64,65). Thus, the microbiome could be an extra component of the equation with a high added value.

Overall, over the past few decades, the surge of infertile couples has skyrocketed. As a result, the race to develop a test that accurately determines endometrial receptivity during the active conception cycle in a noninvasive, simple, cost-efficient, and painless way continues to be a top priority for society.

REFERENCES

1. Zinaman M, Clegg E, Brown C, O'Connor J, Selevan S. Estimates of human fertility and pregnancy loss. *Fertil Steril.* 1996;65(3):503–9.
2. Wang H, Dey S. Roadmap to embryo implantation: Clues from mouse models. *Nat Rev Genet.* 2006;7(3):185–99.
3. Hertig A, Rock J, Adams E. A description of 34 human ova within the first 17 days of development. *Am J Anat.* 1956;98(3):435–93.
4. Wilcox A, Baird D, Weinberg C. Time of implantation of the conceptus and loss of pregnancy. *N Engl J Med.* 1999;340(23):1796–9.
5. Aplin J. The cell biological basis of human implantation. *Baillieres Best Pract Res Clin Obstet Gynaecol.* 2000;14(5):757–64.
6. Beier H. Oviductal and uterine fluids. *Reproduction.* 1974;37(1):221–37.
7. Garrido-Gomez T, Dominguez F, Lopez J et al. Modeling human endometrial decidualization from the interaction between proteome and secretome. *J Clin Endocrinol Metab.* 2011;96(3):706–16.
8. Noyes R, Hertig A, Rock J. Dating the endometrial biopsy. *Fertil Steril.* 1950;1(1):3–25.
9. Shoupe D, Mishell D, Lacarra M et al. Correlation of endometrial maturation with four methods of estimating day of ovulation. *Obstet Gynecol* 1989;73(1):88–92.
10. Balasch J, Fábregues F, Creus M, Vanrell J. The usefulness of endometrial biopsy for luteal phase evaluation in infertility. *Hum Reprod.* 1992;7(7):973–7.
11. Creus M, Ordi J, Fábregues F et al. αvβ3 integrin expression and pinopod formation in normal and out-of-phase endometria of fertile and infertile women. *Hum Reprod.* 2002;17(9):2279–86.
12. Ordi J, Creus M, Quintó L, Casamitjana R, Cardesa A, Balasch J. Within-subject between-cycle variability of histological dating, αvβ3 integrin expression, and pinopod formation in the human endometrium. *J Clin Endocrinol Metabol.* 2003;88(5):2119–25.
13. Murray M, Meyer W, Zaino R et al. A critical analysis of the accuracy, reproducibility, and clinical utility of histologic endometrial dating in fertile women. *Fertil Steril.* 2004;81(5):1333–43.
14. Coutifaris C, Myers E, Guzick D et al. Histological dating of timed endometrial biopsy tissue is not related to fertility status. *Fertil Steril.* 2004;82(5):1264–72.
15. van der Gaast M, Beier-Hellwig K, Fauser B, Beier H, Macklon N. Endometrial secretion aspiration prior to embryo transfer does not reduce implantation rates. *Reprod Biomed Online.* 2003;7(1):105–9.
16. Thurin A, Hausken J, Hillensjö T et al. Elective single-embryo transfer versus double-embryo transfer in in vitro fertilization. *N Engl J Med.* 2004;351(23):2392–402.
17. Ciocca D, Asch R, Adams D, Mcguire W. Evidence for modulation of a 24 K protein in human endometrium during the menstrual cycle. *J Clin Endocrinol Metab.* 1983;57(3):496–9.
18. Kumar S, Zhu LJ, Polihronis M et al. Progesterone induces calcitonin gene expression in human endometrium within the putative window of implantation. *J Clin Endocrinol Metab.* 1998;83(12):4443–50.

19. Getsios S, Chen G, Stephenson M, Leclerc P, Blaschuk O, MacCalman C. Regulated expression of cadherin-6 and cadherin-11 in the glandular epithelial and stromal cells of the human endometrium. *Dev Dyn*. 1998;211(3):238–47.

20. Meseguer M. MUC1 and endometrial receptivity. *Mol Hum Reprod*. 1998;4(12):1089–98.

21. Chen G, Xin A, Liu Y et al. Integrins β1 and β3 are biomarkers of uterine condition for embryo transfer. *J Transl Med*. 2016;14(1):303.

22. Peyghambari F, Fayazi M, Amanpour S et al. Assessment of α4, αv, β1 and β3 integrins expression throughout the implantation window phase in endometrium of a mouse model of polycystic ovarian syndromes. *Iran J Reprod Med*. 2014;12(10):687–94.

23. Casals G, Ordi J, Creus M et al. Osteopontin and αvβ3 integrin as markers of endometrial receptivity: The effect of different hormone therapies. *Reprod Biomed Online*. 2010;21(3):349–59.

24. Almquist L, Likes C, Stone B et al. Endometrial BCL6 testing for the prediction of *in vitro* fertilization outcomes: A cohort study. *Fertil Steril*. 2017;108(6):1063–9.

25. Creus M, Balasch J, Ordi J et al. Integrin expression in normal and out-of-phase endometria. *Hum Reprod*. 1998;13(12):3460–8.

26. Bentin-Ley U, Sjogren A, Nilsson L, Hamberger L, Larsen J, Horn T. Presence of uterine pinopodes at the embryo endometrial interface during human implantation *in vitro*. *Hum Reprod*. 1999; 14(2):515–20.

27. Thie M, Fuchs P, Denker HW. Epithelial cell polarity and embryo implantation in mammals. *Int J Dev Biol*. 1996;40(1):389–93.

28. Achache H, Revel A. Endometrial receptivity markers, the journey to successful embryo implantation. *Hum Reprod Update*. 2006;12(6):731–46.

29. Godbole G, Modi D. Regulation of decidualization, interleukin-11 and interleukin-15 by homeobox A 10 in endometrial stromal cells. *J Reprod Immunol*. 2010;85(2):130–9.

30. Dominguez F, Galan A, Martin JJL, Remohi J, Pellicer A, Simón C. Hormonal and embryonic regulation of chemokine receptors CXCR1, CXCR4, CCR5 and CCR2B in the human endometrium and the human blastocyst. *Mol Hum Reprod*. 2003;9(4):189–98.

31. Dorostghoal M, Ghaffari H, Shahbazian N, Mirani M. Endometrial expression of β3 integrin, calcitonin and plexin-B1 in the window of implantation in women with unexplained infertility. *Int J Reprod Biomed*. 2017;15(1):33–40.

32. Gezginc S, Celik C, Dogan N, Toy H, Tazegul A, Colakoglu M. Expression of cyclin A, cyclin E and p27 in normal, hyperplastic and frankly malignant endometrial samples. *J Obstet Gynaecol*. 2013;33(5):508–11.

33. Zapiecki K, Manahan KJ, Miller GA, Geisler JP. Cyclin E is overexpressed by clear cell carcinomas of the endometrium and is a prognostic indicator of survival. *Eur J Gynaecol Oncol*. 2015;36(2):114–6.

34. Kliman H, Honig S, Walls D, Luna M, McSweet J, Copperman A. Optimization of endometrial preparation results in a normal Endometrial Function Test (EFT) and good reproductive outcome in donor ovum recipients. *J Assist Reprod Genet*. 2006;23(7–8):299–303.

35. Dubowy R, Feinberg R, Keefe D et al. Improved endometrial assessment using cyclin E and p27. *Fertil Steril*. 2003;80(1):146–56.

36. van der Gaast M, Macklon N, Beier-Hellwig K et al. The feasibility of a less invasive method to assess endometrial maturation-comparison of simultaneously obtained uterine secretion and tissue biopsy. *BJOG*. 2008;116(2):304–12.

37. Riesewijk A, Martín J, van Os R et al. Gene expression profiling of human endometrial receptivity on days LH+2 versus LH+7 by microarray technology. *Mol Hum Reprod*. 2003;9(5):253–64.

38. Ponnampalam A, Weston G, Trajstman A, Susil B, Rogers P. Molecular classification of human endometrial cycle stages by transcriptional profiling. *Mol Hum Reprod*. 2004;10(12):879–93.

39. Talbi S, Hamilton A, Vo K et al. Molecular phenotyping of human endometrium distinguishes menstrual cycle phases and underlying biological processes in normo-ovulatory women. *Endocrinology*. 2006;147(3):1097–121.

40. Niederberger C, Pellicer A. Introduction: IVF's 40th world birthday. *Fertil Steril*. 2018;110(1):4.

41. Yanaihara A, Otsuka Y, Iwasaki S et al. Differences in gene expression in the proliferative human endometrium. *Fertil Steril*. 2005;83(4):1206–15.

42. Mirkin S, Arslan M, Churikov D et al. In search of candidate genes critically expressed in the human endometrium during the window of implantation. *Hum Reprod*. 2005;20(8):2104–17.

43. Franchi A, Zaret J, Zhang X, Bocca S, Oehninger S. Expression of immunomodulatory genes, their protein products and specific ligands/receptors during the window of implantation in the human endometrium. *Mol Hum Reprod.* 2008;14(7):413–21.
44. Gaide Chevronnay H, Galant C, Lemoine P, Courtoy P, Marbaix E, Henriet P. Spatiotemporal coupling of focal extracellular matrix degradation and reconstruction in the menstrual human endometrium. *Endocrinology.* 2009;150(11):5094–105.
45. Díaz-Gimeno P, Horcajadas J, Martínez-Conejero J et al. A genomic diagnostic tool for human endometrial receptivity based on the transcriptomic signature. *Fertil Steril.* 2011;95(1):50–60.e15.
46. Ruiz-Alonso M, Blesa D, Simón C. The genomics of the human endometrium. *Biochim Biophys Acta.* 2012;1822(12):1931–42.
47. Ruiz-Alonso M, Blesa D, Díaz-Gimeno P et al. The endometrial receptivity array for diagnosis and personalized embryo transfer as a treatment for patients with repeated implantation failure. *Fertil Steril.* 2013;100(3):818–24.
48. Vilella F, Moreno-Moya J, Balaguer N et al. Hsa-miR-30d, secreted by the human endometrium, is taken up by the pre-implantation embryo and might modify its transcriptome. *Development.* 2015;142(18):3210–21.
49. Campoy I, Lanau L, Altadill T et al. Exosome-like vesicles in uterine aspirates: A comparison of ultracentrifugation-based isolation protocols. *J Transl Med.* 2016;14(1):180.
50. Burns G, Brooks K, Wildung M, Navakanitworakul R, Christenson L, Spencer T. Extracellular vesicles in luminal fluid of the ovine uterus. *PLOS ONE.* 2014;9(3):e90913.
51. Burns G, Brooks K, Spencer T. Extracellular vesicles originate from the conceptus and uterus during early pregnancy in sheep. *Biol Reprod.* 2016;94(3).
52. Ruiz-González I, Xu J, Wang X, Burghardt R, Dunlap K, Bazer F. Exosomes, endogenous retroviruses and toll-like receptors: Pregnancy recognition in ewes. *Reproduction.* 2015;149(3):281–91.
53. Ng Y, Rome S, Jalabert A et al. Endometrial exosomes/microvesicles in the uterine microenvironment: A new paradigm for embryo-endometrial cross talk at implantation. *PLOS ONE.* 2013;8(3):e58502.
54. Simon C, Greening D, Bolumar D, Balaguer N, Salamonsen L, Vilella F. Extracellular vesicles in human reproduction in health and disease. *Endocr Rev.* 2018;39(3):292–332.
55. Burns G, Brooks K, O'Neil E, Hagen D, Behura S, Spencer T. Progesterone effects on extracellular vesicles in the sheep uterus. *Biol Reprod.* 2018;98(5):612–22.
56. Greening D, Nguyen H, Elgass K, Simpson R, Salamonsen L. Human endometrial exosomes contain hormone-specific cargo modulating trophoblast adhesive capacity: Insights into endometrial-embryo interactions. *Biol of Reprod.* 2016;94(2):38.
57. Desrochers L, Bordeleau F, Reinhart-King C, Cerione R, Antonyak M. Microvesicles provide a mechanism for intercellular communication by embryonic stem cells during embryo implantation. *Nat Commun.* 2016;7:11958.
58. Bidarimath M, Khalaj K, Kridli R, Kan F, Koti M, Tayade C. Extracellular vesicle mediated intercellular communication at the porcine maternal-fetal interface: A new paradigm for conceptus-endometrial cross-talk. *Sci Rep.* 2017;7(1):40476.
59. Salomon C, Yee S, Scholz-Romero K et al. Extravillous trophoblast cells-derived exosomes promote vascular smooth muscle cell migration. *Front Pharmacol.* 2014;5:175.
60. Homer H, Rice G, Salomon C. Review: Embryo- and endometrium-derived exosomes and their potential role in assisted reproductive treatments–liquid biopsies for endometrial receptivity. *Placenta.* 2017;54:89–94.
61. Altmäe S, Koel M, Võsa U et al. Meta-signature of human endometrial receptivity: A meta-analysis and validation study of transcriptomic biomarkers. *Sci Rep.* 2017;7(1):10077.
62. Chan C, Virtanen C, Winegarden N, Colgan T, Brown T, Greenblatt E. Discovery of biomarkers of endometrial receptivity through a minimally invasive approach: A validation study with implications for assisted reproduction. *Fertil Steril.* 2013;100(3):810–7.e8.
63. Vilella F, Ramirez L, Berlanga O et al. PGE2 and PGF2α concentrations in human endometrial fluid as biomarkers for embryonic implantation. *J Clin Endocrinol Metabol.* 2013;98(10):4123–32.
64. Moreno I, Codoñer F, Vilella F et al. Evidence that the endometrial microbiota has an effect on implantation success or failure. *Am J Obstet Gynecol.* 2016;215(6):684–703.
65. Moreno I, Cicinelli E, Garcia-Grau I et al. The diagnosis of chronic endometritis in infertile asymptomatic women: A comparative study of histology, microbial cultures, hysteroscopy, and molecular microbiology. *Am J Obstet Gynecol.* 2018;218(6):602.e1–e16.

3

Use of GnRHa for Triggering Final Oocyte Maturation during Ovarian Stimulation Cycles

Dalia Khalife, Jad Farid Assaf, and Johnny Awwad

Introduction

The use of gonadotropin-releasing hormone agonist (GnRHa) for the final induction of oocyte maturation in *in vitro* fertilization (IVF) cycles has gained momentum recently over the use of human chorionic gonadotropin (hCG) in women at high risk for ovarian hyperstimulation syndrome (OHSS) (1,2). With increased use of GnRH antagonists for pituitary downregulation and prevention of a premature luteinizing hormone (LH) surge, GnRHa triggering has been advocated as a viable alternative to trigger ovulation by displacement of the antagonist from its receptors, and stimulation of gonadotropin production and release by the anterior pituitary (3,4). Because of the shorter duration of the GnRHa-induced LH surge, earlier demise of the corpus luteum has been observed yielding a significant reduction in the risk for OHSS at the peril of adversely altering embryo implantation (5). Occasionally, a suboptimal LH response to GnRHa has been reported to compromise oocyte yield and/or maturation. For these reasons, the effectiveness of GnRHa triggering has been put to scrutiny, and the quest for the most optimal luteal phase support (LPS) for this type of cycle is also far from being resolved. Earlier studies using this triggering approach were not encouraging because of reportedly high pregnancy losses and low pregnancy rates (6,7). The adoption of a GnRH agonist trigger protocol with segmentation of the IVF cycle has therefore been proposed with the aim of restoring reproductive success without compromising patient safety. When a fresh embryo transfer is planned, however, alternative strategies may be utilized, namely, the prevention of luteal demise by a low-dose hCG rescue or by intensive supplementation of the luteal phase (8–16). It should also be noted that the GnRHa triggering protocol has attracted lots of attention for oocyte and/ or embryo cryopreservation cycles for clinical reproductive applications, such as fertility preservation, oocyte donation, and preimplantation genetic testing (17–19).

Normal Physiology

The mean duration of the physiologic LH surge in a natural cycle has been estimated at 48–50 hours (20). The surge has been described as triphasic in nature, starting with a rapidly ascending 14-hour phase, followed by another 14-hour plateau, and a gradually declining 20-hour arm (20). Because of the short half-life of LH, a bolus of hCG has been traditionally used for the triggering of final oocyte maturation in stimulated cycles. In view of prolonged hCG half-life, the associated LH receptor stimulation extends to about 8 days into the luteal phase. Excessive stimulation of the corpora lutea in an overstimulated cycle predisposes to the development of OHSS (9). In contrast, the GnRHa-induced gonadotropin surge is rather biphasic and short-lived. It lasts for about 24–36 hours with a rapid LH rise reaching maximal levels at 4 hours, followed by a moderate 16-hour descent (21). The reduction in LH exposure associated with the GnRHa trigger does not seem to impede the process of oocyte maturation but appears to yield in a defective corpus luteum (22). The GnRHa-triggered gonadotropin surge is also characterized by the release of endogenous FSH mimicking midcycle events occurring during a natural cycle (23). The FSH surge is believed to promote the formation of LH receptors on luteinizing granulosa cells, the resumption of meiosis, and the expansion of the cumulus oophorus (19,24).

Safety of GnRHa in the Prevention of OHSS

With the introduction of GnRH antagonists for pituitary downregulation in stimulated cycles, interest in the use of GnRHa for triggering ovulation emerged (3,26). Earlier findings suggested that GnRHa used for final oocyte maturation prevented the clinical manifestation of OHSS via a reduction of ovarian steroids (21). This reduction is attributed to the shorter LH activity associated with GnRHa triggering resulting in defective corpora lutea. In a prospective cohort study, vascular endothelial growth factor (VEGF) concentrations were found to be significantly decreased in the follicular fluid of patients triggered with a GnRHa (28). VGEF has been found accountable for increased vascular permeability associated with OHSS (28). GnRHa appears to stimulate ovarian pigment epithelium-derived factor (PEDF) expression on the granulosa cells, mediating an antiangiogenic effect and inducing a reduction in VEGF activity and consequently the risk for OHSS (29).

A case-control study conducted on patients with a previous history of severe OHSS showed that the use of GnRHa to trigger final oocyte maturation prevented the development of OHSS in the following cycle (1). The protective effect of GnRHa triggering against OHSS was also confirmed by a meta-analysis (31,32). Although isolated cases of OHSS have been sporadically reported after GnRHa triggering in GnRH antagonist downregulated cycles, the overall risk remains very low compared to conventional hCG (33).

Clinical Outcomes Associated with the Use of GnRHa for Triggering Final Oocyte Maturation

Oocyte Efficiency Parameters

In a randomized controlled study, Humaidan et al. reported a significantly higher yield of metaphase II (MII) oocytes in cycles triggered with a GnRHa compared to hCG (6). In an oocyte donation model, significantly more oocytes were collected (34) and better-quality embryos obtained (35) when triggering of ovulation was achieved using a GnRHa trigger compared with hCG. Krishna et al. further confirmed the association of the GnRHa group with a significantly higher number of oocytes retrieved, improved fertilization rates, and enhanced embryo quality compared to hCG (36). Increased follicular EGF-like peptide levels have been suggested to be the reason for enhanced oocyte maturation in women after a GnRHa trigger (37).

Despite numerous other studies supporting an overall improvement in oocyte efficiency parameters after GnRHa triggering (6,12,18,37), several reports nonetheless highlighted the occasional association of this triggering approach with partial or complete failure of oocyte collection. Empty follicle syndrome (EFS) in this context has been attributed to a profound downregulation of the hypothalamic axis (38). In a retrospective study of 508 autologous and donor cycles, Kummer et al. (39) demonstrated a positive correlation between the number of oocytes retrieved and the following parameters: peak estradiol levels as well as posttrigger LH and progesterone levels. EFS was more likely to occur when posttrigger LH levels were less than 15 IU/L and progesterone levels less than 3.5 ng/mL (39). These findings were further confirmed in a prospective study that demonstrated a significantly lower oocyte yield when posttrigger LH was 15 IU/L or less (40). It should be noted, nonetheless, that data on 2304 oocyte donation cycles showed similar incidence of EFS between patients triggered with hCG versus GnRHa (41).

Risk factors for a suboptimal response to GnRHa trigger (defined as a posttrigger LH less than 15 IU/L) were evaluated in a retrospective cohort study (42). Women at risk often had suppressed FSH and LH levels on the second day of the cycle and decreased LH levels on the day of the trigger. They were more likely to require a prolonged duration of stimulation, to require an increased dose of gonadotropins, and to present with a history of menstrual irregularities. In addition, women maintained on long-term oral contraception appear to represent a particularly vulnerable group for suboptimal LH response to GnRHa triggering (42). Potential candidates for GnRHa triggering should therefore be screened *a priori* for the presence of risk factors causing hypothalamic dysfunction. In the event of a failed LH surge after a GnRHa trigger, repeating the trigger with hCG has been shown to be successful in retrieving oocytes (38,39).

Reproductive Success

In a randomized controlled trial, Humaidan et al. compared the clinical outcome of normo-gonadotrophic women randomized to a GnRHa trigger protocol versus hCG (6). The investigators reported a significantly higher early pregnancy loss (EPL) rate and a lower clinical pregnancy rate (CPR) in the GnRHa trigger group of women who received a daily dose of micronized progesterone gel 90 mg vaginally and estradiol tablets 4 mg orally. It should be noted that luteal phase support (LPS) was discontinued in all cases on the day of the pregnancy test. Using a similar study design, Kolibianakis et al. (7) reported an ongoing pregnancy rate of 2.9% and an early pregnancy loss of 83.3% in the GnRHa group who was given daily micronized progesterone capsules 600 mg vaginally and estradiol tablets 4 mg orally. LPS was continued in this study until 7 weeks of gestation. It soon became apparent that conventional LPS found for hCG-triggered IVF/intracytoplasmic sperm injection (ICSI) cycles is not equally appropriate for cycles in which a GnRHa was used for triggering of ovulation (7).

Studies on primates showed that the corpus luteum cannot accomplish its full endocrine transformation with an LH surge lasting less than 48 hours (22). These findings were also suggested by clinical studies that demonstrated a profound disruption of corpus luteum function in cycles triggered with a GnRHa (43). They were further elaborated by the significant fall in luteal serum inhibin A, pro Alpha C, estradiol and progesterone levels associated with this triggering strategy (43). Complete and irreversible luteolysis has also been demonstrated with failure of luteal rescue despite rising endogenous hCG in the case of pregnancy (44).

An earlier systematic review confirmed lower CPR (OR = 0.22, 95% CI 0.05–0.85) and higher EPL (OR = 11.5, 95% CI 0.95–138.98) associated with the use of standard luteal support in GnRHa triggered cycles compared to hCG (35). These findings clearly indicate an urgent need to modify luteal phase support when a GnRHa is used to trigger ovulation. Different strategies have been published for this purpose, including the use of intensive estrogen and progesterone luteal supplementation (26,45–47) and the use of low-dose hCG rescue to salvage the corpus luteum and stimulate endogenous sex steroid production (10,12,13,47–49).

Use of Intensive Luteal Phase Support

The use of intensive estrogen and progesterone supplementation to the profoundly deficient luteal phase in cycles triggered with a GnRHa has been the subject of much research (26,43).

In 2008, Engmann et al. (2008) conducted a randomized controlled trial in which women with polycystic ovary syndrome (PCOS) were randomized to receive a GnRHa or hCG for ovulation trigger. The GnRHa group were given for luteal support a daily dose of 50 mg of progesterone intramuscularly (IM) in combination with 0.3 mg of transdermal estrogen patches every other day until 10 weeks of gestation (26). Close monitoring of luteal estrogen and progesterone levels was also performed with dose adjustment of LPS in order to maintain serum progesterone levels above 20 ng/mL and estradiol levels above 200 pg/mL. There were no significant differences in the implantation rates (36.0% versus 31.0%; $p < .05$) and ongoing pregnancy rates (53.3% versus 48.3%; $p < .05$) between the GnRHa and hCG groups, respectively. While 31% of women in the hCG group developed some form of OHSS, none in the GnRHa group had similar manifestations.

In 2013, Iliodromiti et al. (47) retrospectively stratified 620 cycles at risk for OHSS according to the method of ovulation trigger. The luteal phase support of GnRHa triggered cycles comprised 50 mg IM progesterone daily, 90 mg vaginal progesterone twice daily, and 6 mg of oral estradiol valerate daily administered until 7 weeks of gestation. Live birth rates were similar in both groups

(29.8% versus 29.2%; $p = .69$) (47). Comparable findings were reported by other studies (46,49). Cycle predictors for a successful reproductive outcome after GnRHa triggering have been evaluated by Kummer et al. (50). The investigators found significant positive associations between pregnancy occurrence with peak serum E2 levels greater than 4000 pg/mL and LH levels greater than 3.5 IU/L on the day of the trigger (50).

Use of Low-Dose hCG Luteal Rescue

Another alternative to improving the reproductive success of cycles after GnRHa triggering of final oocyte maturation consists of preventing the demise of the corpus luteum by administering a low hCG dose concurrently at the time of ovulation trigger or after oocyte collection (10–13,51). The added benefit of the hCG rescue dose is to avoid luteolysis and support the endogenous hormone production of the corpus luteum (42).

Low-Dose hCG at the Time of a GnRHa Trigger

Dual triggering of final oocyte maturation has been shown to be effective in a proof-of-concept study of 45 patients when a combination of GnRHa and low-dose hCG (1000–2500 IU) was used for triggering ovulation (34). Pregnancy outcomes were satisfactory with 17.2% EPL and 53.3% OPR. A similar study also showed comparable results with 57.7% OPR and a solitary case of severe OHSS (49). In order to assess the risk of OHSS after dual trigger, Griffin et al. (48) conducted a retrospective cohort study in high-responder women in which they compared GnRHa alone and GnRHa/hCG for triggering of ovulation. The dual-trigger group showed significantly higher live birth rates (LBRs) (52.9% versus 30.9%), implantation rate (IR) (41.9% versus 22.1%), and CPRs (58.8% versus 36.8%) compared with the GnRHa alone group. Both groups received intensive LPS consisting of 50 mg IM progesterone daily and 0.3 mg transdermal E2 patches every other day (48). Moreover, the concept of dual trigger (GnRHa + 6500 IU hCG) was successfully evaluated in another retrospective cohort study that included 376 normal responders who received daily progesterone (50 mg IM and 300 mg vaginally) for luteal support. Higher PR and LBR were achieved without an increased risk of OHSS (52).

It should be noted that a retrospective cohort study presented data on 174 patients, demonstrating the incidence of early OHSS to be significantly higher after the dual trigger compared with GnRHa alone (8.6% versus 0%) with four cases of severe OHSS (53).

Low-Dose hCG at the Time of Oocyte Retrieval

It has been shown that luteinized granulosa cells in stimulated cycles with a GnRHa trigger retain the competence to respond to hCG and maintain their secretion of estrogen and progesterone on the day of ovum pickup (OPU) (54). This finding led to the plausibility of administering a single bolus of hCG (1500 IU) 1 hour after the oocyte retrieval in GnRHa triggered cycles for the purpose of maintaining corpus luteum function and enhancing implantation. This strategy was portrayed in different studies by Humaidan and colleagues (10–12). In their cohort pilot study (10), the investigators demonstrated 50% LBRs when high-risk women received a GnRHa trigger followed by 1500 IU hCG after OPU. Using a prospective controlled design, the same investigators randomized normo-gonadotropic women to receive either hCG trigger or GnRHa trigger followed by 1500 IU hCG at 35 hours (12). They found no statistically significant differences in LBR between the two groups (24% versus 31%, respectively) (12). This strategy was reported to be associated with a low incidence of OHSS, with cases of late-onset OHSS described mostly in patients with a high number of growing follicles (25 or more follicles) (47,55). It should be noted, however, that the safety of this protocol in high-responder women has not yet been fully established. A retrospective study of women at high risk for OHSS showed that this protocol was associated with severe early OHSS in 26% of cases (56).

In an attempt to circumvent the risk of OHSS associated with low-dose rescue dose, Haas et al. (57) designed a proof-of-concept study to evaluate the benefits and safety of rescuing the luteal phase with a low-dose hCG delayed until 3 days after OPU. High midluteal progesterone levels were observed (greater than 127 nmol/L) in these patients with no apparent increase in the risk for OHSS (57).

Use of Daily Luteal GnRH-Agonist Doses

Luteal support using repeated daily doses of GnRH agonist following GnRHa triggering was also assessed in a randomized prospective study by Pirard et al. (58). Using 100 micrograms of nasal buserelin three times per day was associated with luteal progesterone levels comparable to patients receiving hCG trigger with standard LPS support (58). Bar-Hava and colleagues also evaluated the use of daily intranasal GnRHa (Nafarelin) for LPS initiated on the evening after OPU in 46 high-responder patients without progesterone supplementation. The OPR was found to be 52.1% with no cases of OHSS reported (59). Well-designed randomized studies are nonetheless needed to confirm these findings.

Segmentation of IVF Cycles and Freeze-All Policy

In order to circumvent the risk of late-onset OHSS, several investigators introduced the concept of cycle segmentation as the safest approach to high-risk women undergoing ovarian stimulation (27). This strategy consists of cryopreserving all embryos in order to replace them in a subsequent cycle. Transferring embryos in a controlled cycle seems to be associated with a reproductive advantage in terms of success rate by avoiding the detrimental effect of high steroid levels on endometrial receptivity (25,27,30).

Conclusion

There is growing interest in GnRHa for the triggering of final oocyte maturation in women undergoing ovarian stimulation for the purpose of achieving an OHSS-free IVF clinic. Despite a high safety record, the GnRHa trigger protocol has been associated with a very low incidence of OHSS, more so when low-dose hCG rescue is used. For fresh embryo transfers, the most suitable luteal phase support strategy that ensures treatment efficacy and safety remains to be determined. Cycle segmentation and cryo-warmed embryo transfer remains a viable option for IVF centers with successful cryopreservation programs.

More research is expected to refine the role of individualization for luteal phase management of cycles with a GnRHa trigger. Individualization may be based on parameters such as the number of growing follicles, peak estradiol levels, LH levels at the time of trigger, and steroid hormone levels during the luteal phase.

REFERENCES

1. Lewit N, Kol S, Manor D et al. Endocrinology: Comparison of gonadotrophin-releasing hormone analogues and human chorionic gonadotrophin for the induction of ovulation and prevention of ovarian hyperstimulation syndrome: A case-control study. *Hum Reprod.* 1996;11(7):1399–402.
2. Segal S, Casper RF. Gonadotropin-releasing hormone agonist versus human chorionic gonadotropin for triggering follicular maturation in in vitro fertilization. *Fertil Steril.* 1992;57(6):1254–8.
3. Itskovitz-Eldor J, Kol S, Mannaerts B. Use of a single bolus of GnRH agonist triptorelin to trigger ovulation after GnRH antagonist ganirelix treatment in women undergoing ovarian stimulation for assisted reproduction, with special reference to the prevention of ovarian hyperstimulation syndrome: Preliminary report. *Hum Reprod.* 2000;15(9):1965–8.
4. Porter RN, Smith W, Craft IL et al. Induction of ovulation for *in-vitro* fertilisation using buserelin and gonadotropins. *Lancet.* 1984;324(8414):1284–5.
5. Youssef MA, Van der Veen F, Al-Inany HG et al. Gonadotropin-releasing hormone agonist versus HCG for oocyte triggering in antagonist-assisted reproductive technology. *Cochrane Database Syst Rev.* 2014;10(10):CD008046.
6. Humaidan P, Ejdrup Bredkjaer H, Bungum L et al. GnRH agonist (buserelin) or hCG for ovulation induction in GnRH antagonist IVF/ICSI cycles: A prospective randomized study. *Hum Reprod.* 2005;20(5):1213–20.

7. Kolibianakis EM, Schultze-Mosgau A, Schroer A et al. A lower ongoing pregnancy rate can be expected when GnRH agonist is used for triggering final oocyte maturation instead of HCG in patients undergoing IVF with GnRH antagonists. *Hum Reprod.* 2005;20(10):2887–92.
8. Bodri D, Sunkara SK, Coomarasamy A. Gonadotropin-releasing hormone agonists versus antagonists for controlled ovarian hyperstimulation in oocyte donors: A systematic review and meta-analysis. *Fertil Steril.* 2011;95(1):164–9.
9. Fauser BC, de Jong D, Olivennes F et al. Endocrine profiles after triggering of final oocyte maturation with GnRH agonist after cotreatment with the GnRH antagonist ganirelix during ovarian hyperstimulation for *in vitro* fertilization. *J Clin Endocrinol Metab.* 2002;87(2):709–15.
10. Humaidan P. Luteal phase rescue in high-risk OHSS patients by GnRHa triggering in combination with low-dose HCG: A pilot study. *Reprod Biomed Online.* 2009;18(5):630–4.
11. Humaidan P, Bungum L, Bungum M et al. Rescue of corpus luteum function with peri-ovulatory HCG supplementation in IVF/ICSI GnRH antagonist cycles in which ovulation was triggered with a GnRH agonist: A pilot study. *Reprod Biomed Online.* 2006;13(2):173–8.
12. Humaidan P, Bredkjær HE, Westergaard LG et al. 1,500 IU human chorionic gonadotropin administered at oocyte retrieval rescues the luteal phase when gonadotropin-releasing hormone agonist is used for ovulation induction: A prospective, randomized, controlled study. *Fertil Steril.* 2010;93(3):847–54.
13. Humaidan P, Polyzos NP, Alsbjerg B et al. GnRHa trigger and individualized luteal phase hCG support according to ovarian response to stimulation: Two prospective randomized controlled multi-centre studies in IVF patients. *Hum Reprod.* 2013;28(9):2511–21.
14. Papanikolaou EG, Verpoest W, Fatemi H et al. A novel method of luteal supplementation with recombinant luteinizing hormone when a gonadotropin-releasing hormone agonist is used instead of human chorionic gonadotropin for ovulation triggering: A randomized prospective proof of concept study. *Fertil Steril.* 2011;95(3):1174–7.
15. Shapiro BS, Daneshmand ST, Restrepo H et al. Efficacy of induced luteinizing hormone surge after "trigger" with gonadotropin-releasing hormone agonist. *Fertil Steril.* 2011;95(2):826–8.
16. Dosouto C, Haahr T, Humaidan P. Gonadotropin-releasing hormone agonist (GnRHa) trigger—State of the art. *Reprod Biol.* 2017;17(1):1–8.
17. Shapiro BS, Daneshmand ST, Garner FC et al. Embryo cryopreservation rescues cycles with premature luteinization. *Fertil Steril.* 2010;93(2):636–41.
18. Reddy J, Turan V, Bedoschi G et al. Triggering final oocyte maturation with gonadotropin-releasing hormone agonist (GnRHa) versus human chorionic gonadotropin (hCG) in breast cancer patients undergoing fertility preservation: An extended experience. *J Assist Reprod Genet.* 2014;31(7):927–32.
19. Oktay K, Türkçüoğlu I, Rodriguez-Wallberg KA. GnRH agonist trigger for women with breast cancer undergoing fertility preservation by aromatase inhibitor/FSH stimulation. *Reprod Biomed Online.* 2010;20(6):783–8.
20. Hoff JD, Quigley ME, Yen SS. Hormonal dynamics at midcycle: A reevaluation. *J Clin Endocrinol Metab.* 1983;57(4):792–6.
21. Itskovitz J, Boldes R, Levron J et al. Induction of preovulatory luteinizing hormone surge and prevention of ovarian hyperstimulation syndrome by gonadotropin-releasing hormone agonist. *Fertil Steril.* 1991;56(2):213–20.
22. Chandrasekher YA, Brenner RM, Molskness TA et al. Titrating luteinizing hormone surge requirements for ovulatory changes in primate follicles. II. Progesterone receptor expression in luteinizing granulosa cells. *J Clin Endocrinol Metab.* 1991;73(3):584–9.
23. Gonen Y, Balakier H, Powell W et al. Use of gonadotropin-releasing hormone agonist to trigger follicular maturation for *in vitro* fertilization. *J Clin Endocrinol Metab.* 1990;71(4):918–22.
24. Andersen CY, Leonardsen L, Ulloa-Aguirre A et al. FSH-induced resumption of meiosis in mouse oocytes: Effect of different isoforms. *Mol Hum Reprod.* 1999;5(8):726–31.
25. Devroey P, Polyzos NP, Blockeel C. An OHSS-free clinic by segmentation of IVF treatment. *Hum Reprod.* 2011;26(10):2593–7.
26. Engmann L, DiLuigi A, Schmidt D et al. The use of gonadotropin-releasing hormone (GnRH) agonist to induce oocyte maturation after cotreatment with GnRH antagonist in high-risk patients undergoing *in vitro* fertilization prevents the risk of ovarian hyperstimulation syndrome: A prospective randomized controlled study. *Fertil Steril.* 2008;89(1):84–91.

27. Fatemi HM, Popovic-Todorovic B. Implantation in assisted reproduction: A look at endometrial receptivity. *Reprod Biomed Online.* 2013;27(5):530–8.
28. Cerrillo M, Rodríguez S, Mayoral M et al. Differential regulation of VEGF after final oocyte maturation with GnRH agonist versus hCG: A rationale for OHSS reduction. *Fertil Steril.* 2009;91(4):1526–8.
29. Miller I, Chuderland D, Ron-El R et al. GnRH agonist triggering modulates PEDF to VEGF ratio inversely to hCG in granulosa cells. *J Clin Endocrinol Metab.* 2015;100(11):E1428–36.
30. Garcia-Velasco JA. Agonist trigger: What is the best approach? Agonist trigger with vitrification of oocytes or embryos. *Fertil Steril.* 2012;97(3):527–8.
31. Fatemi HM, Garcia-Velasco J. Avoiding ovarian hyperstimulation syndrome with the use of gonadotropin-releasing hormone agonist trigger. *Fertil Steril.* 2015;103(4):870–3.
32. Mourad S, Brown J, Farquhar C. Interventions for the prevention of OHSS in ART cycles: An overview of Cochrane reviews. *Cochrane Database Syst Rev.* 2017;(1):CD012103.
33. Gurbuz AS, Gode F, Ozcimen N et al. Gonadotrophin-releasing hormone agonist trigger and freeze-all strategy does not prevent severe ovarian hyperstimulation syndrome: A report of three cases. *Reprod Biomed Online.* 2014;29(5):541–4.
34. Shapiro BS, Daneshmand ST, Garner FC et al. Gonadotropin-releasing hormone agonist combined with a reduced dose of human chorionic gonadotropin for final oocyte maturation in fresh autologous cycles of in vitro fertilization. *Fertil Steril.* 2008;90(1):231–3.
35. Griesinger G, Diedrich K, Devroey P et al. GnRH agonist for triggering final oocyte maturation in the GnRH antagonist ovarian hyperstimulation protocol: A systematic review and meta-analysis. *Hum Reprod Update.* 2005;12(2):159–68.
36. Krishna D, Dhoble S, Praneesh G et al. Gonadotropin-releasing hormone agonist trigger is a better alternative than human chorionic gonadotropin in PCOS undergoing IVF cycles for an OHSS Free Clinic: A randomized control trial. *J Hum Reprod Sci.* 2016;9(3):164.
37. Humaidan P, Westergaard LG, Mikkelsen AL et al. Levels of the epidermal growth factor-like peptide amphiregulin in follicular fluid reflect the mode of triggering ovulation: A comparison between gonadotrophin-releasing hormone agonist and urinary human chorionic gonadotrophin. *Fertil Steril.* 2011;95(6):2034–8.
38. Asada Y, Itoi F, Honnma H et al. Failure of GnRH agonist-triggered oocyte maturation: Its cause and management. *J Assist Reprod Genet.* 2013;30(4):581–5.
39. Kummer NE, Feinn RS, Griffin DW et al. Predicting successful induction of oocyte maturation after gonadotropin-releasing hormone agonist (GnRHa) trigger. *Hum Reprod.* 2012;28(1):152–9.
40. Chen SL, Ye DS, Chen X et al. Circulating luteinizing hormone level after triggering oocyte maturation with GnRH agonist may predict oocyte yield in flexible GnRH antagonist protocol. *Hum Reprod.* 2012;27(5):1351–6.
41. Castillo JC, Garcia-Velasco J, Humaidan P. Empty follicle syndrome after GnRHa triggering versus hCG triggering in COS. *J Assist Reprod Genet.* 2012;29(3):249–53.
42. Meyer L, Murphy LA, Gumer A et al. Risk factors for a suboptimal response to gonadotropin-releasing hormone agonist trigger during in vitro fertilization cycles. *Fertil Steril.* 2015;104(3):637–42.
43. Babayof R, Margalioth EJ, Huleihel M et al. Serum inhibin A, VEGF and TNFα levels after triggering oocyte maturation with GnRH agonist compared with HCG in women with polycystic ovaries undergoing IVF treatment: A prospective randomized trial. *Hum Reprod.* 2006;21(5):1260–5.
44. Nevo O, alia Eldar-Geva T, Kol S et al. Lower levels of inhibin A and pro-αC during the luteal phase after triggering oocyte maturation with a gonadotropin-releasing hormone agonist versus human chorionic gonadotropin. *Fertil Steril.* 2003;79(5):1123–8.
45. Engmann L, Siano L, Schmidt D et al. GnRH agonist to induce oocyte maturation during IVF in patients at high risk of OHSS. *Reprod Biomed Online.* 2006;13(5):639–44.
46. Imbar T, Kol S, Lossos F et al. Reproductive outcome of fresh or frozen–thawed embryo transfer is similar in high-risk patients for ovarian hyperstimulation syndrome using GnRH agonist for final oocyte maturation and intensive luteal support. *Hum Reprod.* 2012;27(3):753–9.
47. Iliodromiti S, Blockeel C, Tremellen KP et al. Consistent high clinical pregnancy rates and low ovarian hyperstimulation syndrome rates in high-risk patients after GnRH agonist triggering and modified luteal support: A retrospective multicentre study. *Hum Reprod.* 2013;28(9):2529–36.
48. Griffin D, Benadiva C, Kummer N et al. Dual trigger of oocyte maturation with gonadotropin-releasing hormone agonist and low-dose human chorionic gonadotropin to optimize live birth rates in high responders. *Fertil Steril.* 2012;97(6):1316–20.

49. Shapiro BS, Daneshmand ST, Garner FC et al. Comparison of "triggers" using leuprolide acetate alone or in combination with low-dose human chorionic gonadotropin. *Fertil Steril.* 2011;95(8):2715–7.
50. Kummer N, Benadiva C, Feinn R et al. Factors that predict the probability of a successful clinical outcome after induction of oocyte maturation with a gonadotropin-releasing hormone agonist. *Fertil Steril.* 2011;96(1):63–8.
51. Humaidan P, Engmann L, Benadiva C. Luteal phase supplementation after gonadotropin-releasing hormone agonist trigger in fresh embryo transfer: The American versus European approaches. *Fertil Steril.* 2015;103(4):879–85.
52. Lin MH, Wu FS, Lee RK et al. Dual trigger with combination of gonadotropin-releasing hormone agonist and human chorionic gonadotropin significantly improves the live-birth rate for normal responders in GnRH-antagonist cycles. *Fertil Steril.* 2013;100(5):1296–302.
53. O'Neill KE, Senapati S, Maina I et al. GnRH agonist with low-dose hCG (dual trigger) is associated with higher risk of severe ovarian hyperstimulation syndrome compared to GnRH agonist alone. *J Assist Reprod Genet.* 2016;33(9):1175–84.
54. Engmann L, Romak J, Nulsen J et al. *In vitro* viability and secretory capacity of human luteinized granulosa cells after gonadotropin-releasing hormone agonist trigger of oocyte maturation. *Fertil Steril.* 2011;96(1):198–202.
55. Radesic B, Tremellen K. Oocyte maturation employing a GnRH agonist in combination with low-dose hCG luteal rescue minimizes the severity of ovarian hyperstimulation syndrome while maintaining excellent pregnancy rates. *Hum Reprod.* 2011;26(12):3437–42.
56. Seyhan A, Ata B, Polat M et al. Severe early ovarian hyperstimulation syndrome following GnRH agonist trigger with the addition of 1500 IU hCG. *Hum Reprod.* 2013;28(9):2522–8.
57. Haas J, Kedem A, Machtinger R et al. HCG (1500 IU) administration on day 3 after oocytes retrieval, following GnRH-agonist trigger for final follicular maturation, results in high sufficient mid luteal progesterone levels-a proof of concept. *J Ovarian Res.* 2014;7(1):35.
58. Pirard C, Loumaye E, Laurent P et al. Contribution to more patient-friendly ART treatment: Efficacy of continuous low-dose GnRH agonist as the only luteal support—Results of a prospective, randomized, comparative study. *Int J Endocrinol.* 2015;2015:727569.
59. Bar-Hava I, Mizrachi Y, Karfunkel-Doron D et al. Intranasal gonadotropin-releasing hormone agonist (GnRHa) for luteal-phase support following GnRHa triggering, a novel approach to avoid ovarian hyperstimulation syndrome in high responders. *Fertil Steril.* 2016;106(2):330–3.

4

Use of Time-Lapse Embryo Imaging in Assisted Reproductive Technology Practice

Fadi Choucair, Chantal Farra, and Johnny Awwad

Introduction

Diverse factors can adversely affect the efficacy of assisted reproductive technologies (ARTs) and the occurrence of a successful pregnancy. Embryo implantation has long been recognized as an important rate-limiting step to more successful pregnancy outcomes. In an attempt to overcome this inherent limitation of human nature, reproductive specialists have traditionally resorted to the replacement of multiple embryos to increase the likelihood of success. Improved pregnancy rates were very soon overshadowed by an unacceptable rise in the incidence of multiple births, with associated neonatal mortality/morbidity, maternal health hazards, and financial/psychological burden (1). Intuitively, the best strategy to avoid this iatrogenic complication is to restrict the number of embryos transferred at any one time to a single embryo. A recent meta-analysis demonstrated that although the chances of multiple births are significantly reduced after one cycle of fresh single embryo transfer (SET), concomitantly the likelihood of live birth is also significantly decreased (2). The ultimate challenge in *in vitro* fertilization (IVF)/intracytoplasmic sperm injection (ICSI) cycles then becomes to implement a SET policy while maintaining high live birth rates. It was proposed that embryo quality is a predictive prognostic tool for live birth (3). Unfortunately, evidence-based standardized morphologic variables for the selection of embryos with the greatest chance of implantation are lacking. The conventional methodology is to perform isolated and static assessments of cultured embryos, and to compare observed annotations to ones relevant to the stage of development before final selection of the "ideal" embryo. Various embryo scoring models are used in clinical practice, and for this matter, a consensus was established in 2011 on static morphologic assessments of embryos in culture (4). The conventional scoring approach, however, does not account for the dynamic nature of embryo development and may therefore miss out on interval events deemed critical to the selection process. To solve this shortcoming, time-lapse technology was developed and adapted to the IVF laboratory environment to monitor embryo development in real time at well-defined time intervals within the confinement of an incubator.

Time-lapse cinematography was initially used by Payne et al. in 1997 to monitor embryonic development events (5). A decade later, Lemmen et al. identified embryonic kinetic markers correlated with implantation success (6). Currently, several time-lapse (TL) imaging systems are available for IVF. The three most commonly used ones are the Embryoscope, Primo Vision, and Eeva (Early Embryo Viability Assessment) systems. Technically, the Embryoscope is an incubator unit with an integrated TL system that uses a bright-field illumination with seven focal planes to visualize embryonic intracellular events at high resolution and project them over time. Primo Vision consists of small units that can be placed in a conventional incubator and uses bright-field illumination with 11 focal planes to monitor embryo development. The Eeva System is a microscopic TL system that uses a dark-field illumination with one focal plane to map cytokinetic division patterns of embryos with a very low resolution for intracellular details (7).

Defining Morphokinetic Parameters

The embryo morphokinetic assessment in large-scale clinical practice was initially used by a Spanish group in 2011 to select the "best" embryo (8). Special attention was made to specific embryo developmental events such as dysmorphologic characteristics, cleavage time events, and cleavage intervals.

The likelihood of embryo implantation was correlated with two kinetic events in particular, which are the duration of the second-cell cycle (cc2), defined as the time from division into a two-blastomere embryo to division into a three-blastomere embryo (t3-t2); and the second synchrony (s2), defined as the time from division into a three-blastomere embryo to division into a four-blastomere embryo (t4-t3). Specific morphologic exclusion criteria were also defined and found to be associated with a very low implantation rate of 8%. These criteria include (a) direct cleavage from zygote to three-blastomere embryo, defined as: cc2 = t3-t2 < 5 hours post-ICSI; (b) uneven blastomere size at the two-cell stage during the interphase where the nuclei are visible; and (c) multinucleation at the four-cell stage during the interphase where the nuclei are visible. The investigators also demonstrated tighter distributions of cleavage times for implanting embryos and a prominent tail of lagging distributions for the nonimplanting embryos. In this manner, normal time ranges were established for several kinetic parameters, then entered into a mathematical model and found to be highly predictive of embryo implantation. As a result, the first embryo morphokinetic classification was developed. The newly proposed model algorithm was found to be more predictive than static morphologic assessment (area under the curve [AUC] 0.72 versus 0.64).

It should be noted that one particular kinetic event has attracted much attention in morphokinetic studies—the direct cleavage (DC) of zygotes. The occurrence of direct cleavage was detected in nearly 14% of the total embryonic cohort (9). More importantly, since embryos with DC were found to have much lower implantation rates, deselecting these embryos at the time of uterine transfer could improve the efficiency of the implantation process. It is generally agreed that the following morphokinetic features may be used to discard embryos with low implantation potential: (a) direct cleavage from zygote to three-blastomere embryo; (b) too short second-cell cycle, i.e., duration of two-cell stage embryo (cc2 = t3-t2 < 5 hours); and (c) too long second synchrony, i.e., duration as three-cell stage embryo (s2 = t4-t3 > 1.5 hours).

Time-Lapse Imaging Analysis for the Prediction of Blastocyst Development

Several observational studies have attempted to predict the development of embryos to the blastocyst stage using time-lapse imaging (TLI) analysis of embryo development. In an initial study in 2010, Wong et al. (10) using the Eeva (Early Embryo Viability Assessment) System identified three parameters during the cleavage-stage embryos development that collectively predicted blastocyst formation. These parameters are (a) the duration of the first cytokinesis (the very brief last step in mitosis that physically separates the two daughter cells), (b) the time interval between the end of the first mitosis and the initiation of the second, and (c) the time interval between the second and third mitoses (the time between the appearance of the cleavage furrows of the second and third mitoses). Importantly, the success in progression to the blastocyst stage could be predicted with greater than 93% specificity by measuring these three dynamic noninvasive imaging parameters in the first 2 days following fertilization. Another study by Conaghan et al. in 2013 (11) showed that the Eeva prediction and cell-tracking software correctly predicted by day 3 the embryos that will develop into blastocysts with a specificity of 84.2% and a positive predictive value (PPV) of 54.1%. In parallel, other groups used the dynamic embryoscope system to monitor the timings of cell divisions in human cleavage-stage embryos to predict successful blastulation. While Cruz et al. in 2012 (12) showed significant differences in the temporal patterns of development between embryos that reached the blastocyst stage and embryos that did not, these results were not universally reproducible (13). Dal Canto et al. during the same year (13) evaluated similar time kinetics and failed to confirm the previous findings. Overall, the use of TLI to predict blastocyst formation in clinical studies has been associated with a high specificity and a low sensitivity. The occurrence of high false negatives indicates that TLI analysis may be associated with the serious pitfall of rejecting usable embryos with good implantation potential from consideration for uterine transfer or cryopreservation.

TLI Analysis for the Prediction of Euploidy

TLI has been investigated as a discriminatory tool to select embryos with a euploid complement. In this perspective, the cleavage times were studied in correlation with preimplantation genetic screening patterns. In 2014, Basile et al. noticed that embryos falling within optimal morphokinetic ranges exhibited a significantly greater proportion of euploid profiles than those falling outside this range (14). The proposed model identified t5-t2 (OR 2.853; 95% CI, 1.763–4.616) and cc3 (OR 2.095; 95% CI, 1.356–3.238) as the most relevant variables related to normal chromosomal content. A receiver operating characteristic (ROC) analysis determined the predictive properties with respect to chromosomal normalcy with an AUC value of 0.634 (95% CI, 0.581–0.687) (Level of Evidence: IIB). Similarly, Campbell et al. proposed a risk model for predicting euploidy on the basis of two morphokinetic parameters: the time to blastocoel formation and the time to blastocyst expansion (15). Using the same model, Kramer et al. showed that the incidence of aneuploidy did not differ across risk groups identified previously by Campbell (16). Furthermore, their analysis revealed that all areas under the ROC curves were unable to distinguish the ploidy status of embryos. They also found that patient variability for euploid embryos was so great that it is very difficult to make use of morphokinetic parameters efficiently to select euploid embryos using universal criteria (16).

It can therefore be concluded that there is no sufficient evidence to support a role for embryo morphokinetics in predicting the euploidy status of embryos. The in-between patient variability in embryo kinetic characteristics of euploid embryos is greater than embryo ploidy status so that it will be impossible to use these parameters to select euploid embryos.

Time-Lapse Analysis for the Prediction of Embryo Implantation

Although a correlation between the morphokinetic features of preimplantation embryos and *in vitro* blastocyst development has been demonstrated, the application of TLI to predict embryo implantation and pregnancy success has been challenged. The results of a prospective cohort study conducted by Kirkegaard et al. in 2013 on 571 observed embryos revealed that the duration of the first cytokinesis, the duration of the three-cell stage, and direct cleavage to three cells predicted development to high-quality blastocyst (17). However, none of the suggested time points of cellular divisions differed between pregnant and nonpregnant groups. Interestingly, when taking into account potential confounders and predictors of blastocyst development, logistic regression analysis demonstrated that maternal age was the sole significant predictor of pregnancy outcome. In a large observational study, Motato et al. retrospectively analyzed 7483 monitored zygotes (18). They highlighted that the most predictive parameters for blastocyst formation were the time of morula formation tM and the time of transition of five to eight blastomere embryos (t8-t5) with a ROC value of 0.849 (95% CI, 0.835–0.854) (Level of Evidence: IIB). These parameters were nevertheless much less predictive of implantation success with a ROC value 0.546 (95% CI, 0.507–0.585) (Level of Evidence: IIB).

The findings of randomized controlled trials (RCTs) on the subject have also been controversial. In 2014, Rubio et al. demonstrated a significant improvement in ongoing pregnancy and implantation rates (Level of Evidence: IB) for embryos randomized to the Embryoscope compared to conventional morphologic assessment (19). The Embryoscope group also had a significant reduction in early pregnancy loss. More so, a higher percentage of embryos had a timely kinetic pattern in the TLI group compared with control. It was not clear, however, whether the observed benefit in clinical outcome was solely the result of the choice of embryo selection methodology or whether close incubation conditions in the TLI group had confounded the final outcome. Conversely, results from another RCT conducted by Goodman et al. on 119 monitored embryos revealed that pregnancy and implantation rates were not significantly different between TLI and control groups (Level of Evidence: IB) (20). A more recent pilot RCT by Kaser et al. comparing the adjunctive use of the Eeva System on day 3–5 embryos to day 5 selection with conventional incubation alone, showed no significant differences in the clinical and ongoing pregnancy rates between groups (Level of Evidence: IB) (21). An RCT conducted by Park et al. analyzed the impact of the closed incubation system on embryo quality after 2 days of *in vitro* culture (22). The results showed similar embryo development dynamics and morphologic quality scores in the closed Embryoscope incubator compared with the conventional incubation system (Level of Evidence: IB). Surprisingly, the number of miscarriages was significantly higher in the embryoscope compared to the conventional incubation arm.

A recent meta-analysis by Pribenszky et al. in 2017 which included five RCTs supported a clinical benefit of using TLI for embryo selection, but failed to account for the heterogeneity in study designs and the predictive algorithms utilized (23). In the same perspective, Rakowsky et al. appraised six RCTs while assessing the risks of bias for each. The combined results did not suggest any evidence for a beneficial effect of TLI on the embryo selection process prior to uterine transfer (24).

Taken together, the bulk of the evidence remains inconclusive with respect to the efficacy of TLI technology in predicting embryo implantation and pregnancy success. Available meta-analyses have included flawed studies and failed to take into account important confounders that could have biased profoundly the final conclusions. Confounders such as the type of TLI technology, the algorithm prediction model, the incubation system, and the embryo transfer practice were not factored in for final analysis. It is therefore suggested that it may be premature to recommend the TLI innovation for clinical practice on grounds of improved reproductive outcome.

It should be noted that a sound scientific approach to the adoption of any new intervention should follow well-defined stages of research development, beginning with simple observations, followed by retrospective association and cohort correlation studies, and ending with well-designed randomized controlled trials. The very early adoption of TLI into IVF practice long before the publication of high-quality supportive evidence is nonetheless very disturbing. If anything, it reflects the nature of the high-stakes market competition driving the field of reproduction medicine.

Adoption of Algorithm/Prediction Models

Several nested algorithms were crafted to predict embryological and clinical outcomes on the basis of TLI morphokinetic findings. While many were internally developed, very few were externally validated. When comparing the application of a published algorithm model in two independent laboratories (25), the study of the quantitative timing parameters revealed reduced interlaboratory transferability. In a multicenter retrospective study, a blastocyst prediction model with stringent morphokinetic time intervals (26) achieved a high specificity at the expense of a low sensitivity; in other words, the proposed model offered a substantial increase in implantation at the expense of a high rejection of viable embryos. In 2017, Lagalla et al. retrospectively analyzed the distribution and fate of abnormally cleaved embryos (27). They reported that untimely embryo division patterns were equally distributed among all age groups and therefore did not seem to be age related. Data analysis further revealed that irregularly cleaved embryos arrested before blastulation more often than normally cleaved embryos. But, while a subset of irregularly cleaving embryos succeeded in reaching the blastocyst stage, many of them produced chromosomally normal embryos. When six published TLI algorithms were appraised (28), all achieved an AUC less than 0.60 indicating a reduced predictive capability, and a PPV less than 45% demonstrating a poor diagnostic value. Taken together, we may conclude that the available embryo selection algorithms are not always clinically adaptable and may lose significant diagnostic value when externally applied (Level of Evidence: IB). Storr et al. evaluated the agreements between published time-lapse algorithms as well as between algorithms and embryologists for embryo selection (29). They found the inter- and intra-algorithms agreement to be only fair but highly variable.

In summary, the application of TLI-based algorithms in IVF practice suffers several shortcomings: (a) poor interlaboratory transferability marked by reduced predictive capability when applied externally and (b) high rejection of viable embryos accentuated by tightening of morphokinetic criteria achieving high specificity at the expense of low sensitivity.

Confounding Factors

There are several explanations for the lack of conclusive evidence in favor of a beneficial effect of TLI on reproductive success parameters. A broad range of variables potentially confounding embryo morphokinetics has not been accounted for during clinical studies, including the etiology of infertility, the stimulation protocol, the nature of ovarian response, the culture media, and the laboratory environment. Gurbuz et al., for example, compared embryo morphokinetics using two different ovulation triggering agents (30). Early developmental events were found to be significantly delayed in embryos derived from cycles triggered with human chorionic gonadotrophins (hCG) in comparison with a GnRH agonist (GnRHa). In addition, the percentage of timely developing embryos were significantly higher after a GnRHa trigger. Gryshchenko et al. also analyzed the effect of the stimulation protocol on embryo morphokinetics (31). Data analysis revealed that embryos obtained in protocols downregulated with a GnRH agonist developed more slowly than those suppressed with a GnRH antagonist. The use of a total follicle-stimulating hormone dose in excess of 2500 IU was accompanied by a prolongation of the kinetic time parameters. The method of fertilization was also shown to affect embryonic developmental events. In 2012, Dal Canto et al. suggested that ICSI-derived embryos showed significantly faster morphokinetics than those derived from conventional IVF (13). Likewise, Kim et al. reported similar findings on 1830 embryos (32). Freis et al. (33) noticed that endometriosis-associated infertility altered embryo morphokinetics. The origin of the sperm during ICSI cycles has been shown to influence the kinetics of embryo development (34).

Conclusion

The fallacy of the assumption that kinetics could be the sole predictor of embryo viability has neglected the fact that the parameters of embryo viability are indeed multiple and intertwined. We appraise and rate the quality of evidence with respect to the clinical use of embryo morphokinetic assessment in IVF practice as follows: (a) poor evidence for the prediction of the euploid status of embryos, (b) fair evidence for the prediction of blastocyst development *in vitro*, (c) good evidence for the prediction of unfavorable implantation, and (d) poor evidence for the prediction of favorable implantation and pregnancy success. It appears that while timely embryo kinetic patterns fail to reliably predict a successful implantation, untimely kinetics may better predict failed implantation. Time-lapse embryo morphokinetics may therefore be better construed as a tool to deselect poor-quality embryos than to select good-quality ones for uterine transfer or cryopreservation. It should also be emphasized that the majority of the published embryo selection algorithms are not properly validated and have been shown to be poorly transferrable and reproducible.

There are, nonetheless, other potential benefits for the use of TLI systems in human reproduction. TLI may be used to monitor internal quality control within IVF laboratories and for research and development in industry-driven initiatives. The use of the technology may also help advance the science of embryo biology and early development.

REFERENCES

1. Tallo CP, Vohr B, Oh W et al. Maternal and neonatal morbidity associated with *in vitro* fertilization. *J Pediatr.* 1995;127(5):794–800.
2. Pandian Z, Marjoribanks J, Ozturk O et al. Number of embryos for transfer following *in vitro* fertilisation or intra-cytoplasmic sperm injection. *Cochrane Database Syst Rev.* 2013;(7):CD003416.
3. Schieve LA, Peterson HB, Meikle SF et al. Live-birth rates and multiple-birth risk using *in vitro* fertilization. *JAMA.* 1999;282(19):1832–8.
4. Alpha Scientists in Reproductive Medicine and ESHRE Special Interest Group of Embryology. The Istanbul consensus workshop on embryo assessment: Proceedings of an expert meeting. *Hum Reprod.* 2011;26(6):1270–83.
5. Payne D, Flaherty SP, Barry MF et al. Preliminary observations on polar body extrusion and pronuclear formation in human oocytes using time-lapse video cinematography. *Hum Reprod.* 1997;12(3):532–41.
6. Lemmen J, Agerholm I, Ziebe S. Kinetic markers of human embryo quality using time-lapse recordings of IVF/ICSI-fertilized oocytes. *Reprod Biomed Online.* 2008;17(3):385–91.
7. Kovacs P. Embryo selection: The role of time-lapse monitoring. *Reprod Biol Endocrinol.* 2014;12(1):124.

8. Meseguer M, Herrero J, Tejera A et al. The use of morphokinetics as a predictor of embryo implantation. *Hum Reprod.* 2011;26(10):2658–71.

9. Rubio I, Kuhlmann R, Agerholm I et al. Limited implantation success of direct-cleaved human zygotes: A time-lapse study. *Fertil Steril.* 2012;98(6):1458–63.

10. Wong CC, Loewke KE, Bossert NL et al. Non-invasive imaging of human embryos before embryonic genome activation predicts development to the blastocyst stage. *Nat Biotechnol.* 2010;28(10):1115.

11. Conaghan J, Chen AA, Willman SP et al. Improving embryo selection using a computer-automated time-lapse image analysis test plus day 3 morphology: Results from a prospective multicenter trial. *Fertil Steril.* 2013;100(2):412–9e5.

12. Cruz M, Garrido N, Herrero J et al. Timing of cell division in human cleavage-stage embryos is linked with blastocyst formation and quality. *Reprod Biomed Online.* 2012;25(4):371–81.

13. Dal Canto M, Coticchio G, Renzini MM et al. Cleavage kinetics analysis of human embryos predicts development to blastocyst and implantation. *Reprod Biomed Online.* 2012;25(5):474–80.

14. Basile N, del Carmen Nogales M, Bronet F et al. Increasing the probability of selecting chromosomally normal embryos by time-lapse morphokinetics analysis. *Fertil Steril.* 2014;101(3):699–704e1.

15. Campbell A, Fishel S, Bowman N et al. Retrospective analysis of outcomes after IVF using an aneuploidy risk model derived from time-lapse imaging without PGS. *Reprod Biomed Online.* 2013;27(2):140–6.

16. Kramer YG, Kofinas JD, Melzer K et al. Assessing morphokinetic parameters via time lapse microscopy (TLM) to predict euploidy: Are aneuploidy risk classification models universal? *J Assist Reprod Genet.* 2014;31(9):1231–42.

17. Kirkegaard K, Kesmodel US, Hindkjær JJ et al. Time-lapse parameters as predictors of blastocyst development and pregnancy outcome in embryos from good prognosis patients: A prospective cohort study. *Hum Reprod.* 2013;28(10):2643–51.

18. Motato Y, de los Santos MJ, Escriba MJ et al. Morphokinetic analysis and embryonic prediction for blastocyst formation through an integrated time-lapse system. *Fertil Steril.* 2016;105(2):376–84e9.

19. Rubio I, Galán A, Larreategui Z, Ayerdi F et al. Clinical validation of embryo culture and selection by morphokinetic analysis: A randomized, controlled trial of the EmbryoScope. *Fertil Steril.* 2014;102(5):1287–94e5.

20. Goodman LR, Goldberg J, Falcone T et al. Does the addition of time-lapse morphokinetics in the selection of embryos for transfer improve pregnancy rates? A randomized controlled trial. *Fertil Steril.* 2016;105(2):275–85e10.

21. Kaser DJ, Bormann CL, Missmer SA et al. A pilot randomized controlled trial of Day 3 single embryo transfer with adjunctive time-lapse selection versus day 5 single embryo transfer with or without adjunctive time-lapse selection. *Hum Reprod.* 2017;32(8):1598–603.

22. Park H, Bergh C, Selleskog U et al. No benefit of culturing embryos in a closed system compared with a conventional incubator in terms of number of good quality embryos: Results from an RCT. *Hum Reprod.* 2014;30(2):268–75.

23. Pribenszky C, Nilselid A-M, Montag M. Time-lapse culture with morphokinetic embryo selection improves pregnancy and live birth chances and reduces early pregnancy loss: A meta-analysis. *Reprod Biomed Online.* 2017;35(5):511–20.

24. Racowsky C, Martins WP. Effectiveness and safety of time-lapse imaging for embryo culture and selection: It is still too early for any conclusions? *Fertil Steril.* 2017;108(3):450–2.

25. Liu Y, Copeland C, Stevens A et al. Assessment of human embryos by time-lapse videography: A comparison of quantitative and qualitative measures between two independent laboratories. *Reprod Biol.* 2015;15(4):210–6.

26. Kirkegaard K, Campbell A, Agerholm I et al. Limitations of a time-lapse blastocyst prediction model: A large multicentre outcome analysis. *Reprod Biomed Online.* 2014;29(2):156–8.

27. Lagalla C, Tarozzi N, Sciajno R et al. Embryos with morphokinetic abnormalities may develop into euploid blastocysts. *Reprod Biomed Online.* 2017;34(2):137–46.

28. Barrie A, Homburg R, McDowell G et al. Examining the efficacy of six published time-lapse imaging embryo selection algorithms to predict implantation to demonstrate the need for the development of specific, in-house morphokinetic selection algorithms. *Fertil Steril.* 2017;107(3):613–21.

29. Storr A, Venetis C, Cooke S et al. Time-lapse algorithms and morphological selection of day-5 embryos for transfer: A preclinical validation study. *Fertil Steril.* 2018;109(2):276–83e3.

30. Gurbuz AS, Gode F, Uzman MS et al. GnRH agonist triggering affects the kinetics of embryo development: A comparative study. *J Ovarian Res.* 2016;9(1):22.
31. Gryshchenko MG, Pravdyuk AI, Parashchyuk VY. Analysis of factors influencing morphokinetic characteristics of embryos in ART cycles. *Gynecol Endocrinol.* 2014;30(Suppl 1):6–8
32. Kim HJ, Yoon HJ, Jang JM et al. Evaluation of human embryo development in *in vitro* fertilization- and intracytoplasmic sperm injection-fertilized oocytes: A time-lapse study. *Clin Exp Reprod Med.* 2017;44(2):90–5.
33. Freis A, Dietrich JE, Binder M et al. Relative morphokinetics assessed by time-lapse imaging are altered in embryos from patients with endometriosis. *Reprod Sci.* 2018;25(8):1279–85.
34. Desai N, Gill P, Tadros NN et al. Azoospermia and embryo morphokinetics: Testicular sperm-derived embryos exhibit delays in early cell cycle events and increased arrest prior to compaction. *J Assist Reprod Genet.* 2018;35(7):1339–48.

5

Use of Cryopreservation for All Embryos

**Samuel Santos-Ribeiro, Shari Mackens, Biljana Popovic-Todorovic,
Annalisa Racca, Christophe Blockeel, and Panagiotis Drakopoulos**

Introduction

The early days of assisted reproductive technologies (ARTs) were characterized by a treatment stance best summarized by the expression "the more the merrier," with a great deal of effort being focused on maximizing oocyte retrieval rates and, consequently, the number of embryos available for transfer. Initially, owing to the low success rates, all available embryos were usually transferred fresh following *in vitro* fertilization (IVF). However, consecutive improvements in both the clinical and laboratorial aspects of IVF led not only to an increase in pregnancy rates but also to a higher risk for multiple pregnancies (1). Thus, the need for effective embryo cryopreservation strategies first arose not only from the rapid increase in ART success but also from the surge in ART-related complications.

History of Embryo Cryopreservation in Assisted Reproductive Technologies

The first pregnancy resulting from a transfer of a thawed slow-cooled human embryo was reported in 1983 in Australia (2), followed the year after by the first live birth in the Netherlands (3). However, at these early stages, the embryos with the best morphologic classification were still transferred fresh, given their relatively lower pregnancy rates following cryopreservation (4). The low efficiency was the main reason why embryo cryopreservation was initially perceived merely as an ancillary treatment following a failed fresh embryo transfer only in women with either an excessive ovarian response or those at high risk for multiple pregnancy.

Besides slight modifications, such as the introduction of 1,2-propanediol and sucrose as cryoprotectants (5), slow-freezing laboratory protocols have remained unchanged over the years, despite their extensive use in everyday clinical practice. However, human embryo cryopreservation programs have seen a considerable increase in terms of pregnancy rates over time, especially as slow-freezing has been gradually replaced by vitrification, a method that causes instant cooling without ice crystal formation, resulting in higher embryo postthawing survival rates. Conversely to slow-freezing, vitrification protocols have been optimized extensively as their use became increasingly widespread (6) with reassuring safety data already available (7), even though the first report of a successful human live birth was reported only in 2001 (8).

Multiple Pregnancy Reduction Strategies

Several studies have reported less favorable obstetrical outcomes after IVF when compared to spontaneous conception, including higher risks of prematurity, lower birth weight, and perinatal death (9,10). The higher risk of prematurity is primarily due to the greatly increased rate of multiple births. In European countries, large efforts have been made to reduce multiple pregnancies in ART (Figure 5.1), first by attempting to

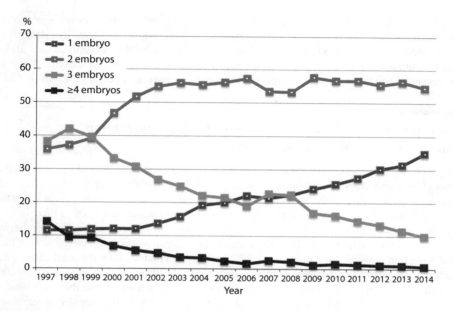

FIGURE 5.1 Number of embryos transferred in ART during fresh cycles in Europe between 1997 and 2014. ART, assisted reproductive technologies. (From De Geyter C et al. *Hum Reprod*. 2018;33[9]:1586–601, with permission.)

reduce high-order multiples (i.e., over two fetuses) by proposing that the "maximum" number of embryos allowed for transfer be two, a recommendation that was followed shortly after by the concept of "elective single embryo transfer" (11). The first multicenter randomized controlled trial (RCT) on this topic was conducted in Scandinavia, comparing the transfer of two fresh embryos with a single fresh embryo transfer followed eventually by a frozen-thawed embryo (12). In this study, no difference in the live birth rates (LBRs) between the two groups was found (43.3% compared with 38.8%), although there was a 33% twin pregnancy rate in the double embryo transfer arm. Following these results, elective single embryo transfer has become government mandated in many European countries, and these policies have shown to dramatically reduce the number of twin and higher-order births without affecting cumulative LBR (13–15). Consequently, while concerns around the usefulness of embryo cryopreservation effectively relayed it initially to a statute of an "adjuvant method," the demand for more efficient strategies to decrease multiple pregnancies have progressively increased its use, with cryopreserved embryos now accounting for up to one-third of all children born after ART in the United States (16).

Vision of a Complication-Free Clinic

Among all the possible issues associated directly with ART, ovarian hyperstimulation syndrome (OHSS) is of major importance, since it is an iatrogenic and potentially life-threatening complication that is almost exclusively related to ovarian stimulation that occurs in women who are frequently otherwise healthy (17). While its incidence is approximately only 2%–3% per cycle, OHSS can ensue in up to a third of all cases of high-risk patients (18).

As a primary preventive measure, the now widely adopted use of the gonadotropin-releasing hormone (GnRH) antagonist protocol has significantly decreased the incidence of OHSS (19). However, besides the use of GnRH antagonists, the option to trigger final oocyte maturation with a GnRH agonist effectively reduced (and even practically abolished) the incidence of early onset severe OHSS (18). However, as the use of a GnRH agonist for triggering hinders IVF pregnancy rates in a fresh embryo transfer attempt (19), several possible rescue strategies had to be studied. The first proposal was the use of enhanced luteal phase support with either an intensified supplementation of progesterone and estradiol (18) or the administration of a low dose of human chorionic gonadotropin (hCG) immediately after oocyte retrieval (20). While these approaches of enhanced luteal phase support seemed initially to significantly increase pregnancy rates after GnRH triggering, they were later found to still perform either suboptimally (21) or to potentially increase the risk of OHSS once more (22). Meanwhile, an alternative strategy that has gained increasing popularity is to intentionally "segment" IVF treatment by cryopreserving all available good-quality embryos to later be replaced in subsequent thawed embryo transfer cycles. This approach has been shown to be the best method until now to reduce the occurrence of early onset severe OHSS (23).

Current Controversial Aspects: The Role of Cryopreservation in Balancing ART Efficiency and Safety

The primary objective of ovarian stimulation in ART is to increase the number of oocytes retrieved and the number of available embryos, enabling the selection of the best embryo for transfer. The generalized use of exogenous gonadotropins has led to a substantial increase in pregnancy rates, from 3%–10% (using no or minimal stimulation) to 20%–50% (24). Several studies have addressed whether there is an optimal number of oocytes following ovarian stimulation, suggesting an independent relationship between the number of oocytes and LBR (25–28). In particular, two large registry studies from the United States and the United Kingdom demonstrated that fresh LBR either reach a plateau (28) or even decline when more than 20 oocytes are retrieved (26), while a further increase in the number of oocytes may only contribute to a rise in the risk of OHSS. However, these studies are limited by the fact that they only analyzed the results of the fresh transfer, not accounting for the potential benefit of the transfer of supernumerary embryos in subsequent frozen-thawed cycles.

New horizons have opened following the development of the segmentation concept in ART (i.e., use of the antagonist protocol combined with GnRH agonist triggering and elective embryo cryopreservation), paving the way for what was coined originally as the "freeze-all strategy" (29). Moreover, an evolution in the understanding of what might be the best balance between efficiency and safety during ART also came from the increasing number of researchers proposing that ART success should be reported using cumulative LBR instead of only fresh embryo transfer LBR (30). Cumulative LBR, in such cases, is defined as the first live born in the fresh or in one of the subsequent frozen cycles following a single ovarian stimulation ART treatment (31). Using the number of women who have at least one live birth as the numerator highlights the outcome for which couples seek treatment, delivering a figure that is more meaningful to patients and also more appropriate for making economic and political decisions in terms of efficacy and cost.

Regarding the relationship between the number of oocytes retrieved and cumulative LBR, the results of two registry analyses referring to historical data demonstrated that cumulative LBR followed the same fresh IVF patterns, reaching a plateau beyond 13–15 oocytes, suggesting that cumulative LBR remain somewhat disappointingly low even in women with high response (32,33). However, another two recent large studies including more homogeneous infertile populations stimulated using GnRH antagonist suppression showed a positive association between the number of oocytes retrieved and cumulative LBR, advocating that the cumulative chances of having a live birth were higher with an increasing ovarian response (34,35). No plateau was detected in cumulative LBR (Figure 5.2), although the increase was more moderate whenever more than 27 oocytes were retrieved (34). In the same context, a large population-based cohort study evaluating exclusively infertile patients with a "freeze-all" strategy showed that LBR improved as the number of oocytes retrieved increased, even beyond 25 oocytes (36). The reasons for the discrepancy between these more recent data and previous studies may be due to two major reasons. First, the initial studies were conducted in a time period in which vitrification had not yet been routinely implemented into clinical practice. Second, several patients may not have used all their supplementary frozen embryos.

These new findings showing that cumulative LBR increase progressively with the number of oocytes retrieved indicate that patients with a higher oocyte yield would have more supernumerary embryos available for transfer, which could further increase the overall success rate. In line with these results, recent genetic studies have also demonstrated that an increase in the number of oocytes not only does not hamper embryo quality, as had previously been suggested by the supporters of mild ovarian stimulation regimens (37), but on the contrary, may even result in a higher yield of euploid embryos (38). Collectively,

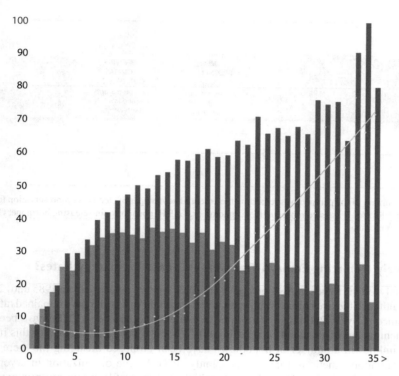

FIGURE 5.2   Cumulative and fresh live birth rates according to the number of oocytes retrieved. Fresh live birth probability (gray bars), cumulative live birth probability (black bars), freeze-all rate (gray line). The analysis was done in an intention to treat fashion. Patients with a freeze-all were considered as not having a live birth in the fresh cycle. (From Polyzos NP et al. *Fertil Steril*. 2018;110[4]:661–70.e1, with permission.)

these results have led to a frequent debate among physicians who now posit that the best approach may be to perform a more intensive stimulation in order to achieve the maximum number of retrievable oocytes followed by the routine use of GnRH agonist triggering and the elective cryopreservation of all embryos. While this concept of intense stimulation seems thought provoking, we would still strongly advocate against a notion of "wild stimulation" (i.e., administering a maximal dose of exogenous gonadotropins to all women, regardless of their predicted ovarian response), given that any benefit in terms of cumulative LBRs in such cases may come at the cost of once more increasing the risk of other ART-related complications (i.e., ovarian torsion/hemorrhage), while the patient's perspective should also be evaluated.

Arguments in Favor of Elective Embryo Cryopreservation

IVF has vastly improved over the last 40 years, from a complicated procedure requiring hospital admission to a fairly simple outpatient technique. Despite these multidirectional improvements, the overall live birth rates have remained disappointingly low. Furthermore, even following increasing safety measures, the use of ovarian stimulation still does not come without risks, and the incidences ART complications have remained relatively stable since the year 2000 (39). Specifically, serious complications such as OHSS may occur at a rate that should not be deemed insignificant, especially in view of the fact that these complications are frequently underreported (40). Moreover, ART is also associated with an increased incidence of other complication such as ectopic pregnancy (41,42) and neonatal morbidity (43), with the optimal strategies to minimize these risks remaining yet to be determined. This delicate balance between ART efficiency and safety is puzzling health-care providers who now consider that the elective cryopreservation of all embryos may play an important role in the future of ART (Figure 5.3).

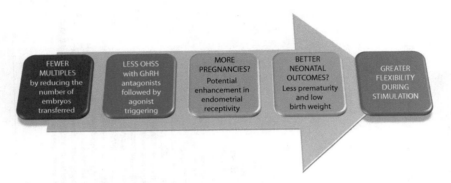

FIGURE 5.3   Summary of the perspectives regarding the potential advantages of elective cryopreservation for all embryos since the dawn of ART. ART, assisted reproductive technologies; GnRH, gonadotropin-releasing hormone; OHSS, ovarian hyperstimulation syndrome.

Does Electively Deferring Embryo Transfers Increase Pregnancy Rates?

A study that analyzed the trends in ART outcomes in a U.S. registry database from 1985 until 2014 (Figure 5.4) noted that although the live born delivery rates after fresh embryo transfer have remained rather stagnant around 30% since the year 2000, live birth after frozen embryo transfers (FETs) have been gradually increasing, reaching approximately 43% in 2014 (44). While the potential reasons for this improvement over time are unknown, a number of hypotheses have been proposed including the more widespread use of preimplantation genetic testing for aneuploidy (PGT-A), the optimization in cryopreservation technologies (i.e., vitrification), and the advent of multiple tools to profile uterine receptivity prior to FET. Moreover, many authors have postulated that the supraphysiologic milieu of hormones produced during ovarian stimulation may affect endometrial receptivity and hinder both embryo implantation and neonatal outcomes. Of all the candidate biomarkers evaluated during the monitoring of ovarian stimulation, the abnormal production of progesterone during the later stages of the follicular phase has been, thus far, proposed most frequently as the best surrogate for endometrial receptivity. Specifically, late-follicular elevated progesterone has been linked to lower pregnancy rates following a fresh embryo transfer (45). Although the complete mechanism behind this hindered pregnancy outcome remains elusive, some investigators consider that this issue may be, at least in part, amenable by elective embryo cryopreservation, given that previous translational studies have shown an abnormal gene expression in the luteal phase of

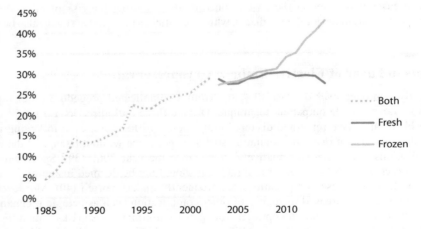

FIGURE 5.4   Live-born delivery rate in autologous cycles by year according to the Society for Assisted Reproductive Technology database. As of 2002, outcomes were divided by fresh versus frozen embryo transfers. (From Toner JP et al. *Fertil Steril.* 2016;106[3]:541–6, with permission.)

endometria exposed prematurely to progesterone (46). This has led many centers to change their clinical practice by measuring serum progesterone levels on the day of ovulation triggering and adopting a freeze-all strategy whenever the production of progesterone during ovarian stimulation is deemed "excessive." The definition of "progesterone overproduction" has itself been a matter of debate, with a large meta-analysis showing that thresholds as low as 0.8 ng/mL could benefit from elective cryopreservation (45). In an attempt to resolve this dilemma, Hill et al. assessed multiple thresholds in terms of efficiency and cost-effectiveness (Figure 5.5), determining that elective embryo cryopreservation was cost effective between 1.50 ng/mL and 2.00 ng/mL, with the number-needed-to-treat (to have one extra live birth) at the threshold of 1.50 ng/mL being 13 (47). Consequently, as the importance of endometrial receptivity after ovarian stimulation gained momentum, elevated late follicular progesterone levels became, along with the risk of OHSS, one of the major indications for elective embryo cryopreservation.

Multiple initial studies have proposed that elective all-embryo vitrification may increase pregnancy rates. However, the first meta-analysis addressing this hypothesis delivered controversial results (48). Specifically, this meta-analysis included the only three available RCTs at the time and found that elective FETs were associated with better ongoing pregnancy rates and similar miscarriage rates. Most (46.0%) data from this review were pooled from a publication that was later retracted based on the results of an investigation that found serious methodologic flaws in the study (49), albeit without affecting too significantly the overall results of the updated meta-analysis that followed (50). However, the remaining two RCTs derived from the same research group varied methodologically in terms of the chosen study population. While one study was performed in predicted normal responders (51), the other was implemented in a group of predicted high responders (52). In the latter trial, the ongoing pregnancy rates did not vary significantly, although this study was limited by the fact that groups varied significantly in terms of day 5 transfer rates and number of supernumerary embryos. The lack of sufficient confirmation of these positive results found in the before-mentioned studies demanded for better-designed RCTs comparing the pregnancy outcomes between fresh embryo transfer and elective FETs in both women with and without an elevated risk of OHSS. To that extent, while a recent clinical trial with over 1500 patients demonstrated that elective FET performs better and was safer in women at high risk for OHSS (53), two other trials published soon after showed no benefit in terms of LBR of this approach in normal responding women (54,55), although it may still reduce the risk of OHSS (55). These results question the overall usefulness of a freeze-for-all policy to enhance ART pregnancy outcomes, especially following a meta-analysis (Figure 5.6) that showed that elective FET does not seem to increase cumulative LBR (56).

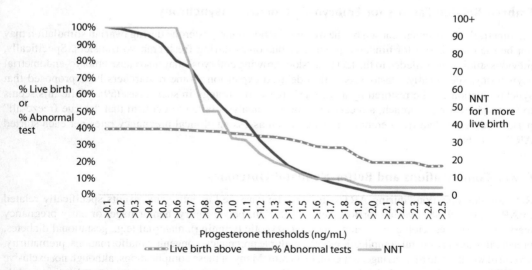

FIGURE 5.5 Demonstration of the relationship between live birth above progesterone thresholds, percentage of the population classified as abnormal above that threshold, and the NNT to obtain one additional live birth at each threshold. NNT, number needed to treat. (From Hill MJ et al. *Fertil Steril.* 2018;110[4]:671–9.e2, with permission.)

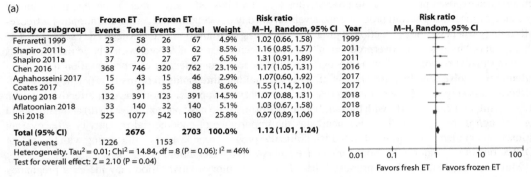

FIGURE 5.6   Forest plots comparing live birth rates after fresh and elective frozen embryo transfers. Intention-to-treat analysis for (a) live birth rates and (b) cumulative live birth rates after 12 months. ET, embryo transfer. (From Roque M et al. *Hum Reprod Update.* 2019;25[1]:2–14, with permission.)

In an attempt to explain these conflicting results, other researchers have posited whether elective embryo cryopreservation may be beneficial only in a clinical setting in which extended culture is performed (57), a result that requires further validation and that, indirectly, was recently challenged in a large registry analysis in which the pregnancy outcomes after cryopreservation also seemed to be worse for poor/normal responders (58).

Embryo-Related Factors for Embryo-Endometrial Asynchrony

Endometrial advancement caused by the overproduction of progesterone during ovarian stimulation may not be the only reason for hindered pregnancy outcomes during fresh embryo transfers. Specifically, previous studies have alluded to the fact that "slow-growing embryos" may also cause embryo-endometrial asynchrony, specifically, blastocysts with a delayed expansion. Some researchers have proposed that synchronization can be restored by a "rescue" freeze-all strategy in such cases (59). While this seems to be an interesting approach, a recent retrospective analysis failed to confirm that "rescue freeze-all" performed better than fresh embryo transfers when assessing clinical pregnancy rates per each started ART cycle (60).

Fewer Complications and Better Neonatal Outcomes

Relevant complications during ART can either be classified as iatrogenic events specifically related to ART (e.g., OHSS, ovarian torsion, pelvic infection, pelvic injury, hemorrhage) or early pregnancy (early miscarriage, ectopic pregnancy, and monozygotic twinning), maternal (e.g., gestational diabetes, preeclampsia), or neonatal complications (e.g., multiple pregnancy, congenital malformations, prematurity, low birth weight, late miscarriage, or perinatal death). Many of these complications, although not exclusive to ART, are more common following it. Among these, two specific early pregnancy complications, while being intrinsically related to ART, are exceedingly difficult to study given their rare occurrence: ectopic pregnancy and monozygotic twinning.

Ever since the first human IVF treatment, which resulted in an ectopic pregnancy (61), ART has been consistently associated with higher ectopic pregnancy rates of up to 8.6% (62). Although the reasons behind this increased incidence of ectopic pregnancy following ART are not completely understood, several studies have demonstrated that this association may be mostly related to the confounding effect of other known risk factors for ectopic pregnancy and infertility such as tubal disease, smoking, and advanced maternal age (63). Following the improvement in cryopreservation techniques, some have postulated that FET cycles may be associated with a slightly lower risk of ectopic pregnancy when compared with fresh cycles (41,42), including a recent population-based study (64). However, another recent register data did not confirm these findings, with FETs failing to show any significant benefit in terms of the prevention of ectopic pregnancy (65).

Regarding the relationship between ART and embryo splitting, although the risk factors and mechanisms responsible remain unclear, it has been argued that specific patient characteristics and ART procedures might play a role in the development of monozygotic twinning. A recent study was the first to propose that FETs may also reduce monozygotic twinning (66). However, this result was recently challenged by two other research groups who showed either no effect (67) or even an increased risk (68). These reports warrant further exploration into this matter, since monozygotic pregnancies are associated with an increased risk of maternal and fetal complications such as fetal growth restriction, preterm delivery, and perinatal mortality (66).

Another potential advantage of the segmentation of IVF treatment may stem from reports that have shown that FETs may significantly reduce the incidence of prematurity and low birth weight (69) (Table 5.1). Although some registry analyses supported a significant decrease in the incidence of prematurity (70), one of the largest nationwide registry analyses, derived from the Society for Assisted Reproductive Technologies (SART) database, demonstrated that prematurity among singletons did not differ significantly after frozen and fresh embryo transfer (71). Despite advances in obstetric care, preterm birth continues to be the leading cause of perinatal morbidity and mortality, and the second largest direct cause of death in children younger than 5 years (72).

The most plausible explanation for these findings appears to be a potentially negative influence of ovarian stimulation on endometrial angiogenesis and embryo implantation. Although the exact mechanism behind this hypothesis is not established, experimental studies in mice have demonstrated that ovarian

TABLE 5.1

Summary of Findings from a Cumulative Meta-Analysis Regarding Neonatal Outcomes Following Frozen Embryo Transfer

Risk of Outcome	Evidence	Evidence Available by Year	No Further Change in Precision, Magnitude, or Direction	More Observational Data Needed
Small for gestational age	Lower in FET	2010	2014	No
Low birth weight	Lower in FET	1997	2014	No
Very low birth weight	Lower in FET	2013	2016	No
Large for gestational age	Higher in FET	2010	2014	No
High birth weight	Higher in FET	2014	2016	No
Very high birth weight	Higher in FET	2013	2014	No
Preterm delivery	Lower in FET	2005	2014	No
Very preterm delivery	Lower in FET	2016	2016	No
Antepartum hemorrhage	No difference	2010	2014	Yes
Admission to NICU	No difference	2012	2013	Yes
Congenital anomalies	No difference	2014	2016	Yes
Perinatal mortality	No difference	2014	2014	Yes
Hypertensive disorders of pregnancy	Higher in FET	2015	2015	Yes

Source: From Maheshwari A et al. *Hum Reprod Update.* 2018;24(1):35–58, with permission.

Abbreviations: FET, frozen embryo transfer; NICU, neonatal intensive care unit.

stimulation, IVF, and embryo culture may alter the fetal and placental development (73). Imprinted genes known for their regulatory role in fetal growth are expressed in significantly higher amounts in superovulated mice compared to nonstimulated controls (74), suggesting that ovarian stimulation may impair fetal growth through an effect on the implanting embryo's trophoblast differentiation and, therefore, placental development. However, the increase in low birth weight infants may be due to epigenetic effects of exogenous stimulation on the oocyte (75). Results from a complementary paired analysis in a population-based study appear to further justify this hypothesis (71). According to this study, sibling comparisons demonstrated that low birth weight was significantly lower in sibling singletons born after frozen transfers when compared with fresh embryo transfers, whereas no difference was observed in siblings born from oocyte donor recipients (in whom no ovarian stimulation was administered either in fresh or frozen cycles).

It is also important to acknowledge that the results from historical data comparing fresh and frozen cycles may not be directly extrapolated to freeze-all cycles, given that most of these studies will suffer from the "second-choice" effect (i.e., the fact that the best embryo available was likely to have been transferred fresh whenever possible). That said, data from three recent RCTs showed either comparable neonatal outcomes results or that, at best, elective embryo cryopreservation had only a modest effect on birth weight or the risk of prematurity (53,54,76).

While the outcomes regarding prematurity and birth weight seem more consistent, the results regarding perinatal/neonatal death are more controversial, with FETs being associated with all possible outcomes ranging from better (69), to similar (77), or even worse (55,78).

Treatment Cycle Scheduling and Other Perceived Advantages

The use of the elective FET policy has gained popularity for other reasons that are not directly related to its potential in terms of ART efficiency and safety. Specifically, since this strategy significantly reduces the incidence of stimulation-related OHSS, it also allows for a greater flexibility in terms of treatment, allowing physicians to prolong ovarian stimulation and schedule oocyte retrievals avoiding holidays and weekends (79). Moreover, given that embryo transfers are electively deferred, procedures that would preclude a fresh embryo transfer can now be performed without concern, thus facilitating the use of more flexible approaches toward ovarian stimulation, including random-day start (80), progestin downregulation (81), and oocyte/embryo accumulation with back-to-back consecutive stimulation cycles (82). While all these approaches are relatively new and require extensive validation prior to widespread use, their emergence was primed by an increased favorable attitude toward the "freeze-all" approach (Figure 5.7).

Potential Reasons for Caution in a Freeze-for-All Era

Macrosomia and Risk of Adverse Intrauterine Programming

For singletons born after FET, significantly higher birth weights and higher rates of macrosomia/large for gestational age (LGA) have been described when comparing to singletons born after fresh cycles or spontaneous conception (43). The most recent meta-analysis reports for an FET (compared to, respectively, fresh cycles and natural conceptions) presented a 1.5- and 1.3-fold increased risk of LGA, and a 1.7- and 1.4-fold increased risk of macrosomia (83). Interestingly, in a large study on perinatal outcomes after single embryo transfer of vitrified embryos, following potential confounder adjustment, no statistically significant difference was withheld for LGA when FET and fresh-cycle singletons were compared (84). Moreover, in the oocyte donation model (thus eliminating the possible influence ovarian stimulation may have on the weight of the newborn infant through its effect on the uterus), no differences were found either at the level of the birth weight, when comparing fresh embryo transfer with FET, or in the function of the cryopreservation method performed (77,85). Finally, three RCTs that recently compared fresh embryo transfers with elective FET showed no increase in overall LGA rates, although two of these trials did report a mean increase in neonatal birth weights in the elective FET arms (53–55).

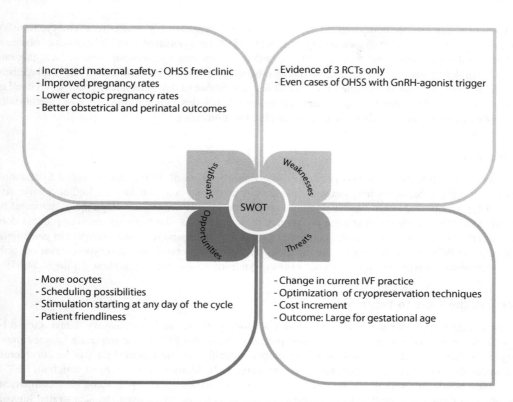

FIGURE 5.7 SWOT analysis of a freeze-all strategy. GnRH, gonadotropin-releasing hormone; IVF, *in vitro* fertilization; OHSS, ovarian hyperstimulation syndrome; RCTs, randomized controlled trials; SWOT, strengths, weaknesses, opportunities, and threats. (From Blockeel C et al. *Hum Reprod.* 2016;31[3]:491–7, with permission.)

The reason why FET could predispose for macrosomia and LGA remains unclear. Although the specific etiology of infertility and treatment type have not been shown to influence birth weight to a large extent, other factors have been described to be linked to adverse outcomes (86). For birth weight specifically, maternal factors such as body mass index (BMI) and parity are significantly influential. However, the increased risk of macrosomia/LGA in FET does not seem to be solely explainable by intrinsic maternal factors as the risk has also been confirmed in sibling cohort studies after adjustment for birth order (87). While the different media used for human embryo culture have been reported to affect birth weight, this is not generally accepted as true (88). It has also been suggested that a longer duration of the embryo culture period might promote LGA (89), but again, this result lacks consistency throughout the available literature (76), and even the opposite, specifically a higher risk of lower birth weight, has been associated with extended culture (90). Adequately powered RCTs are needed to resolve these controversies.

Although macrosomia/LGA per se is frequently associated with an increased risk of stillbirth, cesarean section, shoulder dystocia, fetal hypoxia, hypoglycemia, respiratory distress, and perinatal mortality, the overall perinatal risks are lower for singletons born after FET than after conventional ART with a fresh embryo transfer (43). Finally, whether the increased risk of macrosomia/LGA is associated with health risks in the long term is yet to be determined. A longer follow-up of FET children is needed as it might be possible that epigenetic modifications may have health consequences manifesting only later on during adulthood (91).

Cesarean Section Rates

More cesarean sections are performed following FET than after fresh cycles and spontaneous conception (69,78). This observation is most likely prone to bias as more women in the FET group may have had previous cesarean sections compared to the ones conceiving spontaneously or after fresh embryo transfer, even more given the fact that singleton pregnancies after IVF are associated with higher risks of obstetric and perinatal complications when compared to spontaneous conceptions. Recently, however, a higher rate of postterm delivery and cesarean section has also been described for FET with hormonal replacement treatment compared to natural cycle FET (92). This could be due to the endometrial preparation itself or a selection bias in the hormonal replacement group, which includes a greater proportion of patients with ovulation disorders and at higher risk of adverse obstetric outcomes.

Preeclampsia

A recent cumulative meta-analysis performed by Maheshwari et al. (Table 5.1) included five studies reporting on the outcome of hypertensive disorders of pregnancy and concluded a higher relative risk in the FET group, without a clear biological explanation (43). However, for pregnancies achieved by oocyte donation, known for their high prevalence of preeclampsia, the freezing-thawing process does not seem to confer more risk than fresh embryo transfer in preterm and term preeclampsia or gestational hypertension (93). Moreover, among the recent RCTs assessing elective embryo cryopreservation, only one—performed in women with polycystic ovarian syndrome (53)—confirmed these findings (54,55).

Delay in the Time to Pregnancy

Patients undergoing ART are eager to conceive as soon possible, and unnecessary delays should be avoided whenever possible as they may cause patient distress. An FET per se implies a longer time to pregnancy. However, following a failed fresh embryo transfer, an immediate FET can be considered, as comparable pregnancy outcomes have been reported (94). Moreover, in cycles in which an FET is performed electively, FETs done immediately after the stimulation cycle appear to be have comparable outcomes to those FETs deferred one menstrual cycle or more (95,96). Given the accelerated luteosis following GnRH agonist triggering, the delay in time to pregnancy in such cases could be kept to a minimum if one advances immediately for FET.

Issues Requiring Further Research

Embryo cryopreservation has become an essential therapeutic strategy in ART. With refinements of technology in recent years, the numbers of FET have increased as have pregnancy rates associated with them, to the extent that it has been suggested that the selection of embryos may become less relevant in the future as a means of increasing success rates in ART, as almost all embryos will survive the thawing process (97). Moreover, as the evidence and indications for elective cryopreservation expand to fertility preservation, oocyte/embryo accumulation for poor responders, preimplantation genetic testing (PGT), and recurrent implantation failure, the "decision thresholds" to perform elective FETs have dropped continuously and, in some centers, have even become the norm. However, this trend has occurred despite the existent evidence frequently being graded as low quality and concerns related to eventual risks of the approach. In order to conclusively resolve these issues, multiple trials are needed, and many are currently ongoing not only in the general ART population (ACTRN12612000422820, ACTRN12616000643471, ISRCTN61225414, NCT02570386, NTR3187) but also in specific settings such as repeated implantation failure (NCT02681367), following elective blastocyst transfer (NCT02712840, NCT02746562), in predicted high responders (NCT02148393), in normal/poor responders, and in couples performing PGT (NCT02000349, NCT02133950).

Beyond evaluating the efficiency and safety of this approach, other more practical parameters also require further scrutiny in an elective FET setting. Specifically, the optimal stage for embryo cryopreservation, the best timing for the first FET (NCT03201783), whether both natural and artificial cycle FETs can be performed, how time to pregnancy may be affected, and whether the cost-effectiveness of the approach changes when taking into account the direct and indirect (e.g., neonatal intensive care) costs (50) are all relevant clinical issues lacking robust data at this time.

Finally, further fundamental studies are needed to allow for a better understanding of the potential negative impact of ovarian stimulation on the endometrium and whether it is associated with implantation and subsequent placentation (98,99). Basic research should also attempt to provide clear explanations for the observed increased rates of LGA and hypertensive disorders following FET.

REFERENCES

1. Jones HW, Jr. Twins or more. *Fertil Steril*. 1995;63(4):701–2.
2. Trounson A, Mohr L. Human pregnancy following cryopreservation, thawing and transfer of an eight-cell embryo. *Nature*. 1983;305(5936):707–9.
3. Zeilmaker GH, Alberda AT, van Gent I et al. Two pregnancies following transfer of intact frozen-thawed embryos. *Fertil Steril*. 1984;42(2):293–6.
4. Puissant F, Van Rysselberge M, Barlow P et al. Embryo scoring as a prognostic tool in IVF treatment. *Hum Reprod*. 1987;2(8):705–8.
5. Lassalle B, Testart J, Renard J-P. Human embryo features that influence the success of cryopreservation with the use of 1,2 propanediol. *Fertil Steril*. 1985;44(5):645–51.
6. Cobo A, de los Santos MJ, Castello D et al. Outcomes of vitrified early cleavage-stage and blastocyst-stage embryos in a cryopreservation program: Evaluation of 3,150 warming cycles. *Fertil Steril*. 2012;98(5):1138–46.e1.
7. Belva F, Bonduelle M, Roelants M et al. Neonatal health including congenital malformation risk of 1072 children born after vitrified embryo transfer. *Hum Reprod*. 2016;31(7):1610–20.
8. Mukaida T, Nakamura S, Tomiyama T et al. Successful birth after transfer of vitrified human blastocysts with use of a cryoloop containerless technique. *Fertil Steril*. 2001;76(3):618–20.
9. Schieve LA, Meikle SF, Ferre C et al. Low and very low birth weight in infants conceived with use of assisted reproductive technology. *N Engl J Med*. 2002;346(10):731–7.
10. Helmerhorst FM, Perquin DA, Donker D, Keirse MJ. Perinatal outcome of singletons and twins after assisted conception: A systematic review of controlled studies. *BMJ*. 2004;328(7434):261.
11. De Geyter C, Calhaz-Jorge C, Kupka MS et al. ART in Europe, 2014: Results generated from European registries by ESHRE: The European IVF-monitoring Consortium (EIM) for the European Society of Human Reproduction and Embryology (ESHRE). *Hum Reprod*. 2018;33(9):1586–601.
12. Thurin A, Hausken J, Hillensjo T et al. Elective single-embryo transfer versus double-embryo transfer in *in vitro* fertilization. *N Engl J Med*. 2004;351(23):2392–402.
13. European Society of Human Reproduction Embryology, Kupka MS, D'Hooghe T et al. Assisted reproductive technology in Europe, 2011: Results generated from European registers by ESHRE. *Hum Reprod*. 2016;31(2):233–48.
14. Peeraer K, Debrock S, Laenen A et al. The impact of legally restricted embryo transfer and reimbursement policy on cumulative delivery rate after treatment with assisted reproduction technology. *Hum Reprod*. 2014;29(2):267–75.
15. Saldeen P, Sundstrom P. Would legislation imposing single embryo transfer be a feasible way to reduce the rate of multiple pregnancies after IVF treatment? *Hum Reprod*. 2005;20(1):4–8.
16. Doody KJ. Cryopreservation and delayed embryo transfer-assisted reproductive technology registry and reporting implications. *Fertil Steril*. 2014;102(1):27–31.
17. Papanikolaou EG, Pozzobon C, Kolibianakis EM et al. Incidence and prediction of ovarian hyperstimulation syndrome in women undergoing gonadotropin-releasing hormone antagonist in vitro fertilization cycles. *Fertil Steril*. 2006;85(1):112–20.
18. Engmann L, DiLuigi A, Schmidt D et al. The use of gonadotropin-releasing hormone (GnRH) agonist to induce oocyte maturation after cotreatment with GnRH antagonist in high-risk patients undergoing *in vitro* fertilization prevents the risk of ovarian hyperstimulation syndrome: A prospective randomized controlled study. *Fertil Steril*. 2008;89(1):84–91.
19. Al-Inany HG, Youssef MA, Aboulghar M et al. Gonadotrophin-releasing hormone antagonists for assisted reproductive technology. *Cochrane Database Syst Rev*. 2011;(5):CD001750. https://libguides. jcu.edu.au/ama/articles/cochrane-review.
20. Humaidan P. Agonist trigger: What is the best approach? Agonist trigger and low dose hCG. *Fertil Steril*. 2012;97(3):529–30.

21. Youssef MA, Van der Veen F, Al-Inany HG et al. Gonadotropin-releasing hormone agonist versus HCG for oocyte triggering in antagonist-assisted reproductive technology. *Cochrane Database Syst Rev.* 2014;10(10):CD008046.
22. Iliodromiti S, Blockeel C, Tremellen KP et al. Consistent high clinical pregnancy rates and low ovarian hyperstimulation syndrome rates in high-risk patients after GnRH agonist triggering and modified luteal support: A retrospective multicentre study. *Hum Reprod.* 2013;28(9):2529–36.
23. Bodri D, Guillen JJ, Trullenque M et al. Early ovarian hyperstimulation syndrome is completely prevented by gonadotropin releasing-hormone agonist triggering in high-risk oocyte donor cycles: A prospective, luteal-phase follow-up study. *Fertil Steril.* 2010;93(7):2418–20.
24. Barbieri RL, Hornstein MD. Assisted reproduction-*in vitro* fertilization success is improved by ovarian stimulation with exogenous gonadotropins and pituitary suppression with gonadotropin-releasing hormone analogues. *Endocr Rev.* 1999;20(3):249–52.
25. Briggs R, Kovacs G, MacLachlan V et al. Can you ever collect too many oocytes? *Hum Reprod.* 2015;30(1):81–7.
26. Sunkara SK, Rittenberg V, Raine-Fenning N et al. Association between the number of eggs and live birth in IVF treatment: An analysis of 400 135 treatment cycles. *Hum Reprod.* 2011;26(7):1768–74.
27. Baker VL, Brown MB, Luke B, Conrad KP. Association of number of retrieved oocytes with live birth rate and birth weight: An analysis of 231,815 cycles of *in vitro* fertilization. *Fertil Steril.* 2015;103(4):931–8.e2.
28. Steward RG, Lan L, Shah AA et al. Oocyte number as a predictor for ovarian hyperstimulation syndrome and live birth: An analysis of 256,381 *in vitro* fertilization cycles. *Fertil Steril.* 2014;101(4):967–73.
29. Devroey P, Polyzos NP, Blockeel C. An OHSS-Free clinic by segmentation of IVF treatment. *Hum Reprod.* 2011;26(10):2593–7.
30. Maheshwari A, McLernon D, Bhattacharya S. Cumulative live birth rate: Time for a consensus? *Hum Reprod.* 2015;30(12):2703–7.
31. Zegers-Hochschild F, Adamson GD, Dyer S et al. The international glossary on infertility and fertility care, 2017. *Fertil Steril.* 2017;108(3):393–406.
32. Smith A, Tilling K, Nelson SM, Lawlor DA. Live-birth rate associated with repeat *in vitro* fertilization treatment cycles. *JAMA.* 2015;314(24):2654–62.
33. McLernon DJ, Steyerberg EW, Te Velde ER et al. Predicting the chances of a live birth after one or more complete cycles of *in vitro* fertilisation: Population based study of linked cycle data from 113,873 women. *BMJ.* 2016;355:i5735.
34. Polyzos NP, Drakopoulos P, Parra J et al. Cumulative live birth rates according to the number of oocytes retrieved after the first ovarian stimulation for *in vitro* fertilization/intracytoplasmic sperm injection: A multicenter multinational analysis including approximately 15,000 women. *Fertil Steril.* 2018;110(4):661–70.e1.
35. Drakopoulos P, Blockeel C, Stoop D et al. Conventional ovarian stimulation and single embryo transfer for IVF/ICSI. How many oocytes do we need to maximize cumulative live birth rates after utilization of all fresh and frozen embryos? *Hum Reprod.* 2016;31(2):370–6.
36. Zhu Q, Chen Q, Wang L et al. Live birth rates in the first complete IVF cycle among 20,687 women using a freeze-all strategy. *Hum Reprod.* 2018;33(5):924–9.
37. Verberg MF, Macklon NS, Nargund G et al. Mild ovarian stimulation for IVF. *Hum Reprod Update.* 2009;15(1):13–29.
38. Labarta E, Bosch E, Mercader A et al. A higher ovarian response after stimulation for IVF is related to a higher number of Euploid embryos. *Biomed Res Int.* 2017;2017:5637923.
39. Kawwass JF, Kissin DM, Kulkarni AD et al. Safety of assisted reproductive technology in the United States, 2000-2011. *JAMA.* 2015;313(1):88–90.
40. Delvigne A. Request for information on unreported cases of severe ovarian hyperstimulation syndrome (OHSS). *Hum Reprod.* 2005;20(7):2033.
41. Ishihara O, Kuwahara A, Saitoh H. Frozen-thawed blastocyst transfer reduces ectopic pregnancy risk: An analysis of single embryo transfer cycles in Japan. *Fertil Steril.* 2011;95(6):1966–9.
42. Shapiro BS, Daneshmand ST, De Leon L et al. Frozen-thawed embryo transfer is associated with a significantly reduced incidence of ectopic pregnancy. *Fertil Steril.* 2012;98(6):1490–4.
43. Maheshwari A, Pandey S, Amalraj Raja E et al. Is frozen embryo transfer better for mothers and babies? Can cumulative meta-analysis provide a definitive answer? *Hum Reprod Update.* 2018;24(1):35–58.

44. Toner JP, Coddington CC, Doody K et al. Society for assisted reproductive technology and assisted reproductive technology in the United States: A 2016 update. *Fertil Steril.* 2016;106(3):541–6.

45. Venetis CA, Kolibianakis EM, Bosdou JK, Tarlatzis BC. Progesterone elevation and probability of pregnancy after IVF: A systematic review and meta-analysis of over 60 000 cycles. *Hum Reprod Update.* 2013;19(5):433–57.

46. Labarta E, Martinez-Conejero JA, Alama P et al. Endometrial receptivity is affected in women with high circulating progesterone levels at the end of the follicular phase: A functional genomics analysis. *Hum Reprod.* 2011;26(7):1813–25.

47. Hill MJ, Healy MW, Richter KS et al. Defining thresholds for abnormal premature progesterone levels during ovarian stimulation for assisted reproduction technologies. *Fertil Steril.* 2018;110(4):671–9.e2.

48. Roque M, Lattes K, Serra S et al. Fresh embryo transfer versus frozen embryo transfer in in vitro fertilization cycles: A systematic review and meta-analysis. *Fertil Steril.* 2013;99(1):156–62.

49. JARG Editor-In-Chief. Retraction note to: Can fresh embryo transfers be replaced by cryopreserved-thawed embryo transfers in assisted reproductive cycles? A randomized controlled trial. *J Assist Reprod Genet.* 2013;30(9):1245.

50. Roque M, Valle M, Kostolias A et al. Freeze-all cycle in reproductive medicine: Current perspectives. *JBRA Assist Reprod.* 2017;21(1):49–53.

51. Shapiro BS, Daneshmand ST, Garner FC et al. Evidence of impaired endometrial receptivity after ovarian stimulation for *in vitro* fertilization: A prospective randomized trial comparing fresh and frozen-thawed embryo transfer in normal responders. *Fertil Steril.* 2011;96(2):344–8.

52. Shapiro BS, Daneshmand ST, Garner FC et al. Evidence of impaired endometrial receptivity after ovarian stimulation for *in vitro* fertilization: A prospective randomized trial comparing fresh and frozen-thawed embryo transfers in high responders. *Fertil Steril.* 2011;96(2):516–8.

53. Chen ZJ, Shi Y, Sun Y et al. Fresh versus frozen embryos for infertility in the polycystic ovary syndrome. *N Engl J Med.* 2016;375(6):523–33.

54. Vuong LN, Dang VQ, Ho TM et al. IVF transfer of fresh or frozen embryos in women without polycystic ovaries. *N Engl J Med.* 2018;378(2):137–47.

55. Shi Y, Sun Y, Hao C et al. Transfer of fresh versus frozen embryos in ovulatory women. *N Engl J Med.* 2018;378(2):126–36.

56. Roque M, Haahr T, Geber S et al. Fresh versus elective frozen embryo transfer in IVF/ICSI cycles: A systematic review and meta-analysis of reproductive outcomes. *Hum Reprod Update.* 2019;25(1):2–14

57. Zaca C, Bazzocchi A, Pennetta F et al. Cumulative live birth rate in freeze-all cycles is comparable to that of a conventional embryo transfer policy at the cleavage stage but superior at the blastocyst stage. *Fertil Steril.* 2018;110(4):703–9.

58. Acharya KS, Acharya CR, Bishop K et al. Freezing of all embryos in *in vitro* fertilization is beneficial in high responders, but not intermediate and low responders: An analysis of 82,935 cycles from the society for assisted reproductive technology registry. *Fertil Steril.* 2018;110(5):880–7.

59. Wirleitner B, Schuff M, Stecher A et al. Pregnancy and birth outcomes following fresh or vitrified embryo transfer according to blastocyst morphology and expansion stage, and culturing strategy for delayed development. *Hum Reprod.* 2016;31(8):1685–95.

60. Van Landuyt L, Van De Velde H, Blockeel C et al. Fresh transfer of day 5 slowly developing embryos versus postponed transfer of vitrified fully-developed day 6 blastocysts: What is the best approach? *Reprod Biomed Online.* 2018;37:e10.

61. Steptoe PC, Edwards RG. Reimplantation of a human embryo with subsequent tubal pregnancy. *Lancet.* 1976;1(7965):880–2.

62. Clayton HB, Schieve LA, Peterson HB et al. Ectopic pregnancy risk with assisted reproductive technology procedures. *Obstet Gynecol.* 2006;107(3):595–604.

63. Strandell A, Thorburn J, Hamberger L. Risk factors for ectopic pregnancy in assisted reproduction. *Fertil Steril.* 1999;71(2):282–6.

64. Londra L, Moreau C, Strobino D et al. Ectopic pregnancy after in vitro fertilization: Differences between fresh and frozen-thawed cycles. *Fertil Steril.* 2015;104(1):110–8.

65. Santos-Ribeiro S, Tournaye H, Polyzos NP. Trends in ectopic pregnancy rates following assisted reproductive technologies in the UK: A 12-year nationwide analysis including 160 000 pregnancies. *Hum Reprod.* 2016;31(2):393–402.

66. Mateizel I, Santos-Ribeiro S, Done E et al. Do ARTs affect the incidence of monozygotic twinning? *Hum Reprod.* 2016;31(11):2435–41.
67. Liu H, Liu J, Chen S et al. Elevated incidence of monozygotic twinning is associated with extended embryo culture, but not with zona pellucida manipulation or freeze-thaw procedure. *Fertil Steril.* 2018;109(6):1044–50.
68. Ikemoto Y, Kuroda K, Ochiai A et al. Prevalence and risk factors of zygotic splitting after 937,848 single embryo transfer cycles. *Hum Reprod.* 2018;33(11):1984–91.
69. Maheshwari A, Pandey S, Shetty A et al. Obstetric and perinatal outcomes in singleton pregnancies resulting from the transfer of frozen thawed versus fresh embryos generated through in vitro fertilization treatment: A systematic review and meta-analysis. *Fertil Steril.* 2012;98(2):368–77.e1-9.
70. Pelkonen S, Koivunen R, Gissler M et al. Perinatal outcome of children born after frozen and fresh embryo transfer: The Finnish cohort study 1995–2006. *Hum Reprod.* 2010;25(4):914–23.
71. Kalra SK, Ratcliffe SJ, Coutifaris C et al. Ovarian stimulation and low birth weight in newborns conceived through *in vitro* fertilization. *Obstet Gynecol.* 2011;118(4):863–71.
72. Liu L, Johnson HL, Cousens S et al. Global, regional, and national causes of child mortality: An updated systematic analysis for 2010 with time trends since 2000. *Lancet.* 2012;379(9832):2151–61.
73. Bloise E, Lin W, Liu X et al. Impaired placental nutrient transport in mice generated by *in vitro* fertilization. *Endocrinology.* 2012;153(7):3457–67.
74. Mainigi MA, Olalere D, Burd I et al. Peri-implantation hormonal milieu: Elucidating mechanisms of abnormal placentation and fetal growth. *Biol Reprod.* 2014;90(2):26.
75. Weinerman R, Mainigi M. Why we should transfer frozen instead of fresh embryos: The translational rationale. *Fertil Steril.* 2014;102(1):10–8.
76. De Vos A, Santos-Ribeiro S, Van Landuyt L et al. Birthweight of singletons born after cleavage-stage or blastocyst transfer in fresh and warming cycles. *Hum Reprod.* 2018;33(2):196–201.
77. Vidal M, Vellve K, Gonzalez-Comadran M et al. Perinatal outcomes in children born after fresh or frozen embryo transfer: A Catalan cohort study based on 14,262 newborns. *Fertil Steril.* 2017;107(4):940–7.
78. Wennerholm UB, Henningsen AK, Romundstad LB et al. Perinatal outcomes of children born after frozen-thawed embryo transfer: A Nordic cohort study from the CoNARTaS group. *Hum Reprod.* 2013;28(9):2545–53.
79. Blockeel C, Drakopoulos P, Santos-Ribeiro S et al. A fresh look at the freeze-all protocol: A SWOT analysis. *Hum Reprod.* 2016;31(3):491–7.
80. Cakmak H, Katz A, Cedars MI, Rosen MP. Effective method for emergency fertility preservation: Random-start controlled ovarian stimulation. *Fertil Steril.* 2013;100(6):1673–80.
81. Kuang Y, Chen Q, Fu Y et al. Medroxyprogesterone acetate is an effective oral alternative for preventing premature luteinizing hormone surges in women undergoing controlled ovarian hyperstimulation for *in vitro* fertilization. *Fertil Steril.* 2015;104(1):62-70 e3.
82. Vaiarelli A, Cimadomo D, Trabucco E et al. Double Stimulation in the Same Ovarian Cycle (DuoStim) to maximize the number of oocytes retrieved from poor prognosis patients: A multicenter experience and SWOT analysis. *Front Endocrinol (Lausanne).* 2018;9:317.
83. Berntsen S, Pinborg A. Large for gestational age and macrosomia in singletons born after frozen/thawed embryo transfer (FET) in assisted reproductive technology (ART). *Birth Defects Res.* 2018;110(8):630–43.
84. Kato O, Kawasaki N, Bodri D et al. Neonatal outcome and birth defects in 6623 singletons born following minimal ovarian stimulation and vitrified versus fresh single embryo transfer. *Eur J Obstet Gynecol Reprod Biol.* 2012;161(1):46–50.
85. Galliano D, Garrido N, Serra-Serra V, Pellicer A. Difference in birth weight of consecutive sibling singletons is not found in oocyte donation when comparing fresh versus frozen embryo replacements. *Fertil Steril.* 2015;104(6):1411-8.e1–3.
86. Romundstad LB, Romundstad PR, Sunde A et al. Effects of technology or maternal factors on perinatal outcome after assisted fertilisation: A population-based cohort study. *Lancet.* 2008;372(9640):737–43.
87. Pinborg A, Henningsen AA, Loft A et al. Large baby syndrome in singletons born after frozen embryo transfer (FET): Is it due to maternal factors or the cryotechnique? *Hum Reprod.* 2014;29(3):618–27.
88. De Vos A, Janssens R, Van de Velde H et al. The type of culture medium and the duration of in vitro culture do not influence birthweight of ART singletons. *Hum Reprod.* 2015;30(1):20–7.
89. Makinen S, Soderstrom-Anttila V, Vainio J et al. Does long *in vitro* culture promote large for gestational age babies? *Hum Reprod.* 2013;28(3):828–34.

90. Dar S, Lazer T, Shah PS, Librach CL. Neonatal outcomes among singleton births after blastocyst versus cleavage stage embryo transfer: A systematic review and meta-analysis. *Hum Reprod Update.* 2014;20(3):439–48.

91. Grace KS, Sinclair KD. Assisted reproductive technology, epigenetics, and long-term health: A developmental time bomb still ticking. *Semin Reprod Med.* 2009;27(5):409–16.

92. Saito K, Miyado K, Yamatoya K et al. Increased incidence of post-term delivery and Cesarean section after frozen-thawed embryo transfer during a hormone replacement cycle. *J Assist Reprod Genet.* 2017;34(4):465–70.

93. Blazquez A, Garcia D, Vassena R et al. Risk of pre-eclampsia after fresh or frozen embryo transfer in patients undergoing oocyte donation. *Eur J Obstet Gynecol Reprod Biol.* 2018;227:27–31.

94. Santos-Ribeiro S, Siffain J, Polyzos NP et al. To delay or not to delay a frozen embryo transfer after a failed fresh embryo transfer attempt? *Fertil Steril.* 2016;105(5):1202–7 e1.

95. Santos-Ribeiro S, Polyzos NP, Lan VT et al. The effect of an immediate frozen embryo transfer following a freeze-all protocol: A retrospective analysis from two centres. *Hum Reprod.* 2016;31(11):2541–8.

96. Lattes K, Checa MA, Vassena R et al. There is no evidence that the time from egg retrieval to embryo transfer affects live birth rates in a freeze-all strategy. *Hum Reprod.* 2017;32(2):368–74.

97. Mastenbroek S, van der Veen F, Aflatoonian A et al. Embryo selection in IVF. *Hum Reprod.* 2011;26(5):964–6.

98. Haouzi D, Assou S, Mahmoud K et al. Gene expression profile of human endometrial receptivity: Comparison between natural and stimulated cycles for the same patients. *Hum Reprod.* 2009;24(6):1436–45.

99. Bourgain C, Devroey P. The endometrium in stimulated cycles for IVF. *Hum Reprod Update.* 2003;9(6):515–22.

6

Preimplantation Genetic Screening

M. Yusuf Beebeejaun and Sesh K. Sunkara

Introduction

One in seven couples in the United Kingdom experience difficulty in conceiving. Many of them will require *in vitro* fertilization (IVF) treatment that the National Institute for Health and Care Excellence (NICE) recommends as the effective treatment for prolonged unresolved infertility. In the year 2014, 52,288 women had a total of 67,707 IVF cycles in the United Kingdom. The year 2014 saw a 4.8% increase in the number of IVF treatment cycles performed compared to the year 2013.

Regardless of the increasing trend over time and despite several technological advances, IVF success rates remain low overall (26.5% live birth rate per treatment cycle in the United Kingdom in 2013). IVF success rates are even lower in women of advanced reproductive age. The lower success rate is attributed mainly to the poor quality of the embryos, and the increased embryo aneuploidy rate encountered with increasing female age is thought to be contributory. As per some studies, the embryo aneuploidy rate is reported to be approximately 30% in women aged 30 years and younger and as high as 85% in women aged over 42 years. Embryo aneuploidy is also the main reason for the higher miscarriage rates among older women.

It has been suggested that genetic screening of the embryos by removing few cells (biopsy) and performing genetic analysis, termed *preimplantation genetic screening* (PGS), thereby transferring euploid embryos with the correct number of chromosomes into the uterus during IVF treatment, may lead to improved embryo implantation, fewer miscarriages, and more live births.

Since its implementation over 25 years ago, there has been an increasing trend in its use within IVF cycles. In this chapter, we explore traditional and novel indications, approaches to obtaining cells for pregenetic diagnosis (PGD), and its diagnostic accuracy. With the possibility of exposing an embryo's entire genetic content, PGD obviates certain ethical dilemmas but introduces other novel controversies, and these are also discussed.

Pregenetic Testing

Although usually considered novel, pregenetic testing was first envisioned in 1968 by Gardner and Edwards who biopsied a rabbit blastocyst and performed X-chromatin analysis, suggesting its application to human X-linked recessive traits. Progress in human PGD was unavoidably delayed until the first successful IVF in 1978. The first blastomere biopsy on a day-3 embryo (cleavage stage) was performed by Handyside in 1990, determining sex in a pregnancy at risk for ornithine transcarbamylase (OTC) deficiency, an X-linked disorder. This technique was further adapted for the detection of cystic fibrosis in 1992. At present, chromosomal abnormalities are detected by array comparative genomic hybridization (CGH).

Types of Preimplantation Genetic Testing

With ongoing advancement in the field of PGS, the nomenclature used to describe the various forms of PGS changed. There are three types of preimplantation genetic testing (PGT):

1. *Preimplantation genetic testing for monogenic (single-gene) disorders (PGT-M)*: This aims to identify a pregnancy that is affected by specific genetic characteristics, such as a known heritable genetic mutation carried by one or both biological parents. It can also be used to identify embryos for transfer that can be used as donors, for example, embryos with particular gender or compatible human leukocyte antigen complex type.
2. *Preimplantation genetic testing for structural rearrangements (PGT-SR)*: The goal of PGT-SR is to identify an embryo that is affected by a structural chromosomal abnormality such as translocation, deletion, or duplication.
3. *Preimplantation genetic testing for aneuploidy (PGT-A)*: Formerly known as preimplantation genetic screening (PGS aims to identify embryos with *de novo* aneuploidy), the premise behind PGT-A is that correctly identifying these embryos and their transfer will reduce the risk of miscarriage, avoid the complications related to pregnancy failure, and reduce the time frame from transfer to a viable pregnancy.

Indications for Preimplantation Genetic Screening

The most common reason for PGS is detection of chromosomal abnormalities, most often aneuploidies. Clinically, the main indications for PGS are as follows:

- Single-gene disorders (monogenic disorders), such as autosomal recessive, autosomal dominant, or X-linked disorders)
- Chromosomal structural aberrations (such as a balanced translocation)

In certain conditions, PGS is often offered as a way to increase the chances of an ongoing pregnancy. These conditions can include the following:

- Recurrent miscarriages
- Unsuccessful IVF cycles (more than two)
- Advanced maternal age
- History of chromosomally abnormal child or pregnancy
- Chromosomal translocations
- Family history of structural chromosomal condition
- Family history of X-linked disease
- Inherited genetic disorders

PGS for Chromosomal Aneuploidy

PGD for cytogenetic analysis was first performed through fluorescence *in situ* hybridization (FISH). Through this technique, a limited number of chromosomes were able to be assessed, usually between five and nine. Because of this limitation, multiple cycles of FISH were often needed in order to assess numerous chromosomes. This technique was time consuming and also required expertise.

Array CGH is based on CGH. It is a cytogenetic technique that allows comprehensive analysis of the entire genome. Arrays are also used antenatally through chorionic villus sampling.

Chromosomal Rearrangements

Chromosomal rearrangements include gene translocation or inversion that may result in unbalanced gametes and, hence, an unbalanced zygote. Translocations are often diagnosed as part of recurrent miscarriages. They are often detected through array CGH. In these cases, PGS may be warranted in order to reduce the risk of spontaneous miscarriages secondary to chromosomal abnormalities.

A study by Goddijn et al. in 2004 determined that the mean time for translocation couples to achieve pregnancy naturally is 4–6 years.

The use of PGD in these clinical situations was assessed in 2006 by Otani et al., who concluded that the use of PGS and aneuploidy screening reduced the number of spontaneous miscarriages in this group to 5%. The lifetime cumulative pregnancy rate using PGD was 57.6%, involving an average of only 1.24 cycles.

Single-Gene Disorders

Approximately one-fourth of PGD cases are currently performed to detect a single mutant gene. Genes commonly being investigated include hemoglobinopathies, cystic fibrosis, fragile X syndrome, and Duchenne muscular dystrophy.

Obtaining DNA for Analysis

Developments over the last decade facilitating routine laboratory culture of human embryos to the blastocyst stage (embryo composed of 100–150 cells) have permitted biopsy of the trophectoderm (outer layer of the blastocyst), allowing removal of a small number (5–10) of cells compared to the previously used blastomere biopsy, which allows removal of only one or two cells from a day-3 cleavage-stage (4–8-cell) embryo.

In addition to providing more cells and genetic material for analysis, trophectoderm biopsy has been shown to be safer compared to blastomere biopsy. Furthermore, developments in comprehensive genetic testing techniques allowing analysis of all 23 pairs of chromosomes, in comparison to an earlier FISH technique that had the limitation of analyzing only a few chromosomes, have made PGS more reliable than previously. These advances have led to the recent reinvigorated interest in the use of the new PGS in IVF using trophectoderm biopsy and comprehensive chromosome screening (CCS).

There are three potential approaches to obtaining DNA for analysis. This is based on the age of the embryo and the indication for biopsy:

1. Polar body biopsy
2. Blastomere biopsy from day 3
3. Trophectoderm biopsy from day 5–6

Polar Biopsy

A polar body is often regarded as a by-product of an oocyte during meiotic division. It is therefore possible for the genome content of an oocyte to be deduced by analysis of the first and second polar biopsies. Within human oocytes, polar bodies usually apoptose within 17–24 hours following formation, and the resulting fragments remain entrapped within the zona pellucida.

As part of PGS, polar body biopsy is significantly useful in countries where biopsy of an embryo is not permitted. In these situations, genetic analysis of polar bodies offers an alternative to assess the genetic composition of an embryo, based on the predictive nature of the genetic composition of the oocyte.

Since, by nature, polar bodies are maternally inherited, polar body biopsy (PBB) is limited to the evaluation of maternally inherited mutations or meiotic errors during oocyte development. A polar body diagnosis is therefore unable to assess paternal genotype, thus precluding application if the father has an autosomal dominant disorder. Biopsy of the first and second polar bodies provides information that informally reflects the genetic composition of the oocyte.

If the mother is heterozygous for a known mutant allele, division of the diploid primary oocyte at meiosis I may result in a normal secondary oocyte and a first polar body with the same mutant allele as the mother. Consequently, if a PBB results in a normal allele, genetic makeup can be presumed to be associated with oocytes that have the mutant alleles. Conversely, PBBs demonstrating the mutant alleles are presumed to be associated with oocytes with normal alleles, and these oocytes can then be used for IVF.

Because of its purely maternal origin, PBB has several limitations. Its value is limited if the mother is affected (homozygous) by an autosomal recessive disorder and the father is also a carrier, since all oocytes and polar bodies will display the mutation. Blastocyst biopsy to assess both maternal and paternal genes in the developing embryos will therefore be necessary.

Another limitation is the genetic phenomenon of recombination that can occur during meiosis between homologous chromosomes. The diagnostic potential of PBB is further limited if the genes of interest are close to the telomeric (distal) region of the chromosome, as they are more likely to cross over. In order to counteract this limitation, improved PGT-M protocols that include closely linked markers, short tandem repeats (STRs), or simple sequence repeats (SNRs) may be applied. However, since chromosomal trisomy usually originates in maternal meiosis, a diagnostic PBB will suffice for PGD in 90%–95% of cases.

A further limitation is the fact that the oocyte must either be fertilized or cryopreserved before the results of PBB are available. In so doing, over 30% of oocytes will either not fertilize successfully (i.e., develop two pronuclei) or will not undergo postfertilization development. With regard to genetic limitation, a PBB may diagnose a meiotic anomaly after meosis I that autocorrects itself by meiosis II. Furthermore, PBB has a limited capacity to predict a genetic anomaly that may arise after syngamy. These miotic abnormalities often arise after the fusion of male and female pronucleus.

Cleavage-Stage Embryo (Eight-Cell Blastomere Biopsy)

A cleavage-stage embryo involves a biopsy on day 3, by which time the embryo has around eight cells enveloped within a glycoprotein layer. At this stage, PGT can be achieved by traversing the zona, and extraction of cells can be performed. A D3 biopsy involves the removal of one cell from the blastomere.

Studies by Cohen et al. (1) and DeVos et al. (2) examined the effect of one-cell and two-cell biopsy on embryo survival rate. The reported live birth rates were 37.4% and 22.4% after removal of one versus two cells, respectively.

Because of the one-cell biopsy, one of the limitations of biopsy at the cleavage stage is embryo mosaicism, which is a major diagnostic impediment. Even though tissue mosaicism can occur in a variety of tissues, it is believed that genetic mosaicism within this early embryogenesis stage is secondary to natural genetic self-correction by the embryo.

Trophectoderm Biopsy

The blastocyst, which is the developmental stage achieved 5–6 days following fertilization, usually contains more than 100 cells.

At this stage, more cells can be removed for diagnosis. The trophectoderm is a collection of cells from the outer layer of the blastocyst. Since the trophectoderm is intended to develop into the placenta, embryonic tissue is therefore not technically being biopsied. Trophectoderm cells are extracted using a small pipette or through gentle compression of the blastocyst to extract cells through the opening. A trophectoderm biopsy usually involves five to eight cells in order to limit disruption to the developing placenta. In comparison to other PGS techniques, blastocyst biopsy is regarded as the least disruptive to subsequent development while providing the most DNA for testing, which reduces the possibility of diagnostic errors.

Cryopreservation

Due to the time constraints for a biopsy result to be available, embryos or oocytes are usually vitrified until results of the genetic analysis are available. Of note, if necessary, repeat or confirmatory analysis can be performed. Frozen embryos biopsied at the blastocyst stage can be warmed, re-biopsied, and re-vitrified. However, survival appears to be slightly lower for embryos warmed for a second biopsy.

Limitation of Preimplantation Genetic Screening

Until recently, embryo transfer at day 3 used to be routine practice in IVF. Approximately 50% of embryos survive in culture to day 3 of development, and only around 25% survive to form blastocysts by day 5 or 6. With the limitations around day 3 versus day 5–6 biopsy (as described earlier), if PGS warrants extended blastocyst culture, the percentage of patients who may have no embryos suitable for biopsy or transfer may increase. This may consequently result in fewer embryos available for testing, transfer, or cryopreservation.

Observational studies have also concluded that extended blastocyst culture may result in an increase in the chance of having monozygotic twins and a male child, as well as a potentially higher risk of epigenetic modifications that may lead to an increased risk of adverse neonatal outcomes.

However, the use of day-5 embryos is increasing in IVF programs, even when PGT is not performed. The rationale behind such extended blastocyst culture is the higher rate of live birth that is associated with a day-5 embryo compared to a day-3 embryo. In the United States, approximately 60% of IVF programs transfer embryos to the uterus on day 5 after fertilization, and 30% transfer on day 3.

Chromosomal Mosaicism

Embryo mosaicism is one of the major limitations of PGS and is often regarded as the largest source of false-positive errors. Chromosomal mosaicism is the case whereby different cells within the same embryo having different chromosome numbers are a common finding in IVF-derived human embryos.

Due to its very nature and the risk of aneuploidy being detected, embryo mosaicism may reduce the probability of pregnancy overall from a single-assisted reproductive technology cycle.

Mosaicism may be present in as many as 50% of embryos. It is often secondary to postfertilization mitotic errors, which creates distinct cell populations with both euploid and aneuploid chromosomal constitutions. The proportion of mosaicism within an embryo relates to the stage of development of the embryo at which a mitotic error occurred.

The earlier the stage of the error, the higher is the proportion of abnormal cells. Since aneuploid cell lines divide more slowly than euploid cells, "self-correction" may occur so that the percentage of abnormal cells in an embryo may decrease over time. It is worth noting that around 1%–2% of chorionic villus sampling in pregnancy identifies further mosaicism. Mosaicism may therefore not represent the actual chromosomal constitution of the remainder of the dynamic developing embryo.

Whether normal live births could result from transferring such mosaic embryos is relatively unknown. In a recent study involving biopsy of 3802 embryos at the blastocyst stage, chromosomal mosaicism was detected in 181 (4.8%) embryos. Eighteen women in this study had no euploid blastocysts and consented to have transfer of a mosaic aneuploid embryo that led to eight clinical pregnancies and six singleton term live births.

BIBLIOGRAPHY

1. Cohen J, Wells D, Munné S. Removal of 2 cells from cleavage-stage embryos is likely to reduce the efficacy of chromosomal tests that are used to enhance implantation rates. *Fertil Steril*. 2007;87:496–503.
2. DeVos A, Staessen C, De Rycke M et al. Impact of cleavage-stage embryo biopsy in view of PGD on human blastocyst implantation: A prospective cohort of single embryo transfers. *Hum Reprod*. 2009;24:2988–96.

3. Bolton H, Graham SJ, Van der Aa N et al. Mouse model of chromosome mosaicism reveals lineage-specific depletion of aneuploid cells and normal developmental potential. *Nat Commun.* 2016;7:11165.

4. Carson SA, Gentry WL, Smith AL, Buster JE. Trophectoderm microbiopsy in murine blastocysts: Comparison of four methods. *J Assist Reprod Genet.* 1993;10(6):427.

5. Cieslak-Janzen J, Tur-Kaspa I, Ilkevitch Y et al. Multiple micromanipulations for preimplantation genetic diagnosis do not affect embryo development to the blastocyst stage. *Fertil Steril.* 2006;85:1826–9.

6. Demko ZP, Simon AL, McCoy RC et al. Effects of maternal age on euploidy rates in a large cohort of embryos analyzed with 24-chromosome single-nucleotide polymorphism-based preimplantation genetic screening. *Fertil Steril.* 2016;105:1307–13.

7. Fragouli E, Wells D. Aneuploidy in the human blastocyst. *Cytogenet Genome Res.* 2011;133(2–4):149–59.

8. Franasiak JM, Forman EJ, Hong KH et al. The nature of aneuploidy with increasing age of the female partner: A review of 15,169 consecutive trophectoderm biopsies evaluated with comprehensive chromosomal screening. *Fertil Steril.* 2014;101:656–63.

9. Fritz MA, Schattman G. Reply of the Committee: Parental translocations and need for preimplantation genetic diagnosis? Distorting effects of ascertainment bias and the need for information rich families. *Fertil Steril.* 2008;90:892–3.

10. Gardner RL, Edwards RG. Control of sex ratio at full term in the rabbit by transferring sexed blastocysts. *Nature.* 1968;218:346–9.

11. Goddijn M, Joosten JHK, Knegt AC et al. Clinical relevance of diagnosing structural chromosome abnormalities in couples with repeated miscarriage. *Hum Reprod.* 2004;19:1013–7.

12. Greco E, Minasi MG, Fiorentino F. Healthy babies after intrauterine transfer of mosaic aneuploid blastocysts. *N Engl J Med.* 2015 Nov 19;373(21):2089–90.

13. Griffin DK, Handyside AH, Penketh RJ et al. Fluorescent in-situ hybridisation to interphase nuclei of human preimplantation embryos with X and Y chromosome specific probes. *Hum Reprod.* 1991;6:101–5.

14. Handyside AH. 24-chromosome copy number analysis: A comparison of available technologies. *Fertil Steril.* 2013;100:595–602.

15. Handyside AH, Harton GL, Mariani B et al. Karyomapping: A universal method for genome wide analysis of genetic disease based on mapping crossovers between parental haplotypes. *J Med Genet.* 2010;47:651.

16. Handyside AH, Kontogianni EH, Hardy K, Winston RM. Pregnancies from biopsied human preimplantation embryos sexed by Y-specific DNA amplification. *Nature.* 1990;244:768–70.

17. Harper J. *Preimplantation Genetic Diagnosis.* 2nd ed. Cambridge, UK: Cambridge University Press; 2009.

18. Hu L, Cheng D, Gong F et al. Reciprocal translocation carrier diagnosis in preimplantation human embryos. *EBioMedicine.* 2016;14:139.

19. Human Fertilisation and Embryology Authority. Fertility treatment in 2014: Trends and figures. http://www.hfea.gov.uk/10243.html (accessed March 18, 2018).

20. Kuliev A, Rechitsky S, Verlinsky O. *Atlas of Preimplantation Genetic Diagnosis.* 3rd ed. Boca Raton, FL: CRC Press; 2014.

21. Longo FJ. *Fertilization.* New York, NY: Chapman & Hall; 1997.

22. Moutou C, Goossens V, Coonen E et al. ESHRE PGD consortium data collection XII: Cycles from January to December 2009 with pregnancy follow-up to October 2010. *Hum Reprod.* 2014;29:880–903.

23. National Collaborating Centre for Women's and Children's Health. Fertility: Assessment and Treatment for People with Fertility Problems. *Clinical guideline* 2013. National Institute for Health and Care Excellence. http://www.nice.org.uk/guidance/cg156/evidence (accessed March 15, 2018).

24. Oakley L, Doyle P, Maconochie N. Lifetime prevalence of infertility and infertility in the UK: Results form a population based survey of reproduction. *Hum Reprod.* 2008;23:447–50.

25. Otani T, Roche M, Mizuike M et al. Preimplantation genetic diagnosis significantly improves the pregnancy outcome of translocation carriers with a history of recurrent miscarriage and unsuccessful pregnancies. *Reprod Biomed Online.* 2006;13:879–94.

26. Practice Committees of the American Society for Reproductive Medicine and the Society for Assisted Reproductive Technology. Blastocyst culture and transfer in clinical-assisted reproduction: A committee opinion. *Fertil Steril.* 2013;99(3):667–72.

27. Preimplantation Genetic Screening and Diagnostic Testing Preimplantation Genetic Diagnosis International Society (PGDIS). Guidelines for good practice in PGD: Programme requirements and laboratory quality assurance. *Reprod Biomed Online.* 2008;16:134–47.

28. Scott RT Jr, Upham KM, Forman EJ et al. Cleavage-stage biopsy significantly impairs human embryonic implantation potential while blastocyst biopsy does not: A randomized and paired clinical trial. *Fertil Steril.* 2013;100(3):624–30.

29. Simpson JL. Preimplantation genetic diagnosis at 20 years. *Prenat Diagn.* 2010;30:682–85.

30. Taylor TH, Gitlin SA, Patrick JL et al. The origin, mechanisms, incidence and clinical consequences of chromosomal mosaicism in humans. *Hum Reprod Update.* 2014 Jul;20(4):571–81.

31. Taylor TH, Patrick JL, Gitlin SA et al. Outcomes of blastocysts biopsied and vitrified once versus those cryopreserved twice for euploid blastocyst transfer. *Reprod Biomed Online.* 2014;29(1):59.

32. United States Centers for Disease Control and Prevention. Assisted reproductive technology: National summary report. 2015. https://www.cdc.gov/art/pdf/2015-report/ART-2015-National-Summary-Report. pdf#page=43 (accessed March 21, 2019).

33. Verlinsky Y, Rechitsky S, Verlinsky O et al. Prepregnancy testing for single-gene disorders by polar body analysis. *Genet Test.* 1999;3(2):185.

34. Verlinsky Y, Rechitsky S, Verlinsky O et al. Preimplantation diagnosis for sonic hedgehog mutation causing familial holoprosencephaly. *N Engl J Med.* 2003;348(15):1449.

7

The Use of Single Embryo Transfer

Abha Maheshwari

Background

Over 7 million babies have been born worldwide by the use of *in vitro* fertilization (IVF) in just over 40 years. Though an extremely successful treatment, the biggest complication of IVF has been a high multiple pregnancy rate. This has been due to the transfer of multiple embryos, in the hope that at least one of them will implant. Hence, multiple embryos transferred in the hope of maximizing pregnancy lead to an exponential surge in the proportion of multiples in pregnancies as a result of IVF. It was identified that the only way to reduce multiple pregnancies was to transfer a single embryo. In 1998 (1), data from Human Fertilisation and Embryology Authority (HFEA) showed that by reducing the number of embryos transferred from three to two, the pregnancy rate was not reduced, but the rate of triplets was reduced. This led to widespread use of double embryo transfer as default.

Although triplets were reduced, twins persisted. Even in 2004–2005, twins accounted for 30% of the assisted reproductive technology (ART)-related live births in the United States (2) and 21% in Europe (3) in comparison with 1.6% of all births from naturally conceived pregnancies (4). With the widespread use of IVF, it became clear that twins are in a much higher proportion, and something has to be done about it to reduce the risks associated with multiple births, which can lead to both short- and long-term health problems in the babies born, higher risk to the mother during pregnancy and delivery, as well as significant costs to health care. Single embryo transfer (SET) was suggested as a way forward.

SET is when one embryo is transferred. SET could be an elective single embryo transfer (eSET), when a woman opts to reduce the risk of a multiple birth by having one embryo transferred in a treatment cycle despite having more available. Nonelective single embryo transfer (non-eSET) is when only one embryo is available for transfer. This chapter relates to the use of eSET, and SET is used for all eSET. Double embryo transfer (DET) is when two embryos are transferred to a woman's uterus at the same time.

Although theoretically a sound concept, it has taken a long time for SET to come in practice. There has been a wide global variation in the uptake of SET (5) due to multiple factors. The most important are concerns about a reduction in success (pregnancy) rates.

Evidence of Clinical Effectiveness

There are a variety of ways in which success rates in an IVF program are measured. Measurement of clinical effectiveness depends on both the numerator and the denominator as well as the time period during which clinical effectiveness is being measured (Table 7.1). There are several permutations/ combinations in which these can be used.

There have been several randomized trials comparing single versus double embryo transfer. An individual patient data meta-analysis (6) on eight trials ($n = 1367$) showed that live birth rate in a fresh

TABLE 7.1

Parameters Used in Determining Effectiveness of *In Vitro* Fertilization

Numerator	Denominator	Time Horizon
Pregnancy rate	Per started stimulation	In n number of years
Clinical pregnancy rate	Per embryo transfer episode	
Live birth rate	Per embryo transferred	
Healthy baby rate	Per egg collection	
Cumulative live birth rate		

IVF cycle was lower after single (27%) than double embryo transfer (42%; adjusted odds ratio 0.50, 95% confidence interval 0.39–0.63), as was the multiple birth rate (2% versus 29%). An additional frozen SET, however, resulted in a cumulative live birth rate similar to double embryo transfer (38% versus 42%), with a minimal cumulative risk of multiple birth (1% versus 32%). The odds of term singleton live birth were five times higher after SET as compared to after DET ([6]; these data were published in 2010, but trials were conducted long before then).

Evidence of Cost-Effectiveness

Like clinical effectiveness, there are difficulties with the cost-effectiveness model of single versus double embryo transfer. It depends on whose perspective it is calculated from (health care or patient or clinic providing IVF treatment or society), the time horizon it is measured for (5 years or 10 years or lifelong), and what is being measured. It is important when most IVF treatment is funded by patients themselves, whereas complications and implications of IVF treatment are usually dealt with by the public system (Table 7.2).

There are conflicting results from cost-effectiveness studies, primarily because of variation in what is being measured. Hernandez et al. (2015) suggested that the use of SET followed by single frozen embryo transfer was not a cost-effective strategy when compared to double embryo transfer (7). However, another study showed that there was clear cost-effectiveness for SET policy in the younger age group. Using a decision tree model to evaluate from the health-care provider's perspective, SET followed by an additional frozen-thawed SET if available was less costly and more effective, over DET in women under 32 years (8).

The recent Markov model (9) indicates that when a child's quality adjusted life-years (QALYs) are used as a measure of outcome, it is not cost effective in the long term to replace DET with SET strategies. However, for a balanced approach, a family planning perspective would be preferable, including additional treatment cycles for couples who wish to have another child. It was suggested by the authors that the analysis should be extended to include QALYs of family members. There is continuing debate whether QALY is a good measure of cost-effectiveness when there is a new life created; hence, it should not be used in this context.

Hence, the controversy about cost-effectiveness continues.

TABLE 7.2

Parameters Used to Measure Cost-Effectiveness of Single versus Double Embryo Transfer

Perspective	Time Horizon	What Is Measured
Patient	At live birth	Incremental cost-effectiveness ratio
Health care	At 5 years	Quality adjusted life-years
Societal	At 10 years	Willingness to pay
	Lifelong	

Global Variation in Use of Single Embryo Transfer

Although there is a move toward SET across the world, with obvious advantages in terms of the safety of assisted reproduction, there has been a significant variation in uptake of SET in preference to DET. Several factors have been responsible for this (5).

Lack of Good Prediction Models

In order to maximize the pregnancy rates and minimize the complication rates, it would be ideal if one could predict who would be more likely to have multiple pregnancies. There are no accurate prediction models to identify this. The age of the female partner is the most important predictor of pregnancy rates, so one can argue that women in the younger age group are more likely to have multiple pregnancies. Hence, initial algorithms were based on this (British Fertility Society, Association of Clinical Embryologists guidance). However, using these algorithms, DETs were practiced more in the older age group. This has a double effect, as there are increased obstetric complications in the older age group, and multiple pregnancy will add further to that.

Beliefs

Despite the availability of evidence, practice can only be changed if evidence, beliefs, and expert opinion all coincide (Figure 7.1). It was believed, and still some believe, that putting more than one embryo back is better for pregnancy rates. This belief was not limited to patients alone but to clinicians as well, despite evidence to the contrary (10–13). Hence, it has a taken a long time (more than a decade) to implement the practice of SET preferentially. This is in contrast to the uptake of strategy of the human papillomavirus (HPV) vaccination, where evidence, beliefs, and expert opinion coincided much more rapidly (Figure 7.2). There has always been a struggle between immediate gains (getting pregnant) versus long-term benefits (long-term health of child born, complications in pregnancy).

Cost and Funding of Freezing Spare Embryos

The use of SET is dependent on being able to freeze the spare embryo(s). There is a cost associated with freezing and thawing as well as monitoring for a treatment cycle to use it. There is a cost to the patient as well as to the clinic. With variation in how IVF programs are funded, the freezing of spare embryos may or may not be funded (5). If freezing is not funded, it works as a disincentive for couples, especially when they have only two embryos (i.e., only one to freeze and one to transfer).

Lack of Successful Cryopreservation Program

Not all clinics have had good cryopreservation programs. This has had a major influence on the uptake of SET. If the thaw survival rate is poor, then the benefit of one fresh embryo versus one frozen is

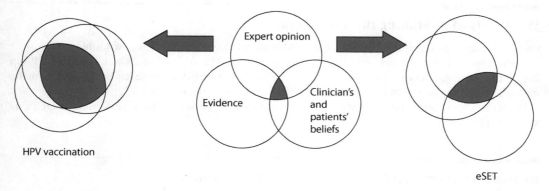

FIGURE 7.1 Preconditions for change in practice.

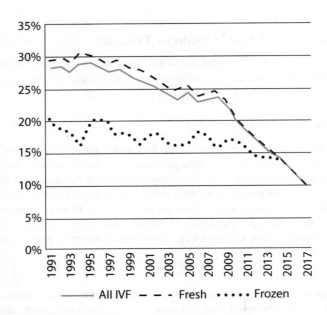

FIGURE 7.2 Multiple birth rates for all *in vitro* fertilization treatment cycles, 1991–2017. (Data from Human Fertilisation and Embryology Authority.)

not available when compared to putting both embryos back in one step. The first baby was born after frozen embryo transfer in 1984; since then there have been significant developments in cryopreservation programs, although there is a learning curve.

Autonomy

The principle of personal autonomy would suggest that patients should be able to choose how many embryos are transferred. Dixon et al. (14) suggested that the choice of embryo transfer strategy is a function of four factors: the age of the mother, the relevance of the SET option, the value placed on a live birth, and the relative importance placed on adverse outcomes. For each patient group, the choice of strategy is a trade-off between the value placed on a live birth and the cost. Hence, there are multiple factors to consider. The clinic's own data, national figures, and appropriate information provided to patients help in exercising autonomy by making an informed choice. As both clinical data and provision of information vary, so does decision-making.

What Helped in Making the Transition?

Over the years and after several debates, the trend of preference toward SET is now visible.

In the United States, the twin rate has been reduced from 33% in 2003 to 28% in 2013 and 13% in 2017 (https://www.sartcorsonline.com). Similarly, in the United Kingdom, there has been a decline in the multiple pregnancy rate from 24% in 2008 to 10% in 2017, as shown in Figure 7.2.

However, a large proportion of embryo transfers in recent years has still been performed as DETs, as shown in Figure 7.3.

Reasons for Increased Use of Single Embryo Transfer

The reason for increased uptake of SET in the last decade is due to the following factors.

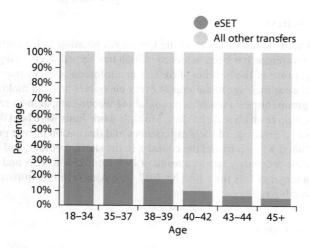

FIGURE 7.3 Elective single embryo transfer as a proportion of all embryo transfers performed in 2014. (Data from Human Fertilisation and Embryology Authority.)

Evidence

Although earlier evidence suggested that there is a reduced pregnancy rate with SET compared to DET (per embryo transfer episode), recent evidence suggests that there is no difference, especially if embryos are transferred at the blastocyst stage (Figure 7.4).

The latest data from HFEA, although not randomized, shows (see Figure 7.4) that SET gives a higher pregnancy rates compared to DET, even when the denominator is per embryo transfer, irrespective of whether the embryo is transferred at cleavage or blastocyst stage.

National and International Guidance

There is good practice guidance from all learned societies (American Society for Reproductive Medicine [15], European Society of Human Reproduction and Embryology [ESHRE Capri Workshop], British Fertility Society), the UK Royal Colleges (Royal College of Obstetricians and Gynaecologists, Royal College of Paediatrics and Child Health, Royal College of Nursing), and other educational institutions about reducing the rate of multiple pregnancies after assisted reproduction.

No. of embryos	eSET		DET	
Stage:	Cleavage	Blastocyst	Cleavage	Blastocyst
Age				
18–34	35.9%	50.7%	38.3%	50.7%
35–37	31.4%	47.4%	33.5%	49.3%
38–39	23.6%	40.9%	25.7%	41.6%
40–42			17.7%	32.8%
43–44	6.8%	30.0%		
45+			7.3%	19.3%
All ages	32.6%	48.5%	30.5%	45.2%

FIGURE 7.4 Comparison of pregnancy rates between single versus double embryo transfers. (Data from Human Fertilisation and Embryology Authority [HFEA] trends and figures 2019).

Education and Awareness

Through initiatives, such as "One at a Time" in the United Kingdom as well as other educational events and materials, a lot of awareness has been achieved, which has helped in changing practices (16). Once the clinic team is fully aware of the benefits of SET, it is reinforced at every opportunity to patients in clinic. A consistent and clear message to patients at every encounter helps in making the decision.

A multidisciplinary group (https://www.hfea.gov.uk/about-us/our-campaign-to-reduce-multiple-births) was set up with membership from all stakeholders. Multiple workshops were held that worked as a forum for clinic staff and allowed exchange of their experiences and discussion of best practices. Targets were set for clinics (in the United Kingdom) and the country, in the short, medium, and long term; these were to bring down the multiple pregnancy rate as a result of IVF from 25% to 15% and to less than 10%. The country has achieved a target of less than 10% by 2017 (17). Although this initiative was led by HFEA, it was not a licensing condition.

Reporting of Success Rates

Although the ideal way to define success rates in IVF has been the subject of much debate, live birth is generally felt to be the most appropriate numerator. There is, however, no consensus regarding the choice of denominator, with suggestions that the results should be presented as live birth per fresh IVF cycle, per oocyte recovery, per embryo transfer, or per woman (18). All IVF clinics are regulated and success rates must be available to all stakeholders. When success rates are reported as per embryo transfer episode (see Table 7.1), it is not a level playing field for SET. However, when success rate is reported per embryo transferred or as cumulative live birth rate, SET performs better. League tables are very important for IVF clinics, as that is how patients choose the clinics. Registries in both the United Kingdom and the United States have changed the reporting systems recently so that there is accountability for safety as well as efficacy. This has had a major impact, as those doing SET are not penalized in the league tables. The United Kingdom now reports headline figures as live birth per embryo transferred. Registries in the United States report cumulative live births.

Freezing Techniques

Improvement in freezing/thawing techniques and confidence that embryos will survive the freezing and thawing mean that clinicians are more comfortable in recommending the freezing of spare embryos rather than transferring them, as there is now evidence that success rates with frozen embryo transfers are at least comparable with fresh embryo transfer. There is now even emerging evidence that frozen embryo transfer may actually be better in terms of pregnancy rates compared to fresh embryo transfers (19).

Embryo Selection

Another reason for putting multiple embryos back was the perception that we cannot select which one will implant. With the ability to extend the culture to the blastocyst, it is now feasible to select the embryo with better implantation potential. In addition, there are other invasive (preimplantation genetic testing) and noninvasive (time lapse, spent culture media) methods to select the best embryo. Some of these methods have proven efficacy, whereas for others more research is needed. However, as embryo selection becomes better, the proportion of SETs is increasing.

Future for Single Embryo Transfer

Twins should no longer be an acceptable risk of assisted reproduction. The multiple pregnancy rate after natural conception is 2%; there is no reason why, if a policy of SET for all is followed, the multiple pregnancy rate should be any more than this. There are still arguments for using SET only for younger women; however, multiple pregnancies in older women will be associated with more obstetric risks, which is all the more reason to avoid multiple pregnancies. Hence, a blanket policy of SET for all is justified in today's world.

Some argue that if the embryos are poor quality, one can put two embryos back. However, what is not clear is whether the implantation of one gets affected by another. What may be better in these cases is that (a) if there are two poor-quality embryos on day 3, to extend to blastocyst and transfer if any of them develop to blastocyst and (b) if there are two poor-quality embryos on day 3, to extend culture to day 6, and if there is a blastocyst it can be frozen and thawed at a later date for transfer. This is important, as a prediction as to which embryo will implant is poor. There have been cases reported with twins when even poor-quality embryos were put back.

With advances in embryo selection, the ability to freeze and thaw embryos successfully with vitrification, and better understanding of IVF programs and embryo-endometrial synchrony, one can argue that there is no indication for transferring more than one embryo at any age and at any embryo quality. Hence, in the future, only SET should be practiced. This is irrespective of whether it is cost effective or not, as this is the only way multiple pregnancy rates can be reduced.

League tables should reflect the success rates per embryo transferred rather than per embryo transfer episode. Funding bodies should take account of this, and patients opting for SET should not have to pay extra. The other measure that league tables must report is cumulative live birth rate per egg collection, which will put all SETs at a level playing field.

It is not only patients and clinics but government, funding bodies, and policymakers who all need to work together for a policy of SET only for all.

There is no need for further research in this area, as it is clear that it is only SET that can prevent multiple pregnancies. Research should be on how best to select these embryos to reduce time to pregnancy.

Conclusion

There is no disputing that SET is safer and equally effective when long-term measures of effectiveness are used. Hence, a uniform policy of SET should be advocated by everyone. Multiple pregnancy rates after ART should not be higher than those following natural conception. For this to happen, there needs to be a joint approach by clinics, policymakers, funders, and patients.

REFERENCES

1. Templeton A, Morris JK. Reducing the risk of multiple births by transfer of two embryos after in vitro fertilization. *N Engl J Med.* 1998;339(9):573–7.
2. Luke B, Brown MB, Grainger DA et al. A Society for Assisted Reproductive Technology Writing Group. Practice patterns and outcomes with the use of single embryo transfer in United States. *Fertil Steril.* 2010;93:490–8.
3. ESHRE. The European IVF monitoring programme (EIM), for the European Society of Human Reproduction and Embryology (ESHRE). Assisted reproductive technology in Europe, 2005. Results generated from European Registers by ESHRE. *Hum Reprod Hum Reprod.* 2009;24:1267–87.
4. ESHRE Capri Workshop Group. Multiple gestation pregnancy. *Hum Reprod.* 2000;15:1856–64.
5. Maheshwari A, Grifiths S, Bhattacharya S. Global variations in the uptake of single embryo transfer. *Hum Reprod.* 2011;17(1):107–20.
6. McLernon DJ, Harrild K, Bergh C et al. Clinical effectiveness of elective single versus double embryo transfer: Meta-analysis of individual patient data from randomised trials. *BMJ.* 2010;341:c6945.
7. Hernandez TE, Navarro-Espigares JL, Clavero A et al. Economic evaluation of elective single-embryo transfer with subsequent single frozen embryo transfer in an in vitro fertilization/intracytoplasmic sperm injection program. *Fertil Steril.* 2015;103(3):699–706.
8. van Loendersloot LL, Moolenaar LM, van Wely M et al. Cost-effectiveness of single versus double embryo transfer in IVF in relation to female age. *Eur J Obstet Gynecol Reprod Biol.* 2017;214:25–30.
9. van Heesch MM, van Asselt AD, Evers JL et al. Cost-effectiveness of embryo transfer strategies: A decision analytic model using long-term costs and consequences of singletons and multiples born as a consequence of IVF. *Hum Reprod.* 2016;(11):2527–40.

10. Gleicher N, Campbell DP, Chan CL et al. The desire for multiple births in couples with infertility problems contradicts present practice patterns. *Hum Reprod.* 1995;10:1079–84.
11. Van Wely M, Twisk M, Mol BW, Van der Veen F. Is twin pregnancy necessarily an adverse outcome of assisted reproductive technologies? *Hum Reprod.* 2006;21:2736–38.
12. Gleicher N, Barad D. The relative myth of elective single embryo transfer. *Hum Reprod.* 2006;21:1337–44.
13. Van Peperstraten AM, Hermens RP, Nelen WL et al. Perceived barriers to elective single embryo transfer among IVF professionals: A national survey. *Hum Reprod.* 2008;23:2718–23.
14. Dixon S, Faghih Nasiri F, Ledger WL et al. Cost-effectiveness analysis of different embryo transfer strategies in England. *BJOG.* 2008;115(6):758–66.
15. American Society of Reproductive Medicine. Practice Committee Opinion. Guidance on limits to the number of embryos to transfer: A Committee opinion. *Fertil Steril.* 2017;107:901–3.
16. Van Peperstraten AM, Hermens RPMG, Nelen WLDM et al. Deciding how many embryos to transfer after in vitro fertilisation: Development and pilot test of a decision aid. *Patient Educ Couns.* 2010;78(1):124–9.
17. Human Fertilisation and Embryology Authority (HFEA). Fertility treatment 2017: Trends and figures, May 2019.
18. Bhattacharya S. Defining success in assisted reproduction. In: *Single Embryo Transfer* eds Gerris J, Adamson GD, Racowsky C. Cambridge UK, Cambridge University Press; 2009: 231.
19. Chen ZJ, Shi Y, Sun Y et al. Fresh versus frozen embryos for infertility in the polycystic ovary syndrome. *N Engl J Med.* 2016;375(6):523–3.

8

Use of Luteal Phase Support

Laura Melado, Barbara Lawrenz, and Human Fatemi

Introduction

The luteal phase of a menstrual cycle is the time between ovulation and, in case of conception, the establishment of a pregnancy or otherwise the onset of menses. In a natural cycle under the influence of LH (luteinizing hormone), formation of the corpus luteum will occur after ovulation. The corpus luteum is characterized by the production of progesterone and also estradiol. Progesterone induces the secretory transformation of the endometrium in the luteal phase and promotes local vasodilatation and relaxation of the uterine muscle (1).

Physiology

Steroid Production of the Ovary in Natural and Stimulated Cycles

Throughout the menstrual cycle, the ovary is producing the steroid hormones estradiol and progesterone. They are essential for embryo implantation, which is demonstrated by the fact that pregnancies with oocyte donation can be achieved after preparation of the endometrium with estradiol and progesterone (2), even in women without ovaries.

In a natural cycle, estradiol synthesis increases progressively from the dominant follicle and initiates LH surge. Even before the LH surge, a small increase in progesterone levels is seen that reflects the increasing LH pulse amplitude and frequency leading up to the surge. A LH surge of 24–36 hours is sufficient to initiate the resumption of oocyte meiosis, luteinization of granulosa cells, ovulation, and the initial phase of corpus luteum (CL) development. Progesterone and 17a-hydroxyprogesterone (17a-OHP) plasma concentrations increase rapidly after the LH surge or administration of human chorionic gonadotropin (hCG) (3), indicating the beginning of granulosa and theca cell luteinization. As well as granulosa cells, the thecal cells produce significant amounts of progesterone. The corpus luteum is producing up to 40 mg of progesterone per day and additionally a significant amount of androgens and estradiol. This is unique to the corpus luteum of many primates, including humans (4).

Progesterone biosynthesis requires two enzymatic steps: first, the conversion of cholesterol to pregnenolone (P5), catalyzed by the enzyme cytochrome P450scc, and second its subsequent conversion to progesterone, which is catalyzed by 3β-hydroxy-steroid-dehydrogenase (3βHSD) (5). Progesterone is further metabolized to androgens by the action of CYP17 in the thecal cells under the influence of LH. This step only takes place in the thecal cell compartment. However, during the early follicular phase, the enzymatic activity necessary to convert 17-OH-progesterone to androstenedione is absent or very low. Therefore, this process leads to increasing concentrations of progesterone and estradiol, as the follicular diameter increases (6).

Whereas in a natural cycle with the development of a single dominant follicle midfollicular FSH levels are declining toward ovulation (7), in ovarian stimulation for *in vitro* fertilization (IVF), multifollicular development is achieved by administration of high daily gonadotropin concentrations. Stimulation dosage usually remains unchanged throughout the stimulation duration, unless the patient's individual response requires a change in the dosage. Therefore, ovarian stimulation will result in a large number of growing follicles, and each follicle contributes to the progesterone in the systemic circulation. Progesterone concentration often reflects the number of preovulatory follicles, and patients with high estradiol concentrations have significantly more oocytes and significantly higher progesterone concentrations (8).

In a natural cycle without conception, luteolysis occurs due to a lack of hCG support. The corpus luteum undergoes a process of regression with the loss of functional and structural integrity (9) leading to a decrease in progesterone production. In case of conception, the trophoblast produces hCG, which prevents the regression of the corpus luteum and stimulates corpus luteum progesterone production, which is necessary for maintenance of the pregnancy until placental progesterone production is adequate. Despite the fact that serum hCG is detectable around the time of implantation on approximately day 8 after ovulation, the hormonal characteristics of conception and nonconception cycles are different from the early luteal phase. Both LH and E2 levels are significantly higher in conception cycles on days 4 and 5 after the LH peak in urine compared to nonconception cycles (10).

Implantation

After conception, the developing embryo will secrete hCG, which has structural similarities with LH and activates the same receptor. The role of hCG is to maintain the corpus luteum and its secretions until the shift of progesterone production from the corpus luteum to the placenta at around 9 weeks of pregnancy has taken place (11).

For a pregnancy to occur, a receptive endometrium, a functional embryo at the blastocyst developmental stage, and synchrony between the embryo and the endometrium are required (12). Failure to achieve receptivity and synchrony results in infertility, and this is also a limiting factor for success in IVF treatment.

Endometrial receptivity is driven by time of progesterone exposure after sufficient exposure to estrogen. The "window of implantation" (WOI), i.e., the time frame in which the endometrium is receptive and able to support trophoblast-endometrial interactions, is very limited. In a natural and idealized 28-day cycle, it is thought to occur sometime around days 22–24 (13). It is assumed that the WOI is constant in time in all women. However, displacement of the WOI might not be a rare cause in infertility patients (Figure 8.1), especially in patients with repeated implantation failure (14).

Influence of Progesterone on Endometrium in Natural and Stimulated Cycles

The physiologic effects of progesterone are primarily mediated by interaction with the progesterone receptor (PR). There are two classic PR isoforms, PR-A and PR-B; PR-A is required for normal ovarian and uterine function (15). They are identical in structure except that the PR-B isoform contains a 164-amino acid *N*-terminal sequence, which is lacking in the PR-A isoform (16). After binding to the nuclear receptors, steroid receptors activate their transcription genes.

The mitogenic effect of progesterone in the stroma is mediated by upregulating PR-A as well as PR-B isoforms of the receptor (17,18).

The different histological appearances of the endometrium, depending on the influence of estrogen or progesterone, have already been studied by Noyes et al. in 1950 (19). Whereas the proliferative phase under the influence of estradiol does not allow recognition of subphases other than early, middle, or late proliferative phase, progressive changes occur in the endometrium of the secretory phase. In the period between 36 and 48 hours after ovulation, no changes of the endometrium are visible. Later, under the influence of progesterone, the epithelial glands and vasculature continue to grow and become spiral, whereas the endometrial thickness is relatively unchanged, resulting in a denser endometrium. The morphologic changes observed on histology for each specific day after ovulation established the classic endometrial dating paradigm that still serves as the gold standard for clinical evaluation of luteal function (20). An endometrial biopsy that shows a difference of more than 2 days between the histologic dating and actual day after ovulation is considered to be "out of phase" (21).

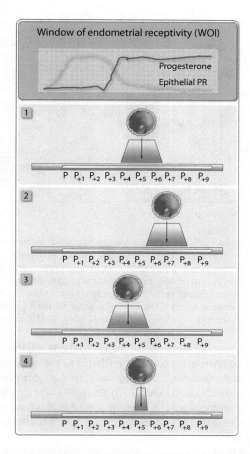

FIGURE 8.1 Displacement of the window of implantation (WOI). It has been assumed that the WOI is constant in time in all women (1). However, the genomic signature of the endometrium demonstrates the existence of a displacement of the WOI in up to 25% of patients that can be delayed (2), advanced (3) or shorter than expected (4). "P+x" refers to the days after progesterone administration (14). (From Galliano D et al. *Hum Reprod Update.* 2015;21[1]:13–8, with permission.)

Comparison of endometrial steroid receptors and proliferation index between natural cycles and gonadotropin-releasing hormone (GnRH)-agonist/human menopausal gonadotropin (hMG)-stimulated cycles for IVF have revealed distinct alterations in endometrial maturation. In stimulated cycles, a more advanced secretory endometrial maturation combined with reduced estrogen receptors (ERs) and PRs and a low proliferation index in glands and stroma has been found on the day of oocyte retrieval, when compared to endometrial maturation in natural cycles on the day of ovulation.

Endometrial biopsies taken 2 days after ovum pick-up (OPU) in stimulated cycles showed a further reduction in steroid receptors and proliferation despite a similar histological maturation as compared to biopsies from natural cycles on day 2 after ovulation (22). It can be assumed that supraphysiologic hormonal levels during stimulation lead to a reduced number of ERs and PRs and a low proliferation index in glands and stroma. Those functional endometrial alterations might affect the proliferative potential of the endometrium (22). However, solely from the serum progesterone concentrations and/or the absolute value of serum progesterone increase, the exact endometrial development on the day of OPU in stimulated cycles cannot be predicted (23).

Besides the aforementioned advancement of endometrial maturation, in patients with a progesterone level above 1.5 ng/mL on the day of hCG administration, differences in endometrial gene expression profile were found, when compared to the gene expression pattern below this threshold (Figure 8.2) (24). These changes might explain the impairment of endometrial receptivity in the presence of elevated progesterone, reflected in the lower pregnancy rates reported in the literature (25).

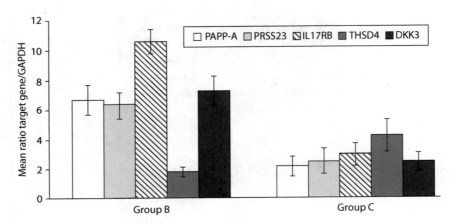

FIGURE 8.2   Validation, using real-time polymerase chain reaction of microarray results on selected genes involved with endometrial receptivity. In patients with a progesterone level above 1.5 ng/mL on the day of human chorionic gonadotropin (hCG) administration (group C), differences in endometrial gene expression profile were found, when compared to the gene expression pattern below this threshold (group B). These changes might explain the impairment of endometrial receptivity in the presence of elevated progesterone, reflected in the lower pregnancy rates. Group B: Patients with progesterone levels 1–1.5 ng/mL on day of hCG administration. Group C: Patients with progesterone levels greater than 1.5 ng/mL on day of hCG administration. (From Van Vaerenbergh I et al. *Reprod Biomed Online*. 2011;22:263–71, with permission.)

The influence of elevated progesterone levels on the endometrial gene expression pattern was also analyzed by Labarta et al. (26) in a study comparing the endometrial dating as well as the endometrium gene expression pattern during the window of implantation in 12 healthy oocyte donors. Six patients had progesterone levels above the progesterone threshold of 1.5 ng/mL. Out of 370 genes, 140 were dysregulated by more than twofold in women with high serum progesterone levels. A large number of those genes represent biological processes like cell adhesion, immune system function, and organ development. Therefore, dysregulation of those genes could affect the endometrium and the implantation process.

Interestingly, at day 7 after trigger, no more endometrial advancement was found in the group with elevated progesterone levels on the day of final oocyte maturation. It was shown previously that no pregnancies are achieved in case of an endometrial advancement of more than 3 days, when the embryo transfer is performed on day 3 (23,27). However, the detrimental effect of elevated progesterone level on the day of final oocyte maturation subsides when the transfer is delayed until the blastocyst stage (28). This suggests that the endometrium could recover during the window of implantation period.

Endocrine Profile in *In Vitro* Fertilization Cycles after Oocyte Retrieval, Depending on Type of Trigger

Ovulation induction in ovarian stimulation for IVF with GnRH-agonist protocols has to be performed by the administration of hCG to mimic the LH surge, whereas with GnRH-antagonist protocols, the use of GnRH-agonist for final oocyte maturation is possible with the advantage of reducing the risk for ovarian hyperstimulation syndrome (OHSS). Due to the different methods of action of hCG and GnRH-agonist, different endocrine profiles are seen after the oocyte retrieval procedure. Patients who were triggered with only hCG or GnRH-agonist plus 1500 IU hCG had lower LH levels compared to patients triggered with GnRH-agonist only. Progesterone levels on day 5 after the oocyte retrieval procedure were highest in patients triggered with either hCG alone or a combination of GnRH-agonist plus 1500 IU hCG and lowest in patients after GnRH-agonist only without any luteal phase support. This difference is caused by the fact that after hCG application, progesterone production of the theca cells is sustained to at least 5 days due to the LH activity and the half-life time of hCG of more than 24 hours (29,30). After GnRH-agonist trigger, severe luteal phase insufficiency occurred due to low levels of endogenous LH and therefore of progesterone (Figure 8.3) (31). There are also differences in endometrial gene expression depending on the type of trigger (Figure 8.4) (32).

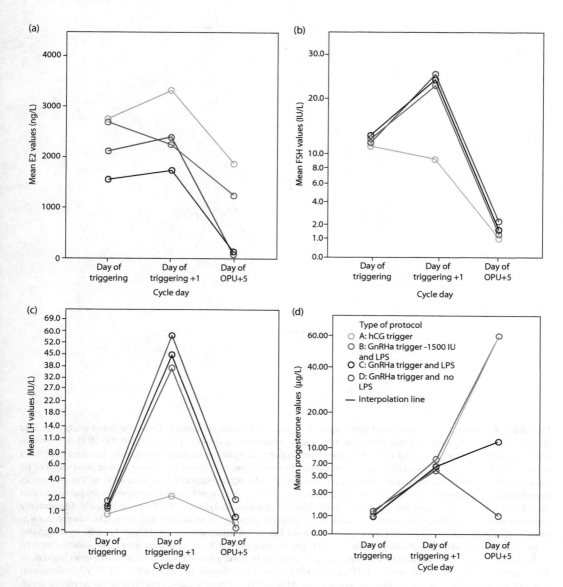

FIGURE 8.3 Early luteal phase endocrine profile, including estradiol, progesterone, luteinizing hormone, and follicle-stimulating hormone, is affected by the mode of triggering final oocyte maturation and the luteal phase support used. The patients have been under ovarian stimulation using recombinant follicle-stimulating hormone and antagonist protocol for *in vitro* fertilization. (From Fatemi HM et al. *Fertil Steril*. 2013;100:742–7, with permission.)

Medication for Luteal Phase Support in Assisted Reproductive Technology

As previously described, progesterone will be produced by the corpus luteum after LH surge in a normal, unstimulated cycle. The correction of a dysfunctional corpus luteum with the symptoms of shortened luteal phase and premenstrual spotting by administration of progesterone was first described in 1949 (33), and a defective luteal phase was defined if the serum midluteal progesterone levels were less than 10 ng/mL (34). The prevalence of a luteal phase defect (LPD) in natural cycles in normo-ovulatory patients with primary or secondary infertility was demonstrated to be about 8.1% (35). However, in 2012, the American Society for Reproductive Medicine stated that there is no reproducible, physiologically relevant,

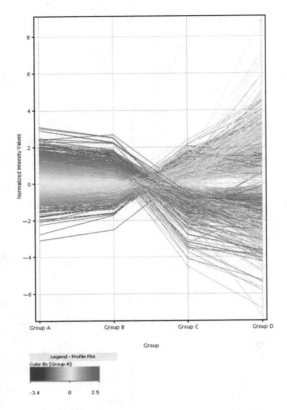

FIGURE 8.4 Study of the endometrial gene expression performed in oocyte donors. The same donor underwent four stimulation protocols with different modes of final oocyte maturation and luteal phase support: (a) 10,000 IU human chorionic gonadotropin (hCG) and standard luteal phase support; (b) agonist gonadotropin-releasing hormone triptorelin 0.2 mg, followed by 1500 IU hCG 35 hours after triggering of final oocyte maturation and standard luteal phase support; (c) triptorelin 0.2 mg with standard luteal phase support; and (d) triptorelin 0.2 mg without luteal phase support. The differences in endometrial gene expression are shown by a profile plot. A profile plot is a graphical data analysis technique to examine the relative behavior of all variables in a multivariate dataset. This data analysis shows all the significantly differentially expressed probe sets or genes, represented by lines. Each line represents a gene, and each line is colored by its expression in group A. The expression of each gene can therefore be followed in the four treatment groups. This analysis shows that groups A and B are similar in gene expression, while groups C and D show more differences in gene expression, when compared with each other and also compared with groups A and B. In group D, some genes show an extreme up- or downregulation. These genes are INHBA (inhibin-ba); MMP1 and MMP3 (matrix metalloproteinases 1 and 3); LEFTY2 (endometrial bleeding associated factor [left-right determination, factor A] transforming growth factor beta [TGF-b] superfamily), which were upregulated in group D; and CXCL13 (chemokine [C-X-C motif] ligand 13), MMP26, and SCGB1D2 (secretoglobin family 1D member 2 or lipophilin B), which were downregulated in group D. (32). (From Humaidan P et al. *Hum Reprod.* 2012;27[11]:3259–72, with permission.)

and clinically practical standard to diagnose LPD or distinguish fertile from infertile women (36). The minimum threshold of progesterone level that is essential for the maintenance of a pregnancy is unknown, and successful pregnancies have been reported even when the concentration of progesterone was never above 15 nmol/L for the first 14 days (37). After ovarian stimulation for IVF/intracytoplasmic sperm injection (ICSI) treatment, it seems that patients having progesterone levels at the day of implantation of more than 30 ng/mL and estradiol levels of more than 100 pg/mL are more likely to have a viable and ongoing pregnancy compared to patients with hormone levels below those thresholds (38).

In stimulated cycles for IVF, a defective luteal phase occurs in almost all patients (23,27,39), and different theories have been discussed (40). However, the reason for the luteal phase insufficiency seen after controlled ovarian stimulation seems to be the multifollicular development achieved during the follicular phase, resulting in supraphysiological luteal levels of P and E2 that inhibit LH secretion by the pituitary via negative feedback actions at the level of the hypothalamic-pituitary axis (41–45). Besides the defective luteal phase due to the supraphysiologic levels of estradiol and progesterone, the window of implantation might be shorter in IVF cycles compared to a natural cycle (46).

To counterbalance the luteal phase insufficiency after ovarian stimulation, different methods of luteal phase support can be applied—either direct substitution of progesterone via different routes of administration or indirect substitution of progesterone via the stimulation of the remaining corpora lutea to sustain progesterone production.

As a consequence of the increasing knowledge of patient-specific characteristics, the old concept of one type of luteal phase support for all IVF patients has to be abandoned and a personalized approach, depending on the type of final oocyte maturation and the ovarian response, should be implemented into daily clinical routine.

Progesterone for Luteal Phase Support

Oral Progesterone

Natural progesterone is rapidly metabolized after oral intake and has been shown to be ineffective in inducing a sufficient secretory transformation. Synthetic progesterone derivates are associated with side effects, especially regarding the impact on the lipids (47) and on the psyche (48), which will limit their use. Micronization of progesterone reduces the particle size and improves absorption and bioavailability (49). After oral digestion of 200 mg micronized progesterone, maximal progesterone concentrations within the range of luteal phase are reached within 2–4 hours and will remain elevated for approximately 6–7 hours (50). Even higher doses of micronized progesterone have failed to induce sufficient secretory transformation. It seems that progesterone metabolites produced by the first liver passage lead to cross-reactions and are therefore responsible for those high progesterone levels.

Intramuscular Progesterone

Progesterone is rapidly absorbed after intramuscular injection. High progesterone plasma concentrations are reached after approximately 2 hours, and peak concentrations will be achieved after around 8 hours. To achieve serum progesterone concentrations that are equivalent to those during the luteal phase in the natural cycle, injection of 25 mg progesterone is required. It has been suggested that the intramuscular site of injection might serve as a depot with progesterone accumulation in the fat tissue, leading to more sustained serum concentrations of progesterone (51). The disadvantage of intramuscular application of progesterone is that injection is painful, and frequent injections are required to sustain sufficient progesterone concentrations. Also, swelling, redness, and even sterile abscess formation are not uncommon side effects.

A rare but more severe and even life-threatening complication after intramuscular progesterone injections for luteal phase support is the development of eosinophilic pneumonia as an allergic reaction to the oil vehicle used as excipient for the substance (52).

Subcutaneous Progesterone

Subcutaneous progesterone injections are well-tolerated and have demonstrated noninferiority in efficacy to vaginal progesterone for luteal phase support in IVF. It could pose an alternative for women who want to avoid intramuscular injections as well as the vaginal route (52).

Vaginal Progesterone

Progesterone plasma concentrations reach maximal levels approximately 3–8 hours after vaginal application and then fall continuously over the next 8 hours. Compared to intramuscular progesterone, it is more quickly cleared out of the circulation. To achieve luteal phase plasma levels, higher dosages of vaginal progesterone are needed; in most cases, 300–600 mg of progesterone is administered daily divided

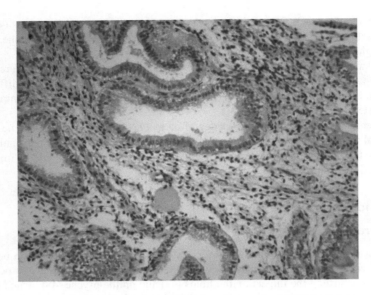

FIGURE 8.5 Endometrial biopsy after vaginal micronized progesterone. Coiled glands with active secretion and minimal residual vacuoles. Stromal edema. Absence of mitotic activity. The maturation corresponds to day 6 of the luteal phase (HES, ×200). (From Fatemi HM. *Facts Views Vis Obgyn*. 2009;1[1]:30–46, with permission.)

into two or three doses (53), depending on the formula, for example, tablets, creams, or suppositories. Vaginal mucosa absorbs proteins and lipids; however, absorption is influenced by the kind of formula preparation, and it is enhanced after previous estrogenization (54).

After vaginal administration of progesterone, the serum levels are lower compared to intramuscular application and sometimes even lower than measured in a natural cycle. However, despite the low serum levels, adequate secretory endometrial transformation was achieved (Figure 8.5) (55). This suggests that vaginally administered progesterone exerts a direct local effect on the endometrium before entering the systemic circulation, the "first uterine pass" effect. The mechanism behind the first uterine pass effect is not fully understood, and different routes of action are discussed: absorption of progesterone into the rich venous or lymphatic vaginal system and/or possibly countercurrent transfer between uterovaginal lymph vessels or veins and arteries, direct drug diffusion through the tissues, or even due to intraluminal transfer from the uterus to the vagina similar to sperm transport. As the vaginal route is effective in providing sufficient luteal phase support and there are minimal side effects, it is a valuable and preferred route of progesterone administration (56).

Finally, it seems, that the route of progesterone administration does not have an impact on ART outcome; therefore, the patient's preference can be considered when choosing the route of progesterone administration for luteal phase support (57).

Human Chorionic Gonadotropin for Luteal Phase Support

With the application of hCG, no luteolysis occurs, as the corpora lutea will be stimulated and will sustain progesterone production. For a long time, hCG administration was the standard luteal phase support; however, the disadvantage of this approach is the possible development of OHSS, especially in the good-responder patients (58).

Derived from the knowledge gathered by providing luteal phase support with low-dose hCG administration after GnRH-agonist trigger, Andersen et al. (59) designed a mathematical model to calculate the daily applied hCG dosage required to maintain sufficient hCG concentrations and, therefore, adequate progesterone levels in the luteal phase. Preliminary results indicate that a daily applied dosage of 100 IU hCG without additional exogenous progesterone seems to be sufficient to maintain the corpora lutea function until endogenous hCG from the developing embryo takes over.

This approach may present a means of further individualizing luteal phase support. Unfortunately, the aforementioned small doses of hCG are not commercially available, rendering it difficult to implement this as a clinical routine.

Timing of Luteal Phase Support with Progesterone

The timing of luteal phase support in ART cycles is crucial, as it has to be initiated before endogenous progesterone levels are decreasing or low. Preovulatory exposure of the endometrium to progesterone may have a negative impact on the endometrial receptivity as already described.

When luteal phase support was started before oocyte retrieval, a decreased likelihood of pregnancy was found when compared to starting on the day of oocyte retrieval. When progesterone was initiated on the evening of oocyte retrieval versus started on days 1–3 after oocyte retrieval, no difference in clinical PR was found. However, when progesterone administration was started on day 6, a decreased likelihood of pregnancy was found. Therefore, initiation of progesterone supplementation between the evening of oocyte retrieval and day 3 after retrieval seems to be ideal (60).

Duration of Luteal Phase Support

In early pregnancy, the embryo is producing a significant and rapidly increasing amount of hCG that will replace a possible lack of endogenous LH after ovarian stimulation. Later in the pregnancy, between 7 and 9 weeks, progesterone production will shift from the corpora lutea toward the placenta. Studies evaluating the duration of progesterone administration after a positive pregnancy test did not find any influence on the miscarriage rate and the delivery rate when progesterone application was continued or discontinued for 3 weeks after positive pregnancy test (61,62).

Luteal Phase Support after GnRH-Agonist Trigger

The use of GnRH-agonist for final oocyte maturation is common in high-responder patients as development of OHSS can almost completely be avoided. Following the introduction of GnRH-agonist for final oocyte maturation in GnRH-antagonist protocols, the first large randomized controlled trials reported a very poor reproductive outcome with this approach. It was assumed that the severity of the induced luteolysis by application of GnRH-agonist cannot be counterbalanced using standard luteal phase support with "only" progesterone administration (63). The administration of hCG or high doses of steroids (64) is considered to be essential to prevent luteolysis.

There is an ongoing debate on the adequate luteal phase support in this scenario.

Luteolysis occurs when LH support from the primate corpus luteum is withdrawn for 3 or more days (65); hence, corpus luteum function can be rescued if LH activity is reinitiated within 3 days, suggesting that corpus luteum viability can be preserved without LH support for at least 72 hours (66). In order to sustain progesterone production from the corpora lutea and therefore rescue the luteal phase, different treatment options have been described.

Following the concept that GnRHa-induced luteolysis can be reverted with the administration of hCG, low doses of hCG can be given during the luteal phase. However, it was found that the rescue of the corpora lutea for up to 3 days of gonadotropin deprivation is hCG dose dependent, i.e., 1500 IU or more (67). The approach of administration of 1500 IU of hCG 35 hours after GnRH-agonist trigger results in comparable pregnancy rates in respect to hCG trigger, but unfortunately with this dosage, OHSS in the high-responder-group occurred (67,68). Other authors (69) applied low-dose HCG in different dosages in the luteal phase after GnRH agonist triggering and could demonstrate that those dosages were effective in normalizing the reproductive outcome. Despite the low dosages of hCG, OHSS could not be completely avoided.

A proof-of-concept study evaluated a luteal phase support by application of daily low hCG dosages (125 IU rec-hCG) from the day of OPU without the use of exogenous progesterone. Significant differences during the luteal phase were observed with progesterone levels being significantly higher in the groups receiving daily low-dose hCG supplementation (70). Hence, even with this low hCG dosage, OHSS occurred in 3% of the patients, and hence, no hospitalization was needed.

OHSS can be almost completely avoided by the use of GnRH-agonist (200 mg of GnRH-agonist nasal spray twice daily; a total of 400 mg/d) for LPS after GnRH-agonist trigger without exogenous progesterone, and midluteal progesterone levels of around 190 nmol/L (approximately 59.7 ng/mL) can be achieved (71).

As a consequence of these findings, it is now recognized that not all patients after GnRH-agonist trigger are in need of an intensive and aggressive luteal phase support and should not be treated with a "one-size-fits-all" approach. The concept of "luteal coasting" is based on the individual luteolysis pattern by applying hCG based on the progesterone levels measured in the early and midluteal phases and can be performed with or even without the additional use of exogenous progesterone (72). Depending on the progesterone level 48 hours after oocyte retrieval, a single hCG dosage between 375 and 1500 IU, given in early luteal phase, can maintain adequate progesterone levels, and this approach may well optimize the chance of pregnancy while reducing the risk of OHSS associated with higher doses of hCG supplementation in the luteal phase (73). The necessity for repeat blood tests to measure progesterone levels poses the most important disadvantage of this approach.

Luteal Phase Support in Insemination Cycles

Intrauterine insemination (IUI) is a frequently applied technique to increase the probability of conception in couples with subfertility or unexplained infertility; however, the necessity of luteal support is addressed in only a few studies.

IUI can be performed in either natural cycles or stimulated cycles by using clomiphene citrate or gonadotropins for stimulation.

In natural IUI cycles, it can be assumed that no luteal phase insufficiency should be present; therefore, there is no biological or empirical evidence that treatment with hCG or progesterone in the luteal phase is necessary or improves the pregnancy rate (74). Nevertheless, the addition of progesterone, hCG, and/ or other substances became established clinical practice even in the absence of any robust evidence of effectiveness (75).

In patients who undergo mild ovarian stimulation for IUI, it can be assumed that due to supraphysiologic hormonal levels, endogenous LH will be low, leading possibly to a luteal phase insufficiency.

However, it is crucial to differentiate between the kind of stimulation done. After clomiphene citrate administration, an increase in LH pulse frequency will result in a significant increase of serum E2 and progesterone levels, with a lengthening of the luteal phase. A study evaluating a beneficial impact of progesterone application in normo-ovulatory patients stimulated with clomiphene citrate for IUI did not find higher ongoing pregnancy rates in patients receiving progesterone after IUI compared to those who had no luteal phase support (76). However, after gonadotropin stimulation, comparable to ovarian stimulation for IVF, supraphysiologic hormonal levels will lead to suppression of endogenous LH, and development of luteal phase insufficiency can be expected. It was shown that after IUI in a gonadotropin-stimulated cycle, the chance of pregnancy and live birth is higher, when progesterone application is done after IUI (77).

Luteal Phase Support in Frozen Embryo Transfer Cycles

Due to the improvement of the cryoconservation techniques in the IVF laboratory with the introduction of vitrification, more and more frozen embryo transfer (FET)—or warmth oocyte embryo transfer—cycles are performed worldwide (78). This move toward frozen embryo transfer is the result of an ongoing debate on the impact of supraphysiologic hormonal levels on endometrial receptivity, particularly in the case of progesterone elevation. In addition, frozen embryo transfer facilitates preimplantation genetic testing for aneuploidy (PGT-A) at the blastocyst stage, which prevents a timely transfer on day 5 after oocyte retrieval.

TABLE 8.1

Results of the Study Designed to Compare the Pregnancy Rates between Natural Cycles (Spontanous Luteinizing Hormone [LH] Group) and Modified Natural Cycles (Human Chorionic Gonadotropin [hCG] group) Showed Significantly Higher Pregnancy Rates in the Natural Cycle with the Detection of LH Surge

	Spontaneous LH ($n = 61$)	hCG Group ($n = 63$)	Difference, %(95% CI)	P Value
Ongoing pregnancy rate-ET (%)	31.1 (19)	14.3 (9)	16.9 (2.1–30.9)	0.025
Miscarriage rate-ET (%)	0 (0)	3.2 (2)	−3.2 (−10.9 to 3.2)	NS
Biochemical rate-ET (%)	3.3 (2)	3.2 (2)	0.1 (−7.9 to 8.3)	NS
Positive hCG-ET (%)	34.4 (21)	20.6 (13)	13.8 (−1.9 to 28.7)	NS

Source: From Fatemi HM et al. *Fertil Steril.* 2010;94:2054–8, with permission; Le Lannou D et al. *Reprod Biomed Online.* 2006;13:368–75.

Note: hCG administration to end the follicular phase resulted in significantly lower pregnancy rates compared to natural cycles.

Abbreviations: CI, confidence interval; ET, embryo transfer; hCG, human chorionic gonadotropin; LH, luteinizing hormone; NS, not significant.

To optimize the pregnancy rates, synchronization of the embryo development and the endometrium is crucial. There are different ways to prepare and synchronize the endometrium:

- *Natural cycle*: A simple way to prepare endometrium is to use the natural cycle with endogenous production of estradiol of the growing follicle. In this scenario, the LH surge has to be detected in order to plan correct timing for embryo thawing and embryo transfer. Another option is to use an injection of hCG to trigger the ovulation (modified natural cycle). A study designed to compare the pregnancy rates between natural cycles and modified natural cycles showed significantly higher pregnancy rates in the natural cycle with the detection of LH surge (78). The administration of hCG to end the follicular phase resulted in significant lower pregnancy rates compared to natural cycles. It is assumed that hCG may have a negative effect on endometrium receptivity (79,80) (Table 8.1).

- *Hormonal-replacement cycle*: This is a more common approach with the administration of exogenous estradiol and progesterone. The advantages of this approach are that disturbances due to cycle variation can be avoided, and also planning of the embryo transfer is possible, which will smooth the workflow for the IVF laboratory. The hormonal replacement cycle can be performed with or without cotreatment with GnRH-agonists (81).

Until now, the best approach for FET is still under discussion, and there is an urgent need for randomized controlled trials to compare the correctly conducted natural cycle with correct determination of LH surge and the hormonal replacement cycle.

Conclusion

It is the task of the reproductive medicine specialist to individualize luteal phase support according to the patient's specific characteristics, needs, and desires and the type of treatment performed.

After the use of hCG for final oocyte maturation, exogenous progesterone administration in the form of vaginal tablets, creams or suppositories is the gold standard and seems to be sufficient to maintain an adequate luteal phase support. Oral medication might be an alternative, yet more data are required to rely on this approach. Daily application of hCG in low dosages represents a progesterone-free alternative; however, until now, this is not a patient-friendly approach, as the low hCG dosages recommended are not presently commercially available.

The greatest indication for individualization of the luteal phase is following GnRH-agonist triggers in high-responder patients in order to tailor luteal phase support to the patient-specific pattern of luteolysis and minimize the risk of causing OHSS with unnecessary high hCG dosages. Case series have demonstrated that reducing the hCG dosage according to a patient's progesterone level or even foregoing luteal phase support is feasible. Future studies should develop an algorithm that provides the minimal-required hCG dosage, depending on the systemic progesterone levels.

REFERENCES

1. Bulletti C, de Ziegler D. Uterine contractility and embryo implantation. *Curr Opin Obstet Gynecol.* 2005;17:265–76.
2. Csapo AI, Pulkkinen MO, Ruttner B et al. The significance of the human corpus luteum in pregnancy maintenance. I. Preliminary studies. *Am J Obstet Gynecol.* 1972;112:1061–7.
3. Simon C, Martín JC, Pellicer A. Paracrine regulators of implantation. *Baillieres Best Pract Res Clin Obstet Gynaecol.* 2000;14:815–26.
4. Bergh PA, Navot D. The impact of embryonic development and endometrial maturity on the timing of implantation. *Fertil Steril.* 1992;58:537–42.
5. Ruiz-Alonso M, Galindo N, Pellicer A, Simón C. What a difference two days make: "Personalized" embryo transfer (pET) paradigm: A case report and pilot study. *Hum Reprod.* 2014;29:1244–7.
6. Devroey P, Pados G. Preparation of endometrium for egg donation. *Hum Reprod Update.* 1998;4:856–61.
7. Christenson LK, Devoto L. Cholesterol transport and steroidogenesis by the corpus luteum. *Reprod Biol Endocrinol.* 2003;10:90.
8. Devoto L, Fuentes A, Kohen P et al. The human corpus luteum: Life cycle and function in natural cycles. *Fertil Steril.* 2009;92:1067–79.
9. Chaffin CL, Dissen GA, Stouffer RL. Hormonal regulation of steroidogenic enzyme expression in granulosa cells during the peri-ovulatory interval in monkeys. *Mol Hum Reprod.* 2000;6:11–8.
10. Yding Andersen C, Bungum L, Nyboe Andersen A, Humaidan P. Preovulatory progesterone concentration associates significantly to follicle number and LH concentration but not to pregnancy rate. *Reprod Biomed Online.* 2011;23:187–95.
11. Fleming R, Jenkins J. The source and implications of progesterone rise during the follicular phase of assisted reproduction cycles. *RBMonline.* 2010;21:446–9.
12. Kyrou D, Al-Azemi M, Papanikolaou EG et al. The relationship of premature progesterone rise with serum estradiol levels and number of follicles in GnRH antagonist/recombinant FSH-stimulated cycles. *Eur J Obstet Gynecol Reprod Biol.* 2012;162:165–8.
13. Stocco C, Tellerias C, Gibori G. The molecular control of corpus luteum formation, function and regression. *Endocr Rev.* 2007;28:117–49.
14. Chen J, Oiu O, Lohstroh PN et al. Hormonal characteristics in the early luteal phase of conceptive and nonconceptive menstrual cycles. *J Soc Gynecol Investig.* 2003;10:27–31.
15. Kastner P, Krust A, Turcotte B et al. Two distinct estrogen-regulated promoters generate transcripts encoding the two functionally different human progesterone receptor forms A and B. *EMBO J.* 1990;9:1603–14.
16. Wei LL, Gonzalez-Aller C, Wood WM et al. "5"-Heterogeneity in human progesterone receptor transcripts predicts a new amino-terminal truncated "C"-receptor and unique A-receptor messages. *Mol Endocrinol.* 1990;4:1833–40.
17. Salmi A, Pakarinen P, Peltola AM, Rutanen EM. The effect of intrauterine levonorgestrel use on the expression of c-JUN, oestrogen receptors, progesterone receptors and Ki-67 in human endometrium. *Mol Hum Reprod.* 1998;4:1110–5.
18. Tseng L, Zhu HH. Regulation of progesterone receptor messenger ribonucleic acid by progestin in human endometrial stromal cells. *Biol Reprod.* 1997;57:1360–6.
19. Noyes RW, Hertig AT, Rock J. Dating the endometrial biopsy. *Fertil Steril.* 1950;1:3–25.
20. Noyes RW, Hertig AT, Rock J. Dating the endometrial biopsy. *Am J Obstet Gynecol.* 1975;122:262–3.
21. Wentz AC. Endometrial biopsy in the evaluation of infertility. *Fertil Steril.* 1980;33:121–4.
22. Bourgain C, Ubaldi F, Tavaniotou A et al. Endometrial hormone receptors and proliferation index in the periovulatory phase of stimulated embryo transfer cycles in comparison with natural cycles and relation to clinical pregnancy outcome. *Fertil Steril.* 2002;78:237–44.
23. Ubaldi F, Bourgain C, Tournaye H et al. Endometrial evaluation by aspiration biopsy on the day of oocyte retrieval in the embryo transfer cycles in patients with serum progesterone rise during the follicular phase. *Fertil Steril.* 1997;67:521–6.

24. Van Vaerenbergh I, Fatemi HM, Blockeel C et al. Progesterone rise on HCG day in GnRH antagonist/rFSH stimulated cycles affects endometrial gene expression. *Reprod Biomed Online*. 2011;22:263–71.

25. Bosch E, Valencia I, Escudero E et al. Premature luteinization during gonadotropin-releasing hormone antagonist cycles and its relationship with in vitro fertilization outcome. *Fertil Steril*. 2003;80:1444–9.

26. Labarta E, Martínez-Conejero JA, Alamá P et al. Endometrial receptivity is affected in women with high circulating progesterone levels at the end of the follicular phase: A functional genomics analysis. *Hum Reprod*. 2011;26:1813–25.

27. Kolibianakis EM, Devroey P. The luteal phase after ovarian stimulation. *Reprod Biomed Online*. 2002a;5:26–35.

28. Papanikolaou EG, Kolibianakis EM, Pozzobon C et al. Progesterone rise on the day of human chorionic gonadotropin administration impairs pregnancy outcome in day 3 single-embryo transfer, while has no effect on day 5 single blastocyst transfer. *Fertil Steril*. 2009;91:949–52.

29. Damewood MD, Shen W, Zacur HA et al. Disappearance of exogenously administered human chorionic gonadotropin. *Fertil Steril*. 1989;52:398–400.

30. Yen SS, Llerena O, Little B et al. Disappearance rates of endogenous luteinizing hormone and chorionic gonadotropin in man. *J Clin Endocrinol Metab*. 1968;28:1763–7.

31. Fatemi HM, Polyzos NP, van Vaerenbergh I et al. Early luteal phase endocrine profile is affected by the mode of triggering final oocyte maturation and the luteal phase support used in recombinant follicle-stimulating hormone–gonadotropin-releasing hormone antagonist in vitro fertilization cycles. *Fertil Steril*. 2013;100:742–7.

32. Humaidan P, Van Vaerenbergh I, Bourgain C, Alsbjerg B, Blockeel C, Schuit F, Van Lommel L, Devroey P, Fatemi H. Endometrial gene expression in the early luteal phase is impacted by mode of triggering final oocyte maturation in recFSH stimulated and GnRH antagonist co-treated IVF cycles. *Hum Reprod*. 2012;27(11):3259–72.

33. Jones GES. Some new aspects of management of infertility. *JAMA*. 1979;141:1123.

34. Jordan J, Craig K, Clifton DK, Soules MR. Luteal phase defect: The sensitivity and specificity of diagnostic methods in common clinical use. *Fertil Steril*. 1994;62:54–62.

35. Rosenberg SM, Luciano AA, Riddick DH. The luteal phase defect: The relative frequency of, and encouraging response to, treatment with vaginal progesterone. *Fertil Steril*. 1980;34:17–20.

36. Practice Committee of the American Society for Reproductive Medicine. Current clinical irrelevance of luteal phase deficiency: A committee opinion. *Fertil Steril*. 2015;103:e27–32.

37. Csapo AI, Pulkkinen M. Indispensability of the human corpus luteum in the maintenance of early pregnancy. Luteectomy evidence. *Obstet Gynecol Surv*. 1978;33:69–81.

38. Liu HC, Pyrgiotis E, Davis O, Rosenwaks Z. Active corpus luteum function at pre-, peri- and postimplantation is essential for a viable pregnancy. *Early Pregnancy*. 1995;1:281–7.

39. Macklon NS, Fauser BC. Impact of ovarian hyperstimulation on the luteal phase. *J Reprod Fertil*. 2000;55:101–8.

40. Fatemi HM, Popovic-Todorovic B, Papanikolaou E et al. An update of luteal phase support in stimulated IVF cycles. *Hum Reprod Update*. 2007;13:581–90.

41. Beckers NG, Macklon NS, Eijkemans MJ et al. Nonsupplemented luteal phase characteristics after the administration of recombinant human chorionic gonadotropin, recombinant luteinizing hormone, or gonadotropin-releasing hormone (GnRH) agonist to induce final oocyte maturation in in vitro fertilization patients after ovarian stimulation with recombinant follicle-stimulating hormone and GnRH antagonist cotreatment. *J Clin Endocrinol Metab*. 2003;88:4186–92.

42. Fatemi HM. The luteal phase after 3 decades of IVF: What do we know? *Reprod Biomed Online*. 2009;19:4331.

43. Fauser BC, Devroey P. Reproductive biology and IVF: Ovarian stimulation and luteal phase consequences. *Trends Endocrinol Metab*. 2003;14:236–42.

44. Tavaniotou A, Devroey P. Effect of human chorionic gonadotropin on luteal luteinizing hormone concentrations in natural cycles. *Fertil Steril*. 2003;80:654–5.

45. Tavaniotou A, Albano C, Smitz J, Devroey P. Comparison of LH concentrations in the early and mid-luteal phase in IVF cycles after treatment with HMG alone or in association with the GnRH antagonist Cetrorelix. *Hum Reprod*. 2001;16:663–7.

46. Bourgain C, Devroey P. The endometrium in stimulated cycles for IVF. *Hum Reprod Update*. 2003;9:515–22.

47. Hirvonen E, Mälkönen M, Manninen V. Effects of different progestogens on lipoproteins during postmenopausal replacement therapy. *N Engl J Med.* 1981;304:560–3.
48. Dennerstein L, Burrows GD, Hyman GJ, Sharpe K. Hormone therapy and affect. *Maturitas.* 1979;1:247–59.
49. Norman TR, Morse CA, Dennerstein L. Comparative bioavailability of orally and vaginally administered progesterone. *Fertil Steril.* 1991;56:1034–9.
50. Nillius SJ, Johansson ED. Plasma levels of progesterone after vaginal, rectal, or intramuscular administration of progesterone. *Am J Obstet Gynecol.* 1971;110:470–7.
51. Bouckaert Y, Robert F, Englert Y et al. Acute eosinophilic pneumonia associated with intramuscular administration of progesterone as luteal phase support after IVF: Case report. *Hum Reprod.* 2004;19(8):1806–10.
52. Baker VL, Jones CA, Doody K et al. A randomized, controlled trial comparing the efficacy and safety of aqueous subcutaneous progesterone with vaginal progesterone for luteal phase support of *in vitro* fertilization. *Hum Reprod.* 2014;29(10):2212–20.
53. Devroey P, Palermo G, Bourgain C et al. Progesterone administration in patients with absent ovaries. *Int J Fertil.* 1989;34:188–93.
54. Villanueva B, Casper RF, Yen SS. Intravaginal administration of progesterone: Enhanced absorption after estrogen treatment. *Fertil Steril.* 1981;35:433–7.
55. Fatemi HM. Assessment of the luteal phase in stimulated and substituted cycles. *Facts Views Vis Obgyn.* 2009;1(1):30–46.
56. Tavaniotou A, Smitz J, Bourgain C, Devroey P. Comparison between different routes of progesterone administration as luteal phase support in infertility treatments. *Hum Reprod Update.* 2000;6:139–48.
57. van der Linden M, Buckingham K, Farquhar C et al. Luteal phase support for assisted reproduction cycles. *Cochrane Database Syst Rev.* 2015 Jul 7;(7):CD009154.
58. Ludwig M, Diedrich K. Evaluation of an optimal luteal phase support protocol in IVF. *Acta Obstet Gynecol Scand.* 2001;80:452–66.
59. Andersen CY, Fischer R, Giorgione V, Kelsey TW. Micro-dose hCG as luteal phase support without exogenous progesterone administration: Mathematical modelling of the hCG concentration in circulation and initial clinical experience. *J Assist Reprod Genet.* 2016;33(10):1311–8.
60. Connell MT, Szatkowski JM, Terry N et al. Timing luteal support in assisted reproductive technology: A systematic review. *Fertil Steril.* 2015;103:939–46.
61. Nyboe AA, Popovic-Todorovic B, Schmidt KT et al. Progesterone supplementation during early gestations after IVF or ICSI has no effect on the delivery rates: A randomized controlled trial. *Hum Reprod.* 2002;17:357–61.
62. Schmidt KL, Ziebe S, Popovic B et al. Progesterone supplementation during early gestation after *in vitro* fertilization has no effect on the delivery rate. *Fertil Steril.* 2001;75:337–41.
63. Humaidan P, Bredkjaer HE, Bungum L et al. GnRH agonist (buserelin) or hCG for ovulation induction in GnRH antagonist IVF/ICSI cycles: A prospective randomized study. *Hum Reprod.* 2005;20:1213–20.
64. Engmann L, Benadiva C. Agonist trigger: What is the best approach? Agonist trigger with aggressive luteal support. *Fertil Steril.* 2012;97:531–3.
65. Hutchison JS, Zeleznik AJ. The rhesus monkey corpus luteum is dependent on pituitary gonadotropin secretion throughout the luteal phase of the menstrual cycle. *Endocrinology.* 1984;115:1780–6.
66. Hutchison JS, Zeleznik AJ. The corpus luteum of the primate menstrual cycle is capable of recovering from a transient withdrawal of pituitary gonadotropin support. *Endocrinology.* 1985;117:1043–9.
67. Dubourdieu S, Charbonnel B, Massai MR et al. Suppression of corpus luteum function by the gonadotropin-releasing hormone antagonist Nal-Glu: Effect of the dose and timing of human chorionic gonadotropin administration. *Fertil Steril.* 1991;56:440–512.
68. Humaidan P. Luteal phase rescue in high-risk OHSS patients by GnRHa triggering in combination with low-dose HCG: A pilot study. *Reprod Biomed Online.* 2009;18:630–4.
69. Seyhan A, Ata B, Polat M et al. Severe early ovarian hyperstimulation syndrome following GnRH agonist trigger with the addition of 1500 IU hCG. *Hum Reprod.* 2013;28:2522–8.
70. Castillo JC, Dolz M, Bienvenido E et al. Cycles triggered with GnRH agonist: Exploring low-dose HCG for luteal support. *Reprod Biomed Online.* 2010;20:175–81.
71. Andersen CY, Elbaek HO, Alsbjerg B et al. Daily low-dose hCG stimulation during the luteal phase combined with GnRHa triggered IVF cycles without exogenous progesterone: A proof of concept trial. *Hum Reprod.* 2015;30:2387–95.

72. Bar-Hava I, Mizrachi Y, Karfunkel-Doron D et al. Intranasal gonadotropin-releasing hormone agonist (GnRHa) for luteal-phase support following GnRHa triggering, a novel approach to avoid ovarian hyperstimulation syndrome in high responders. *Fertil Steril.* 2016;106:330–3.

73. Kol S, Breyzman T, Segal L, Humaidan P. "Luteal coasting" after GnRH agonist trigger—Individualized, HCG-based, progesterone-free luteal support in "high responders": A case series. *Reprod Biomed Online.* 2015;31:747–51.

74. Lawrenz B, Samir S, Garrido N et al. Luteal coasting and individualization of human chorionic gonadotropin dose after gonadotropin-releasing hormone agonist triggering for final oocyte maturation—A retrospective proof-of-concept study. *Front Endocrinol.* 2018;9:33.

75. Ragni G, Vegetti W, Baroni E et al. Comparison of luteal phase profile in gonadotrophin stimulated cycles with or without a gonadotrophin-releasing hormone antagonist. *Hum Reprod.* 2001;16:2258–62.

76. ESHRE Capri Workshop Group. Intrauterine Insemination. *Hum Reprod Update.* 2009;15:265–77.

77. Kyrou D, Fatemi HM, Tournaye H, Devroey P. Luteal phase support in normo-ovulatory women stimulated with clomiphene citrate for intrauterine insemination: Need or habit? *Hum Reprod.* 2010;25:2501–6.

78. Oktem M, Altinkaya SO, Yilmaz SA et al. Effect of luteal phase support after ovulation induction and intrauterine insemination. *Gynecol Endocrinol.* 2014;30:909–12.

79. Le Lannou D, Griveau JF, Laurent MC, Gueho A, Veron E, Morcel K. Contribution of embryo cryopreservation to elective single embryo transfer in IVF-ICSI. *Reprod Biomed Online.* 2006;13:368–75.

80. Fatemi HM, Kyrou D, Bourgain C, Van den Abbeel E, Griesinger G, Devroey P. Cryopreserved-thawed human embryo transfer: Spontaneous natural cycle is superior to human chorionic gonadotropin-induced natural cycle. *Fertil Steril.* 2010;94:2054–8.

81. Montagut M, Santos-Ribeiro S, De Vos M et al. Frozen-thawed embryo transfers in natural cycles with spontaneous or induced ovulation: The search for the best protocol continues. *Hum Reprod.* 2016;31:2803–10.

9

Measuring Safety and Efficiency in In Vitro Fertilization

Nicole C. Michel, Natalie Shammas, and Shima Elbakhit Albasha

Advent of a Controversy

In recent years, there has been a marked increase in regulations governing assisted reproduction facilities. Likewise, accrediting bodies have been more stringent in implementing peer-based schemes for improving quality. These circumstances have primarily been brought on by two major influences:

- The rapid innovation of assisted reproductive technology (ART)
- Ubiquitous media attention to the mishaps that can transpire in *in vitro* fertilization (IVF) clinics

This chapter is valuable for keeping up with modern mentalities, as it will highlight the most current effective strategies for running a clinic. Of note, the writing of this chapter has tremendously benefited from the work of Mortimer and Mortimer in establishing benchmarks that can be applied globally (1).

Currently Contested Aspects

Lately, the controversial theme surrounding safety and efficiency in an IVF laboratory concerns which management methodologies are constructive, and which are unhelpful.

Prior to examining the assorted methodologies in depth, it is helpful to distinguish some vocabulary, principally with regard to the concepts of quality and risk. This is important, considering that if anyone is to argue whether particular methodologies are superior to others, then the core elements being managed must first be clarified.

Commentary on Quality and Risk

In medicine, "quality" can be defined as *duty of care* and has been associated with the attainment of best practice. Essentially, quality of care is an intricate notion with many facets, including treatment efficacy and influence on well-being of both patients and progenies. In addition, the concept of quality acknowledges the monetary and physical costs of attaining the desired result (2).

In a laboratory, quality control (QC) is about ensuring tasks are done properly, instruments are working, and assays are run accurately. This guarantees that results come close to what is predicted. However, *quality assurance* (QA) ensures that a system is designed in such a way that it will increase the probability that the process will go exactly as planned, increasing consistency and overall performance.

While the goal of "quality" is to fulfill requirements, these change with consumers' growing expectations. Within the realm of IVF, services should be more readily accessible and provided in a pleasant setting with personalized attention. The part of the quality system that is dedicated to constantly increasing efficiency is called *quality improvement* (QI).

Total quality management (TQM) assimilates quality control, assurance, and improvement into one cohesive management philosophy. For many experts, TQM is simply the *scientific way of doing business* and, therefore, apt for operating an IVF clinic (3).

Since TQM is a comprehensive quality system integrating QC, QA, and QI into a repetitious process, it is not an ephemeral undertaking. It is an endless pursuit for development. There are no shortcuts for its enactment. In essence, an organization must

- Promote a concise, long-term approach that is cohesive with all of the organization's other business plans.
- Craft an all-encompassing set of policies attending to the needs of all areas within the organization. These policies form the basis of TQM and will include ambitions and supplies. They should be established together with those who will be responsible for transforming the plans into realizations.
- Install these policies through all ranks of the organization.
- Perform systems analysis of all processes at the most fundamental levels.
- Foster prevention-based activities. This often requires a cultural shift from faultfinding to acknowledging honest slip-ups as chances for improvement.
- Commence targeted quality assurance processes so that QI can follow.

To enhance quality, it is essential to confirm that the team has the required proficiencies, expertise, and equipment to complete objectives (2). Furthermore, competent and effective management—and leadership—are essential (3–6). Studies have shown that a style of leadership that focuses on encouraging and empowering the staff to change services locally and work in a more patient-centered manner is the most significant factor in influencing patient centeredness (7). Overall, the improvement team should be composed of various leaders, or stakeholders. A stakeholder is one who has an enthusiasm in a specific endeavor and can sway its success or failures. Effective stakeholders split the work accordingly, fulfilling the following positions: team lead, technical experts, clinical leader, improvement advisor, and executive sponsor (8).

Moving forward, the other element to be discussed is "risk." Risk can be defined as vulnerability to peril, injury, or loss. In a clinic, risk entails any concern about a prospective incident that might jeopardize routine operations. *Risk management* utilizes foresight of fiscal and physical risks to evade or mitigate their impact. It incorporates tactics for spotting and defying such hazards (3,9–11).

In recent years, IVF clinics have had to face more convoluted risk issues, necessitating stricter management (9–12). Successful risk management teams habitually detect, scrutinize, and eradicate potential threats. This way, complications are thwarted before they arise. For example, preceding execution of any novel procedure, all involved personnel must complete training and demonstrate proficiency. Equipment must be authenticated prior to handling; it must be dependable and be operative if ever in suboptimal surroundings. However, factors such as temperature, osmolarity, pH, and contamination must be stringently regulated as much as possible on every sliver of equipment utilized. Moreover, it is vital that these factors are measured at the precise locality where the embryos are maneuvered. Taking precautionary measures in such ways is all part of effective risk management (2).

Again, there are various methodologies that can be chosen to implement quality and risk management. Next, an evaluation of these methods is presented. Specifically, a synopsis on how they each work and what their advantages are is provided. Subsequently, a brief assessment is made on each of their disadvantages.

Supporting Evidence for Each Method

Achieving Accreditation

Accreditation is a synergistic series of actions whereby an organization is acknowledged for being in compliance with *standards*. *Standards* are meticulous criteria that guarantee that practices are functioning at an adequate level.

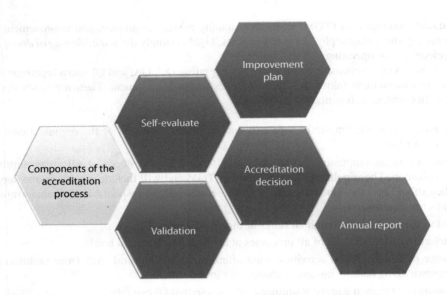

FIGURE 9.1 Depiction of the accreditation process, once enrolled. This process typically takes 3 years.

Accreditation programs have been found to be the most significant element in stimulating patient-centeredness. In particular, it has been confirmed that if accreditation bolsters compliance to evidence-based standards, then it is instrumental in achieving superior care for patients (7). Furthermore, accrediting bodies are important for ensuring a quality-controlled environment. In one instance, where an accrediting body recommended that IVF candidates receive standardized precycle counseling, success rates increased by 15% (13).

As of now, achieving accreditation is a choice. It ascertains a laboratory's compliance with prearranged criteria via self and peer assessments (3). It has to be a dynamic document, because our knowledge transforms over time and with practice. Effective accreditation schemes are composed of these basic characteristic stages (alternatively summarized in Figure 9.1):

Stage 1: A self-assessment of all facets of the organization. Objectives of the self-assessment process include the following:

- Determining fulfillment of accreditation conditions
- Judging the organization's alignment with its own beliefs
- Appraising outcomes and effectiveness
- Itemizing areas for improvement

Stage 2: Peer survey. A team visits the property, convenes with management, interviews personnel, and scrutinizes data to weigh compliance with the accrediting body's prearranged criteria.

Stage 3: Report and recommendations. Advice is given to facilitate improvement in areas of weakness and to develop areas of strength.

Quality Cycle

In the "plan-do-study-act" (PDSA) *quality cycle* (Figure 9.2), a problem is recognized. Then, a solution is identified, put into effect, and the outcome checked to confirm that the matter has been resolved. Scientists will instantly recognize the PDSA cycle as a simple manifestation of the basic scientific method. Implementation of the PDSA cycle within health-care systems has been shown to increase safety measures by up to 12% (14).

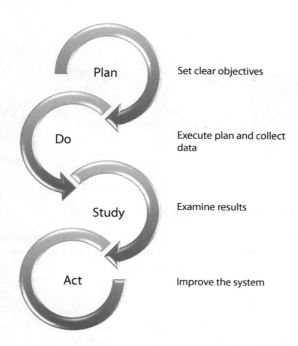

FIGURE 9.2   The plan-do-study-act cycle.

Rapid Cycle Change

Although most core change teams are familiar with the PDSA approach, it was widely unknown, until recently, precisely how to conduct more minute tests of change and convey advancement. McQuillan et al. have proposed a way of doing so by coalescing a sequence of PDSA cycles in a process called *rapid cycle change*. This is a continual process, whereby the first cycle produces results that guide the next cycle, and so on, until attainment of the ultimate goal (Figure 9.3). This method is exceedingly sensible in comparison to blindly executing numerous interventions, which could equate to unwarranted spending and inadvertent consequences (15).

Model for Improvement

PDSA and rapid cycle change are both integral components of a larger model, the Model for Improvement. The Model for Improvement is intended as a means for attaining an objective at any extent through

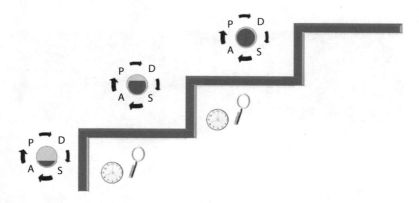

FIGURE 9.3   Rapid cycle change. Several plan-do-study-act cycles are applied to transform a thought into a concrete result.

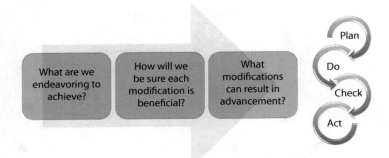

FIGURE 9.4 A visual diagram of the Model for Improvement.

learned experience and decisive action. This model condenses quality improvement into three queries presented in Figure 9.4. The fundamental principle of the Model for Improvement is that not all change is improvement, but all improvement necessitates change (8).

System Mapping Approaches

To understand systems, it is easiest if one first understands processes. A *process* is a sequence of transformations that lead to an outcome. It is a solitary, simple progression. A *system* is an assembly of numerous elements interacting to construct a methodical run of events. A system is larger in scale compared to a process and is classically made up of a set of processes that transpire either successively, or concurrently, with other processes. The output of one is an input to another.

Nonetheless, to appreciate an entire system, one must be familiar with both the individual processes and the extrinsic factors acting on each process. To better grasp the risks in any system, knowledge needs to be accessible through modes, such as (a) understanding of people, (b) incident reports, and (c) system mapping approaches (SMAs) (16). This analysis is often undertaken in a diagrammatic fashion, via *process mapping*. In this case, the system is sketched as a flowchart, with every step clearly elucidated. The benefit of this method is refinement and automatization of the existing process (17). Process maps also have been proven useful for strengthening the risk identification processes of failure modes and effects analysis (FMEA) (16). The volume of detail in the IVF process is certainly extensive, and even Figure 9.5 is just brief synopsis of the substantial steps involved. Though these paradigms have been exemplified

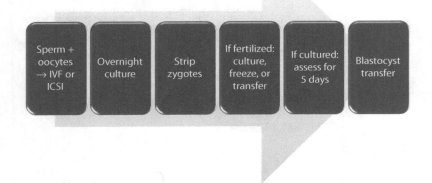

FIGURE 9.5 A map of the *in vitro* fertilization laboratory process. ICSI, intracytoplasmic sperm injection.

using the familiar tool of *flowcharting*, several other intricate tools exist, such as *swim lane analysis* or *top-down process mapping* (3) that are each appropriate for distinctive scenarios. For example, while swim lane analysis helped participants understand the roles and responsibilities in a given system, a top-down process map is an exceptional means for creating a standard operating procedure (SOP) from the ground up. Evaluation showed that the most useful SMA tool in risk identification is a system diagram. *System diagrams* convey interplay between the various constituents in a system. While the evaluation indicated that the system diagram is the most instrumental SMA in risk identification, it can also be surmised that using a mixture of several maps is an effective means for determining risks (16).

A solid process map will yield the subsequent outcomes:

- Forming collective protocols for patient care
- Promoting adherence to protocols and thereby minimizing complications due to faulty exchange of information
- Noting abnormalities and flaws and thus early identifying problems that could lead to unprevented errors
- Understanding the information flow and thus identifying requirements and specifications for information system reengineering and interoperability (17)

Once a process-mapping exercise has concluded, knowledge will be revealed and made accessible to the entire organization. Corporate knowledge can then be divulged to the subsequent generation without any inconsistencies or misinterpretations.

Process Control Charts

Process control is a method that was built to oversee the operation of processes. Essentially, process control methods let us distinguish whether or not a system is "under control" in relation to its usual level of functioning. The most commonly used tool for this is the *process control chart*, where the measurement of concern is termed an *indicator* (Figure 9.6).

Provided that the input of a process control chart stays within the control limits, the process is thought to be under control. Conversely, additional action is needed if any of the following circumstances arise:

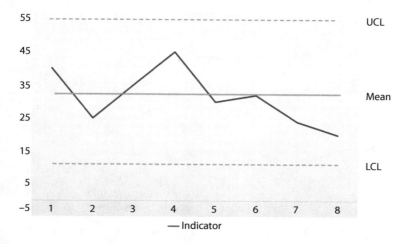

FIGURE 9.6 A model of a control chart for a generic process. The outcome is measured using an indicator. Baseline data are required to give an accurate picture. The mean and standard deviation (SD) are calculated. They are used to form a "control mean," upper control limit (UCL), and lower control limit (LCL). UCL and LCL = the mean $\pm$ 3 SD. The amount of baseline data required to calculate the control limits is not randomly preset. The number used must be adequate enough to give a decent indication of variability. However, it should not be so many that the control limits become too narrow.

- *The indicator surpasses its control limit in the opposing direction*: Urgent action must be taken to establish whether there is an authentic problem and, if so, to resolve it.
- *The indicator surpasses its warning limit in the opposing direction*: Action must be taken to establish if a problem is occurring or might be emerging.
- *The indicator displays three successive changes in the opposing direction but does not surpass the warning or control limit*: Action must be taken to establish whether a problem might be emerging.
- *The indicator surpasses its control limit in the favorable direction*: The system must be inspected to understand why it happened and whether the development is authentic and fixed (Figure 9.7).

While pregnancy rate is a meaningful indicator of general performance, it is not specific enough. The most suggestive measure of output quality is implantation rate, versus pregnancy rates (2). Therefore, laboratory performance indicators (LPIs) that each oversee a distinct process via a control chart are mandatory (3,18). For example, a more appropriate indicator might be the proportion of embryos reaching developmental milestones at predefined time points of embryo culture (2). Keeping an inclusive panel of LPIs helps a clinic to swiftly respond to any issues. If all LPIs are within control limits, it signifies that no changes have been detected. If an issue surfaces, then the lab will promptly be able to spot it because of the LPIs.

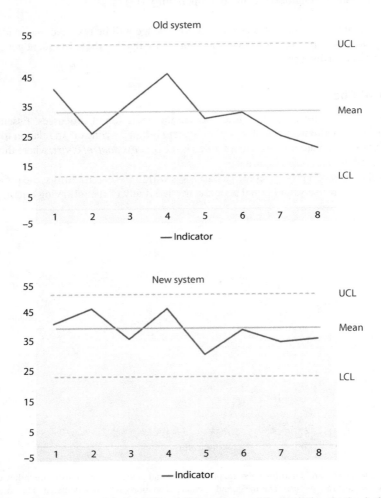

FIGURE 9.7 Control charts can be useful to compare whether or not a modification to a system has had a positive impact. An increase in the value of the control mean in the new system suggests a systematic improvement. Additionally, a narrowing of the control limits illustrate improved stability of the new system.

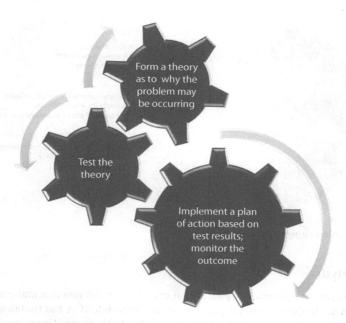

FIGURE 9.8   The troubleshooting process, once a problem has been identified.

Troubleshooting

Figure 9.8 displays a basic troubleshooting process and demonstrates how the scientific method is central to conducting the process successfully (3,11). In the event of a problem, regular documentation allows parameters to be compared during different time periods (19). Furthermore, formalizing the process helps less seasoned personnel to apply the same technique, while also providing the framework whereby it is documented.

Failure Modes and Effects Analysis

FMEA is a dynamic tool that assists in identifying and offsetting defects in process designs. It uses coordinated tactics to detect segments in need of upgrading. It does so based on severity and on how often failure is expected. Its applicability has made it a broadly used tool that can be used to advance processes globally.

Piloting an FMEA entails taking the following actions:

1. *Chart the process*: Identify all the operations that are intended to ensue.
2. *Identify failure modes*: Identify the ways in which any of the operations could go awry.
3. *Realize the effects*: Become aware of the ramifications of each failure mode.
4. *Identify contributory factors*: Identify these factors or consider all potential root causes of each failure mode.
5. *Rate the likelihood of each failure mode and the gravity of its consequence*: Use customary rating scales (e.g., Figure 9.9).
6. *Compute the criticality of each failure mode*: This is done by multiplying the likelihood and consequence ratings.
7. *Chart the scores into a risk matrix*: Section the criticality scores into the following classifications: diminutive, significant, or severe risk.
8. *Recognize any existing controls*: Dissect the process map. Identify any observational systems, and gauge their effect on the given criticality scores.
9. *Formulate an action plan*: It is important that there is a system in place for assessing the influence of every change that is introduced.

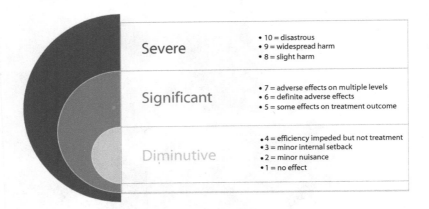

FIGURE 9.9   Failure effect ratings for FMEA analysis.

Root Cause Analysis

Root cause analysis (RCA) is a series of phases that can pinpoint the fundamental causes of an adverse effect with the aim of stopping it from happening again. Although RCA has traditionally been used in health care to examine the source of medical mistakes, it has lately focused more on abating the gaps in quality of health care and advancing quality outcomes. Of note, resistance to change can be lessened by utilizing the rapid cycle change method—by beginning with slight modifications, then ascertaining what works from what does not (15). According to Mortimer and Mortimer, *resistance to change* derives from an innate human aversion to change. They then go on to justify that self-assured, astute folks appreciate that change can be positive. They know that the challenges that accompany it can promote prosperity (1). Thus, RCA is an indispensable instrument for quality improvement. The use of RCA is centered on the notion that a specific outcome may be elucidated by investigating the underlying elements that may be partly responsible for that outcome. The objectives of RCA are delineating what is transpiring, establishing the cause of the outcome's occurrence, and formulating a strategy to avoid the outcome from recurring (20).

Running an RCA is virtually a retrospective FMEA. It can be summarized by the following steps:

1. *Uncover the facts of the matter*: Find out everything possible about the incident, concentrating on the elements that might have caused the event to occur.
2. *Create a graphical representation of the contributory factors*: Inquire "why?" or "how?" so that each can be designated as either "contributory" or "noncontributory."
3. *Initiate an action plan*: The plan should have at least one enhancement for each known contributory factor.
4. *Execute the plan*: Carry out the corrective actions.
5. *See it through to completion*: Utilize the monitoring processes to assess the efficacy of the corrective actions. If the problem has not been entirely settled, fine-tuning and repetition of the process may be needed.

Once more, it is important to keep in mind that the aim is to learn as much as possible about the event, and to deter repeated happenings. Each causative factor that cannot be derived any further is deemed a "root cause." An RCA reporting table should include the subsequent plans for each root cause:

- Make restorative actions.
- Appoint individuals who will carry out these actions. Delegating oversight over each task should ensure they will be carried out to completion, and will boost the prospects of having a favorable outcome.

- Set an action deadline. A temporal agenda will mitigate indolence and help the process to seem tangible.
- Identify a measurement technique. One should be able to discern if the change has made any impact. The following list outlines the ways in which quality improvement is often measured (8,15):
  - *Outcome Measures*: Assess the clinical impact of the corrective action on patients
  - *Process Measures*: Assess system efficacy and possible changes
  - *Balancing Measures*: Check for inadvertent ramifications of the corrective action
- Appoint individuals to follow-up on each corrective action.
- Set a date to reassess. By this point, one may anticipate that substantial strides have been taken.

Opposing Evidence for Each Method

Achieving Accreditation

An increasing number of clinics have pursued certification under the ISO 9001:2000 standard for quality management and the ISO 15189 standard for medical laboratories (1,4,21,22). Although these standards have made remarkable headway in refining systems, they do not necessarily cultivate quality assurance. In fact, a clinic may theoretically attain ISO9001:2000 certification even if they were unsuccessful in yielding offspring.

Also, since accreditation is devised and imposed by means of legislation, it comprehensibly differs across the globe. This makes for a high volume of inconsistencies. And while licenses are typically granted once an inspection proves that a laboratory is in compliance with codes, it is still recommended that thought be given to earning a Quality Management System (QMS) certification (23,24). By obtaining a QMS certification, it suggests that the management system of this laboratory meets requirements defined under an international norm (25).

Quality Cycle

On first glance, it does not take long to realize that this method provides the reader with only an oversimplification of the quality improvement process. As a result, many details will go neglected. Furthermore, this method does not account for the modified process. Hence, the ultimate fate of the project is often left unknown (26).

Rapid Cycle Change

If the system was manufacturing poorly designed products to begin with, it may possibly make them even faster now. In addition, since changes are made so hastily, there is not copious time to fully gauge the scope of each new development. Thus, each successive decision made after that may inadvertently be driving project efforts in the wrong direction.

Model for Improvement

As to be expected, the shortcomings of this model are virtually identical to those of the quality cycle: primarily, the fact that there is no part of the process that addresses follow-up for the outcome.

System Mapping Approaches

In order to utilize this method, it requires arduous work of breaking down the system to its basic components, so that the influences affecting each component may be explored. For example, although IVF can be portrayed as an uncomplicated process, it cannot be analyzed wholly through this way due to the considerable amounts of constituent subprocesses.

Process Control Charts

Indicators are key to the expansion and upholding of a quality system. After all, one must be able to measure in order to control. However, laborious, consistent measurement of indicators is necessary to articulately validate the key role of data systems in a prosperous IVF clinic.

Troubleshooting

Since troubleshooting is such a basic, rudimentary process, it is not as applicable when dealing with complex, multifaceted matters. Furthermore, any given step is dependent on, and must wait on, the step prior to it. Consequently, decision-making is recurrently stalled.

Failure Modes and Effects Analysis

FMEA does not resolve issues, as it is merely a tool for assessment. Also, it is difficult to ever deem it complete, since there is a nearly endless amount of possible failure modes to consider.

Root Cause Analysis

RCAs will often detect more contributory factors than anticipated. This can present financial issues if there are so many factors identified that the budget is unable to address them all. In addition, while this method focuses on triggers, it does not assign anyone responsibility for effectively addressing what can be done to remedy each cause (27).

Areas for Further Research

In conclusion, TQM is a necessity in IVF laboratories. As Mortimer and Mortimer stated, the method evolves once the tenets are implemented (1). Though TQM is unable to promise rewards, it can promise smooth operation and productivity. A properly regulated organization expedites the acknowledgement of complications. Then, TQM can offer the means for stamping out the causative factors. Finally, it is evident that risk management is akin to quality management and that both synchronize with each other. Those who have witnessed a correct practice of TQM can confirm its universally versatile advantages.

However, further investigation could be helpful to elucidate which specific methods are most valuable to employ within a practice of TQM. An area for future research could involve a meta-analysis comparing the various methodologies mentioned in this chapter. A key advantage to using a meta-analysis approach is that it will result in a high statistical power, leading us to feel more assured in knowing which methods are most beneficial to running an IVF laboratory.

REFERENCES

1. Mortimer D, Mortimer ST. Quality and risk management in the IVF laboratory. In: *Infertility and Assisted Reproduction*. New York, NY: Cambridge University Press; 2008:548–61.
2. Banker M, Olofsson J, Sjoblom L. Quality management systems for your *in vitro* fertilization clinic's laboratory: Why bother? *J Hum Reprod Sci*. 2013;6(1):3–8.
3. Centola GM. Quality and risk management in the IVF laboratory: by Mortimer D, Mortimer ST, Cambridge, United Kingdom: Cambridge University Press. *J Androl*. 2005:232 p.
4. Buchta C, Coucke W, Mayr WR, Müller MM, Oeser R, Schweiger CR, Körmöczi GF. Evidence for the positive impact of ISO 9001 and ISO 15189 quality systems on laboratory performance—Evaluation of immunohaematology external quality assessment results during 19 years in Austria. *Clin Chem Lab Med (CCLM)*. 2018;56(12):2039–46.
5. Weintraub P, Mckee M. Leadership for innovation in healthcare: An exploration. *Int J Health Policy Manag*. 2018;8(3):138–44.

6. Antes AL, Mart A, Dubois JM. Are leadership and management essential for good research? An interview study of genetic researchers. *J Empirical Res Hum Res Ethics.* 2016;11(5):408–23.

7. Hijazi HH, Harvey HL, Alyahya MS, Alshraideh HA, Abdi RM, Parahoo SK. The impact of applying quality management practices on patient centeredness in Jordanian public hospitals: Results of predictive modeling. *INQUIRY. J Health Care Organ Provision Financing.* 2018;55:1–15.

8. Silver SA, Harel Z, Mcquillan R, Weizman AV, Thomas A, Chertow GM, Chan CT. How to begin a quality improvement project. *Clin J Am Soc Nephrol.* 2016;11(5):893–900.

9. Ziegler DD, Gambone JC, Meldrum DR, Chapron C. Risk and safety management in infertility and assisted reproductive technology (ART): From the doctors office to the ART procedure. *Fertil Steril.* 2013;100(6):1509–17.

10. Kennedy CR, Mortimer D. Risk management in IVF. Best practice and research. *Clin Obstet and Gynaecol.* 2007;21(4):691–712.

11. Mortimer D. Setting up risk management systems in in-vitro fertilization laboratories. *Clin Risk.* 2004;10: 128–37.

12. Alper MM. Experience with ISO quality control in assisted reproductive technology. *Fertil Steril.* 2013;100(6):1503–8.

13. Salam M. Success of in vitro fertilization: A researched science or a performance indicator. *J Clin Gynecol Obstet.* 2017;6(3–4):53–7.

14. Demirel A. Improvement of hand hygiene compliance in a private hospital using the Plan-Do-Check-Act (PDCA) method. *Pak J Med Sci.* 2019;35(3):721–5.

15. Mcquillan RF, Silver SA, Harel Z, Weizman A, Thomas A, Bell C, Nesrallah G. How to measure and interpret quality improvement data. *Clin J Am Soc Nephrol.* 2016;11(5):908–14.

16. Simsekler MC, Ward JR, Clarkson PJ. Evaluation of system mapping approaches in identifying patient safety risks. *Int J Qual Health Care.* 2018;30(3):227–33.

17. Bonacina S, Pozzi G, Pinciroli F, Marceglia S, Ferrante S. A design methodology for medical processes. *Appl Clin Inform.* 2016;07(01):191–210.

18. Neuburger J, Walker K, Sherlaw-Johnson C, Meulen JV, Cromwell DA. Comparison of control charts for monitoring clinical performance using binary data. *BMJ Qual Saf.* 2017;26(11):919–28.

19. Elder K, Van de Bergh M, Woodward B (n.d.). Troubleshooting ICSI Procedures. In: *Troubleshooting and Problem-Solving in the IVF Laboratory* (Vol. 1). 2015: 171–88. doi:10.1017/CBO9781107294295

20. Harel Z, Silver SA, Mcquillan RF, Weizman AV, Thomas A, Chertow GM, Bell CM. How to diagnose solutions to a quality of care problem. *Clin J Am Soc Nephrol.* 2016;11(5):901–7.

21. Alsan, D. Which skills are needed and how they should be gained by laboratory medicine professionals for successful ISO 15189 accreditation. *EJIFCC,* 2018;29(4), 264–73.

22. Schneider F, Maurer C, Friedberg RC. International Organization for Standardization (ISO) 15189. *Ann Lab Med.* 2017;37(5):365–70.

23. Carey RB, Bhattacharyya S, Kehl SC, Matukas LM, Pentella MA, Salfinger M, Schuetz AN. Implementing a quality management system in the medical microbiology laboratory. *Clin Microbiol Rev.* 2018;31(3):1–17.

24. Grizzle WE, Gunter EW, Sexton KC, Bell WC. Quality management of biorepositories. *Biopreserv Biobank.* 2015;13(3):183–94.

25. Vendrell X, Carrero R, Alberola T, Bautista-Llácer R, García-Mengual E, Claramunt R, Pérez-Alonso M. Quality management system in PGD/PGS: Now is the time. *J Assist Reprod Genet.* 2009;26(4):197–204.

26. Reed JE, Card AJ. The problem with Plan-Do-Study-Act cycles. *BMJ Qual Saf.* 2015;25(3):147–52.

27. Peerally MF, Carr S, Waring J, Dixon-Woods M. The problem with root cause analysis. *BMJ Qual Saf.* 2016;26(5):417–22.

10

To Flush Follicles during Egg Collection or Not

Hans-Peter Steiner

Introduction

There is no doubt that the egg collection technique is an important part of *in vitro* fertilization (IVF). The question of whether to flush follicles during egg collection or not is still a controversial topic that has been hotly discussed since the introduction of IVF 40 years ago. In this chapter, an attempt is made to provide an answer to this question, providing evidence that supports flushing follicles in the proper way. Millions of oocytes could have been harvested, and thousands of babies could have been born, if the proper egg collection techniques had been used and a few simple rules of physics had been followed.

History of Egg Collection in *In Vitro* Fertilization

The first approach to ovum pickup (OPU) for IVF was taken using transabdominal laparoscopy (1). This approach was followed by the use of transabdominal, ultrasound-guided, oocyte retrieval (2). Suzan Lenz was the first physician to perform ultrasound-guided OPU in IVF in December 1980. She chose to use the transvesical follicle aspiration technique and conducted it at Rigs Hospital, Copenhagen, Denmark. Information about transvaginal oocyte retrieval with transvaginal aspiration under transabdominal ultrasound guidance was published in 1984 (3). Transvaginal OPU under transvaginal ultrasound guidance was introduced and reported in 1985 by Wikland and Hamberger (4) and has remained a standard of care for OPU since that time.

Brinsden remarked in 1992: "We believe that the use of vaginal ultrasound has enabled the technique of oocyte recovery to be refined down to the least invasive, least painful, most accurate, and most simple method that we are likely to be able to achieve in the foreseeable future" (5).

Since that time, the technique of using manual aspiration with syringes has been supplanted by that of electronic aspiration with pumps, which can maintain a steady aspiration pressure of about 120 mm Hg. Remarkably, the Rigs Hospital in Copenhagen is one of the few IVF centers at which a syringe instead of an aspiration pump is still used in OPU. Double-lumen needles or single-lumen needles with three-way valves have been widely used to optimize oocyte retrieval rates while flushing follicles.

A series of studies conducted over the past 30 years have compared the efficiency of single-lumen needles to double-lumen needles with the same outer diameter in terms of flushing follicles. The authors, however, did not consider the effects of the dramatically narrowed inner diameter of the inner needle on aspiration and the surrounding space required for flushing the double-lumen needles (6–11). Knight et al. (9) examined the effects of flushing and not flushing follicles on the total number of oocytes collected and pregnancy rates. Over 1139 treatment cycles, the authors found no statistical difference in the total number of oocytes collected or on pregnancy rates, but instead noted that increased operation time and anesthesia were required for the flushing group. On the basis of these observations, Knight concluded that flushing was "superfluous." For this reason, 80% of IVF doctors today use a single-lumen needle, and most do not flush follicles during egg collection.

State of the Art in Egg Collection

While 80% of researchers at IVF centers today "do not believe" in flushing follicles, 20% "do believe in the efficacy of flushing." As stated earlier, however, these beliefs—a mode of expression that is more accurately used in a religious or philosophic context—are based on a faulty conclusion that neglects the basic considerations of fluid dynamics that are taking place inside these needles. It is important to mention that a famous IVF clinic in Belgium, which has a noted reputation worldwide, routinely uses a 17-gauge single-lumen needle to flush follicles manually, injecting a flushing fluid into the silicone stopper of the needle system. This is a basis for concern, because the cumulus oocyte complex, which is already situated close to silicone stopper during this process, may be flushed back into that collapsed follicle if this technique is used (12).

Important Aspects of Fluid Dynamics Regarding Aspiration and Flushing Fluids in Pipes

In 1989, Reeves made an important statement regarding the behavior of fluids inside needles used in IVF during egg collection:

> The laws of physics applicable to a device such as an ovum pick up needle are those relating to the flow of fluid through pipes, in particular Poiseuillès law. This law takes in consideration the lumen diameter and the length of the conduit, in this case the length of the needle and the tube carrying the egg to the collecting container. The other parameters are the viscosity of the fluid and the force applied, in this case vacuum. Obviously, the success of the exercise is judged by the number of eggs, collected in relation to the number of follicles available; however, the law of physics used to collect the eggs are frequently ignored or not considered. (13)

The Poiseuillè law refers to the fact that at a constant driving pressure, the flow rate of a liquid through a capillary tube is directly proportional to the fourth power of the radius of the tube and inversely proportional to the length of the tube and viscosity of the liquid (Figure 10.1). For this reason, it is important for IVF doctors to carefully consider the implications of this law while flushing follicles for egg collection using either single- or double-lumen needles.

Another important consideration that must be taken is the *Reynolds number*. Described in the branch of physics concerned with the mechanics of fluids, the Reynolds number is a dimensionless number that gives a measure of the ratio of the inertial forces to the viscous forces and, consequently, quantifies the relative importance of these two types of forces for given flow conditions.

With regard to follicle flushing and egg collection, IVF physicians must consider both the Poiseuillè law and the Reynolds number, because a proper flushing effect can only be achieved if the effects of the flow rate and viscosity of the liquid being flushed *in relation to* the radius and the length of the needle

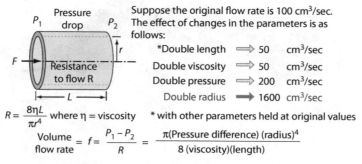

FIGURE 10.1 The Poiseuillè law. (From Hyperphysics, http://hyperphysics.phy-astr.gsu.edu, with permission.)

are considered *and* the effects of the inertial forces on the viscous forces in the particular flushing environment (i.e., the needle and the follicle being flushed). This flushing environment is defined by the needle used (ideally with an optimal inner diameter), the characteristics of the liquid being flushed, and the pulsating movement of the flushing syringe, which is activated either by hand or with the assistance of a mechanical or electronic flushing pump activated by the physician's foot. Because flushing has been summarily dismissed as "superfluous" by many physicians, this area of research has been neglected, and important possibilities for the optimization of egg collection in IVF have been overlooked (14).

Evidence in Favor of an Optimized Egg Collection System

By carefully considering the factors described earlier, an optimized egg collection system has been developed for use in my practice, which is based on considerations of physics. Specifically, this system includes the following components:

- A unique, single-lumen needle (STEINER-TAN needle) that enables follicles to be flushed through an opening as narrow as possible in order to minimize the patient's pain and the incidence of bleeding, but also achieve an optimal flushing effect. Details are shown below.
- A three-way stopcock is located close to the silicone stopper, which can be operated to change the direction of the fluid flow by changing its position from "aspiration" to "flushing." This stopcock is handled by an assistant manually or operated at a flushing pump, enabling the physician to change its position by activating a foot pedal without the need of assistance.
- The dead space present in the system has been minimized by 7 cm or the maximum length of the needle.
- A STEINER mechanical flushing pump (Figure 10.2) that can be activated by the physician's foot or a STEINER electronic aspiration and flushing pump that is combined in a single device (Figure 10.3) can be used. These pumps include an integrated warming element that ensures the constant temperature of the flushing fluid and prevents contamination and loss of temperature, which can occur if the flushing syringe is handheld.

Additional considerations that are involved with the use of the system include convincing colleagues that acoustic communication between the laboratory and operating room must be ensured. The biologist should have the ability to communicate commands in the case of poor responders, i.e., to continue flushing as long as granulosa cells are still found in the specimen.

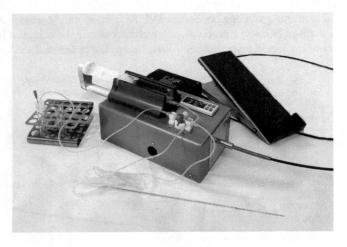

FIGURE 10.2 STEINER Mechanical Flushing Pump with Warming Element, shown here with STEINER-TAN needle, 17-gauge, with three-way valve clicked at pump.

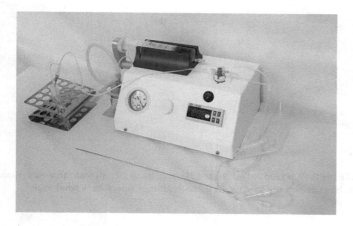

FIGURE 10.3 STEINER Combi Pump, shown here with STEINER-TAN needle 17-gauge classic.

There is sometimes confusion regarding the exact meaning of the term *flushing*. Flushing means completely refilling the follicle over a period of a few seconds. Flushing with a predefined volume, such as 3 cc as is performed in some centers, makes no logical sense because each flushing environment is inherently different. All follicles, even if there are 20 or more, should be flushed at least once to increase the chances of success (i.e., obtaining viable oocytes), which is currently not the standard in most IVF centers. The cumulative pregnancy rate resulting from the use of fresh or frozen oocytes should be the measure of IVF success.

STEINER-TAN Needle, a New Needle Technology

A single-lumen needle is inserted in plastic tubing starting at a position located 7 cm from the needle tip. After the follicle has collapsed, the flushing fluid is allowed to flow along the outside of the needle, passes through two drilled holes, and enters the lumen of the needle to refill the collapsed follicle (Figure 10.4). This needle optimizes the fluidic turbulence during both the aspirating and flushing processes (15) (Figure 10.5). In addition, the amount of dead space in the needle has been minimized to allow scientists to investigate the fluid of each follicle separately (16). The needle is optimally sharp (back bevel angle) and has an echo tip (Figure 10.6).

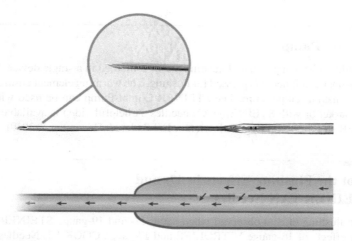

FIGURE 10.4 STEINER-TAN needle. For further information, please see the animation available on YouTube using the key words: Steiner computer animation.

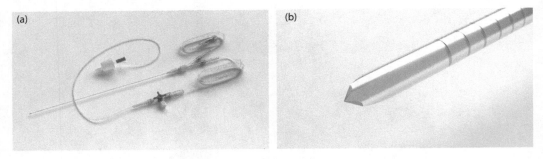

FIGURE 10.5   (a) STEINER-TAN needle: 17-, 19-, and 21-gauge quasi-DL, all with three-way stopcocks located close to the silicone stopper, to be used with a *special* needle guide (b). *Note*: Optimal back bevel angle.

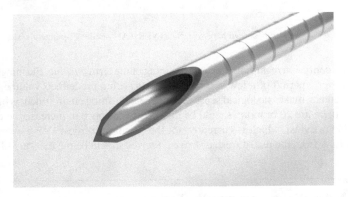

FIGURE 10.6   STEINER-TAN Needle CLASSIC. Dead space length of needle (can be used with *any* needle guide).

STEINER Mechanical Flushing Pump

By activating the pedal, the physician can choose the velocity and amount of the flushing fluid by pressing a pedal with his or her foot. The warming element ensures that the flushing fluid is held at a constant temperature. This pump can be used with any DL needle available on the market or with STEINER-TAN needles.

STEINER Combi Pump

This is an electronic aspiration pump and flushing pump combined in a single device. The right pedal is pressed for aspiration; the left pedal is pressed for flushing. The warming element ensures that the flushing fluid is held at a constant temperature. The STEINER Combi Pump can be used with any DL needle available on the market or with STEINER-TAN needles. A helpful video is available on YouTube with the title "STEINER Combi Pump Egg Collection in IVF" (dated: December 7, 2019).

Comparison of the Flushing Effects in 17- and 19-Gauge STEINER-TAN Needles

We compared the flushing effects observed when using 17- and 19-gauge STEINER-TAN SL needles as to the flushing effects of 16-gauge VITROLIFE and 17-gauge COOK DL Needles (Figure 10.7). In order to obtain comparable results, we used the flushing line for aspiration. The comparison was carried out under conditions of constant vacuum (120 mm Hg), and an aspiration time of 20 seconds was used.

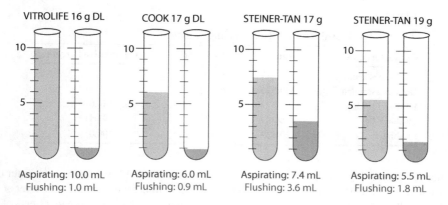

VITROLIFE 16 g DL   COOK 17 g DL   STEINER-TAN 17 g   STEINER-TAN 19 g

Aspirating: 10.0 mL   Aspirating: 6.0 mL   Aspirating: 7.4 mL   Aspirating: 5.5 mL
Flushing: 1.0 mL   Flushing: 0.9 mL   Flushing: 3.6 mL   Flushing: 1.8 mL

FIGURE 10.7   Comparison of the flushing effect in 17- and 19-gauge STEINER-TAN needles.

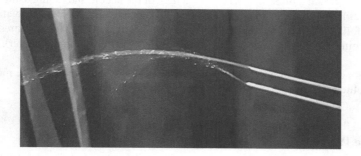

FIGURE 10.8   Comparison of flow characteristics between two needles: Upper needle: 17-gauge STEINER-TAN; lower needle: COOK 17-gauge DL. No linear flow was observed for the COOK 17-gauge DL due to technical characteristics of the needle. (For further information, please see the videos available on YouTube using the key words: Steiner, flushing.)

The 17-gauge STEINER-TAN SL needle demonstrated a nearly fourfold higher flushing capacity as compared to the 17-gauge COOK or 16-gauge VITROLIFE DL needles. The flushing capacity of the 19-gauge STEINER-TAN SL needle was twice that of the COOK DL 17-gauge and VITROLIFE DL 16-gauge needles. The flow characteristics for these needles were also compared and found to be extremely different (Figure 10.8).

How to Categorize the Flushing Effects of Different Needles

Before choosing to adopt a new needle technology, a flushing check can be easily performed so that an optimal decision can be made.

Empirical Flushing Check for Any SL or DL Needle
    A horizontal flow of at least 15–20 cm is created using a 50 cc syringe filled with water (upper needle), ensuring that the collapsed follicle (diameter 18–20 mm) will be refilled (flushed) within approximately 5 seconds.

Pilot Study of Flushing versus Not Flushing Follicles

We conducted the first comparative study worldwide on the effects of flushing or not flushing follicles, with the primary goal to examine the flushing effects using a single needle with a single follicle. Studies that had been conducted previously had always compared the flushing effects of different needles and not

TABLE 10.1

Pilot Study—Flushing versus Not Flushing Follicles

Characteristics	Number	Percent (%)	Cumulative Percentage
No oocytes aspirated	204/543	(37.6)	
Oocytes aspirated	339/536	(62.4)	
Without flushing	152/339	(44.8)	(44.6)
Flushing 2×	158/339	(46.6)	(91.4)
Flushing 4×	29/339	(8.6)	(100.0)

nonflushing versus flushing per se. We used an 18-gauge STEINER-TAN needle with an outer diameter of 1.2 mm and an inner diameter of 0.8 mm, as well as 90 cm of tubing with an inner diameter of 1.5 mm. Because the needle had a dead space of needle of only 7 cm, it was possible to compare effects of flushing versus not flushing the follicle with a single needle for the first time. After the follicle had collapsed, it was possible to flush the proximal three-quarters of the length of the needle and tubing using a gentle flushing method without refilling follicle using this STEINER-TAN needle. At the same time, the aspiration was turned on. Each follicle was aspirated and flushed quasi-selectively (16). We punctured 543 follicles in 31 patients (averaging 17.5 follicles per patient, DM of follicles were 10 mm and larger), and 339 oocytes were aspirated.

Table 10.1 shows the results of the study: the number of oocytes retrieved could be more than doubled by flushing the follicle two times.

Case Report—Ultrasoft Stimulation IVF: Ovarian Hyperstimulation Syndrome Free IVF in Future PCO Patients?

Patients with polycystic ovary syndrome (PCO) are one of most important challenges in assisted reproductive technology (ART) due to the high incidence of severe side effects like ovarian hyperstimulation syndrome (OHSS). This case report demonstrates how we can perhaps avoid this sometimes life-threatening complication for our patients.

The patient was aged 29 years, with severe PCO, anti-Müllerian hormone (AMH) 7.5 ng/mL right ovary approximately 50, left ovary at least 30 antral follicles.

Treatment was as follows: (**Previous cycle**: Oral contraceptive)

Cycle day 3: 150 Mikrogramm Elonva (Corifollitropin alfa)

Day 9: 1. Egg Collection: Canceling egg collection after aspiration and flushing half of follicles at right ovary due to sporadic granulosa cells only and 3 retrieved immature oocytes (1 M I, 2× GV)

Evening of day 9: Agonist triggering ovulation with 2 Amp. DECAPEPTYL 0.1 mg/1 mL (100 Mikrogramm Triptorelinacetat)

Day 11: 2. Egg Collection: 36 hours after agonist trigger. Out of both ovaries 16 oocytes, <u>13 MII for intracytoplasmic sperm injection (ICSI)</u>.

(**Result of 1. Egg collection**: 1× *in vitro* maturation (IVM) ICSI after 24 hours IVM: 1× 3PN
Result of 2. Egg Collection: out of 13× ICSI on day of Egg Collection: 10× 2PN)

Day 5: 5 Blastocysts

Day 6: 2 more Blastocysts

Freeze-all policy due to unsynchronized endometrium.

Egg Collection Technique as follows: Under mild sedation, STEINER-TAN needle 19-gauge for flushing two times each follicle, STEINER Scraper (110° automatically rotating "scraping" movement of needle during aspiration). Please watch YouTube video STEINER Scraper.

Hypothesis: Using Corifollitropin 150 as the only medication for ultrashort stimulation in PCO patients in combination with early "triggering ovulation" with agonist using flare-up effect of pituitary gland

and freeze-all policy is a promising solution in order to avoid any degree of OHSS. Alternatively, in countries where Elonva is not yet approved by the food and drug regulatory agency: recombinant follicle-stimulating hormone 150 from day 3 until day 8.

This case report of ultrasoft stimulation IVF with 7 blastocysts out of 10 fertilized oocytes should be the trigger to replace conventional IVF and IVM in PCO patients in the future and should inspire further studies.

Conclusion

Through extensive practical experience and scientific research, we can conclude that physicians working in the field of IVF should focus on developing new reproductive technologies and products to improve the pregnancy rates of the clients.

Vaughn et al. (17) stated that IVF physicians can increase cumulative pregnancy rates (from fresh and frozen cycles) in IVF by 8% with every additional egg harvested. This finding is noteworthy and should encourage all physicians working in this field to invest efforts in optimizing the percentage of harvested eggs/follicles by exploring such technological advances. Physicians should critically rethink the standard egg collection technique used in their clinics and use optimized egg collection systems, rather than investing more money in technologies that have not been shown to improve the clinical pregnancy rate. In the words of Albert Einstein, "We cannot solve our problems with the same level of thinking that created them."

Disclosure

The author of this chapter founded the company IVFETFLEX.COM with the brand name *IVF-future* to develop and market the optimized egg collection technology mentioned in this chapter.

Addendum

Protocol for Economic Flushing Medium

Note: Pre-warm overnight in an incubator.

Version (a)

500 mL Minimum Essential Medium (MEM) with Earle's Balanced Salts with L-glutamine
VWR (0043 1 97002444) Art. L0415–500
0.5 mL penicillin G-natrium, 1 MEGA IE
(amp. with 5 mL dissolved in aqua bidest; use 0.5 mL and the remainder can be frozen in portions)
0.125 mL heparin immuno 5000 I.E./mL (pharmacy)
11 mL aqua bidest
L-glutamine, penicillin, heparin, and sterile aqua bidest are combined, filtered, and mixed with MEM.

Version (b)
500 mL NaCl + 0.125 mL heparin

REFERENCES

1. Steptoe PC, Edwards RG. Laparoscopic recovery of preovulatory human oocytes after priming of ovaries with gonadotrophins. *Lancet*. 1970;1(7649):683–9.
2. Lenz S, Lauritsen JG, Kjellow M. Collection of human oocytes for *in vitro* fertilisation by ultrasonically guided follicular puncture. *Lancet*. 1981;1(8230):1163–4.

 3. Gleicher N, Friberg J, Fullan N, Giglia RV, Mayden K, Kesky T, Siegel I. Egg retrieval for *in vitro* fertilisation by sonographically controlled vaginal culdocentesis. *Lancet.* 1983;2(8348):508–9.
 4. Wikland M, Enk L, Hamberger L. Transvesical and transvaginal approaches for the aspiration of follicles by use of ultrasound. *Ann N Y Acad Sci.* 1985;442:182–94.
 5. Brinsden PR, Rainsbury PA. (editors.) *In Vitro Fertilization and Assisted Reproduction.* New York, NY: Parthenon Publishing Group; 1992.
 6. Scott RT, Hofmann GE, Muasher SJ, Acosta AA, Kreiner DK, Rosenwaks Z. A prospective randomized comparison of single- and double-lumen needles for transvaginal follicular aspiration. *J In Vitro Fert Embryo Transf.* 1989;6(2):98–100.
 7. Kingsland CR, Taylor CT, Aziz N, Bickerton N. Is follicular flushing necessary for oocyte retrieval? A randomized trial. *Hum Reprod.* 1991;6(3):382–3.
 8. Waterstone JJ, Parsons JH. A prospective study to investigate the value of flushing follicles during transvaginal ultrasound-directed follicle aspiration. *Fertil Steril.* 1992;57(1):221–3.
 9. Knight DC, Tyler JP, Driscoll GL. Follicular flushing at oocyte retrieval: A reappraisal. *Aust N Z J Obstet Gynaecol.* 2001;41(2):210–3.
10. Levens ED, Whitcomb BW, Payson MD, Larsen FW. Ovarian follicular flushing among low-responding patients undergoing assisted reproductive technology. *Fertil Steril.* 2009;91(4 Suppl):1381–4.
11. Bagtharia S, Haloob AR. Is there a benefit from routine follicular flushing for oocyte retrieval? *J Obstet Gynaecol.* 2005;25(4):374–6.
12. Méndez Lozano DH, Fanchin R, Chevalier N, Feyereisen E, Hesters L, Frydman N, Frydman R. [The follicular flushing duplicate the pregnancy rate on semi natural cycle IVF] [Article in French]. *J Gynecol Obstet Biol Reprod (Paris).* 2007;36(1):36–41.
13. Reeves G. Letters to the editor. *J In Vitro Fert Embryo Transf.* 1989;6(6):353–4.
14. Sunkara SK, Rittenberg V, Raine-Fenning N, Bhattacharya S, Zamora J, Coomarasamy A. Association between the number of eggs and live birth in IVF treatment: An analysis of 400 135 treatment cycles. *Hum Reprod.* 2011;26(7):1768–74.
15. Steiner HP. Optimizing technique of follicular aspiration and flushing. In: Chávez-Badiola A, Allahbadia GN, editors. *Minimal Stimulation IVF—Milder, Mildest or Back to Nature.* New Delhi: Jaypee Brothers Medical Publishers; 2011: 98–102.
16. Schenk M, Huppertz B, Obermayer-Pietsch B, Kastelic D, Hörmann-Kröpfl M, Weiss G. Biobanking of different body fluids within the frame of IVF—A standard operating procedure to improve reproductive biology research. *J Assist Reprod Genet.* 2017;34(2):283–90.
17. Vaughan DA, Leung A, Resetkova N, Ruthazer R, Penzias AS, Sakkas D, Alper MM. How many oocytes are optimal to achieve multiple live births with one stimulation cycle? The one-and-done approach. *Fertil Steril.* 2017;107(2):397–404.

11

Use of Blastocyst Culture

Mohamed A. Aboulghar and Mona M. Aboulghar

Introduction

In vitro fertilization (IVF) and intracytoplasmic sperm injection (ICSI) have become procedures used throughout the world and are expanding for the treatment of female and male subfertility. It is well recognized that assisted reproductive technology (ART) is associated with higher fetal and maternal risks. The first IVF pregnancy was achieved after day 2 embryo transfer (1). Since then, scientific research continued to improve the outcome of IVF. Improvement of ovarian stimulation using gonadotropin-releasing hormone agonist (GnRHa) (2) or GnRh-antagonist (3) protocols helped to increase pregnancy rates. Modification of embryo transfer techniques and development of softer catheters were steps forward toward better results (4). The improvement of laboratory standards and modifications of the culture media helped to achieve high-quality embryos (5).

Sequential media was developed for extended culture to develop blastocyst transfer (6), and later, single culture media was used to achieve culture to blastocyst (7). During the past decade, there was an increased trend for conducting embryo transfer at the blastocyst stage. Advantages and possible increased risks of extended culture were evaluated by several studies with some controversial data (8).

Many centers worldwide are culturing embryos up to the blastocyst stage. In the United Kingdom, 34% of embryos were transferred at the blastocyst stage (8). Extended culture was created with the objective of obtaining the best available embryos for transfer (9). The regulatory bodies were pushing for the routine single embryo transfer whenever feasible (10). The objective was to avoid multiple pregnancies with the accompanying serious maternal and fetal complications, which resulted in a heavy burden on health-care budgets (11).

Why Extend Culture to Blastocyst?

Extended culture allowed embryo transfer at the stage of blastocyst, which was believed to result in higher pregnancy rates (12). The development of a blastocyst encouraged clinicians to transfer one embryo, which satisfied the request of the regulatory bodies to avoid multiple pregnancies.

Blastocyst transfer is considered advantageous because it mimics the natural physiology of a blastocyst reaching the uterine cavity on days 5–6; hence, it may provide better embryo-endometrium synchrony. This may increase implantation rates (13).

One additional advantage is that the extended culture to blastocyst means that the activation of the embryonic genome at the eight-cell stage was successfully achieved, which assures the IVF team that they are transferring an embryo with high probability of implantation (14).

In Vitro Fertilization/Intracytoplasmic Sperm Injection Outcome after Blastocyst Transfer

The first prospective randomized study of infertile women (below 36 years) comparing embryo transfer (ET) at cleaved embryo versus blastocyst transfer showed significantly higher pregnancy and delivery rates after the blastocyst stage; 32% versus 21.6% (relative risk [RR] 1.48, 95% confidence interval [CI] 1.04–2.11) (14). Several randomized studies showed no difference in clinical pregnancy rate between day 3 and day 5 embryo transfer (6,15).

In a Cochrane review that included 18 studies, it was found that there is a significant increase in the live birth rate in blastocyst versus cleaved embryo transfer. These results are only valid in young patients with good prognoses with higher numbers of eight-cell embryos on day 3 (16). Table 11.1 lists randomized studies comparing pregnancy rate and live birth rate in cleaved versus blastocyst embryo transfers.

A Cochrane review comparing blastocyst and cleavage embryo transfer (17) which included 12 randomized controlled trials (RCTs) including 1510 women, reported higher live birth rates after blastocyst transfer (odds ratio [OR] 1.40, 95% CI 1.13–1.74) but reported that cumulative pregnancy rates were significantly higher in cleavage stage (OR 1.59, 95% CI 1.11–2.25). However, in the update

TABLE 11.1

Randomized Studies Comparing Pregnancy Rate and Live Birth Rate in Cleaved versus Blastocyst Embryo Transfers

Authors	Study Type	Clinical Pregnancy Rate	Live Birth Rate	Comments
Utsunomiya et al. (15)	RCT 480 women	Ongoing pregnancy rate no significant difference 29.2% versus 29%		
Papanikolaou et al. (12)	RCT 351	Significantly higher in blastocyst $P = .02$	Significantly higher in blastocyst 32% versus 21.6% (RR 1.48; 95% CI 1.04–2.11)	
Blake et al. (16)	Cochrane review of 18 RCTs		In 9 RCTs significantly higher LBR in blastocyst (OR 1.35, 95% CI 1.05–1.74)	Young patients with good prognoses
Glujovsky et al. (17)	Cochrane review 1510 women 23 studies, 12 RCT reported LBR	OR 1.14; 95% CI 0.99–1.32 No significance	Significantly higher LBR in cleaved embryo transfer Blastocyst ET significantly higher LBR (OR 1.4, 95% CI 1.13–1.74)	
Aziminekoo et al. (9)	RCT 118 women	No significant difference in clinical PR 33/3% in blastocyst versus 27.9% $P = .519$		
Glujovsky et al. (19)	Cochrane review 275 RCT 4031 women	OR 1.3, 95% CI 1.14–1.47	LBR higher in blastocyst transfer OR 1.48, 95% CI 1.20–1.82 Cumulative pregnancy rate 0.89, 95% CI 0.64–1.22 (no significant difference)	Low-quality evidence; more cryo embryos at cleaved stage; more cycles of blastocysts with no transfers
Martins et al. (20,30)	Meta-analysis 12 studies 1200 women	No significant difference (0.89, 95% CI 0.67–1.16)	No significant difference (RR 1.11, 0.95% CI 0.92–1.35)	

Abbreviations: CI, confidence interval; LBR, live birth rate; OR, odds ratio; RCT, randomized controlled trial; RR, relative risk.

of the same review, there was no significant difference in the cumulative pregnancy rate between the two groups.

In a small randomized study that included 118 infertile women, there was no significant difference between blastocyst and cleaved embryo transfer (9). In a retrospective study comparing blastocyst versus cleaved embryo transfer, the live birth rate was significantly lower in the cleaved embryo transfer (31.3% and 37.8%), $P = .041$. The cumulative live birth rates were 52.6% for cleaved stage versus 52.5% for blastocyst stage ($P = .989$) (18).

In a recent Cochrane review that included 27 randomized studies (4031 women) (19), the live birth rate following fresh embryo transfer was shown to be higher in the blastocyst stage (OR 1.48, 95% CI 1.20–1.82). The researchers concluded that if 29% of women achieved live birth after the fresh cleavage stage, between 32% and 42% will achieve live birth after blastocyst transfer. The authors stated that the difference between live birth rates was low-quality evidence. It also showed that there are more embryos cryopreserved after the cleavage stage as compared to the blastocyst stage. Failure to transfer any embryos was higher in the blastocyst stage (OR 2.50, 95% CI, 1.76–3.55). The conclusion of the Cochrane review was that there is low-quality evidence for higher live births after blastocyst transfer; however, there was no evidence of a difference between the two groups in cumulative pregnancy rates after a one-cycle retrieval (OR 0.89, 95% CI 0.64–1.22).

The most recent systematic review and meta-analysis of blastocyst versus cleavage-stage embryo transfer included 12 studies including 1200 women undergoing blastocyst transfer and 1218 undergoing cleavage transfer (20). There was no significant difference in the live birth rate between blastocyst and cleaved embryos (RR 1.11, 95% CI 0.92–1.35). There was also no significant difference between the two groups in the cumulative pregnancy rate (0.89, 95% CI 0.67–1.16).

A recent large study included 388 women, 38 years or younger who were undergoing IVF with more than three oocytes fertilized on day 1 after oocyte collection. Patients were randomized to blastocyst versus cleavage-stage transfer. There was no significant difference between the clinical pregnancy rate per started cycle between both groups (36.06% for blastocyst versus 38.66% for cleaved embryos) (21).

In routine practice, many IVF centers continue culture to the blastocyst stage if there are four or more good-quality cleaved embryos. So, patients with poor prognoses are excluded from extended culture and blastocyst transfer. In several cycles, extended culture will not result in a blastocyst, and the embryo transfer is canceled. But, as *in vitro* culture conditions are different from those *in vivo*, cleaved day-3 embryos may fail to reach the blastocyst stage at *in vitro* culture media. The same embryo may survive and proceed normally in *in vivo* conditions.

No clear data are available in the literature to show the number of embryos that failed to reach the blastocyst stage in *in vitro* culture. Again, any figure will not represent accurate data, because only patients with good prognoses are selected to extended culture in real practice.

Type of Media and Extended Culture

Culture of preimplantation-stage embryos has always been a key element of laboratory embryology and has contributed substantially to the success of many assisted reproduction procedures. In spite of the scientific and commercial challenge stimulating research worldwide to optimize embryo culture conditions, a consensus is missing even in the basic principles, including composition and exchange of media, the required physical and biological environment, and even the temperature of incubation. Although some researchers suppose that the efficiency of the presently applied *in vitro* culture systems has already approached the biological limits, the authors are confident that substantial improvements may be achieved that may considerably expand the possibilities of future assisted reproduction in humans (22).

In a large prospective study, continuous embryo culture elicits higher blastulation but similar cumulative delivery rates similar to that of sequential media (23).

A Cochrane review (24) included 32 studies: 17 studies of randomized women (total 3666), 3 randomized cycles (total 1018), and 12 randomized oocytes (over 15,230). It was not possible to pool any of the data because each study compared different culture media. Only seven studies reported live birth or ongoing pregnancy. Four of these studies found no evidence of a difference between the media compared, for either day 3 or day 5 embryo transfer. Most studies (22/32) failed to report their source of funding, and none described their methodology in adequate detail. The overall quality of the evidence was rated as very low for nearly all comparisons. The authors' conclusions were that an optimal embryo culture medium is important for embryonic development and, subsequently, the success of IVF or ICSI treatment. There has been much controversy about the most appropriate embryo culture medium. Numerous studies have been performed, but no two studies compared the same culture media, and none of them found any evidence of a difference between the culture media used. We conclude that there is insufficient evidence to support or refute the use of any specific culture medium. Properly designed and executed randomized trials are necessary.

A meta-analysis evaluated if single medium is better than sequential medium at improving ongoing pregnancy rates in patients undergoing ART procedures. The data were extracted from randomized studies. The primary endpoint was ongoing pregnancy rate. There was no significant difference between single and sequential mediums for clinical pregnancy (RR = 1.09; 95% CI = 0.83–1.44; P = .530, ongoing pregnancy (RR = 1.11, 95% CI = 0.87–1.40; P = .39), or miscarriage rates (RR = 0.89; 95% CI = 0.44–1.81, P = .74). No significant difference was found for ongoing pregnancy rates between single or sequential media. The authors concluded that the choice of embryo culture approach did not affect the ongoing pregnancy rates (25).

An RCT of low 5% versus 2% ultra-low oxygen for extended culture was performed using embryos donated for research. Embryos in the 2% group were less likely to arrest at the cleavage stage and more likely to blastulate (26).

A prospective study underwent embryo culture in either continuous single-culture media (CSCM, n = 972) or sequential media (Quinn's Advantage, n = 514), respectively. ICSI, blastocyst culture in either standard (MINC) or undisturbed (Embryoscope) incubation, transfer, and pregnancy follow-up were performed. Subanalyses and logistic regression corrected for confounders were performed. Continuous embryo culture resulted in a higher overall blastocyst rate per inseminated oocyte than sequential (n = 2211/5841, 37.9% versus 1073/3216, 33.4%; p < .01). However, the cumulative delivery rates per ended cycle (i.e., delivery achieved or no blastocyst produced or left; greater than 90%) were comparable in the two groups (n = 244/903, 27.0% versus 129/475, 27.2%). The neonatal outcomes were similar. Continuous culture involves better embryological but similar clinical outcomes than sequential. This large prospective study supports the absence of clinical disparity among the two approaches (23).

Embryos were randomly allocated into two study arms to compare embryo development on a time-lapse system using a single-step medium or sequential media. The percentage of day 5 good-quality blastocysts was 21.1% SD ± 21.6 and 22.2% SD ± 22.1 in the single-step time-lapse medium (G-TL) and the sequential media (G-1/G-2) groups, respectively. Single-step culture medium supports blastocyst development equivalently to established sequential media (27).

A prospective randomized study compared two commercially available types of human embryo culture media: G1-PLUS/G2-PLUS sequential medium (Vitrolife) and the GL BLAST sole medium; there was no significant difference when comparing patients divided into higher and lower fertility age. No significant statistical difference was noted between the fertilization rates (P = .59), cleavage (P = .91), evolution to blastocyst (P = .33), and total pregnanciesy (P = .83) when comparing the embryos cultured in the different media analyzed (28).

In a meta-analysis and a systematic review, no differences were observed between single and sequential media for either ongoing pregnancy per randomized woman (RR = 0.9, 95% CI = 0.7–1.3); or clinical pregnancy per randomized woman (RR = 1.0, 95% CI = 0.7–1.4); or miscarriage per clinical pregnancy (RR = 1.3, 95% CI = 0.4–4.3). The overall quality of the evidence was very low. Although using a single medium for extended culture has some practical advantages, and blastocyst formation rates appear to be higher, there is insufficient evidence to recommend either sequential or single-step media as being superior for the culture of embryos to days 5/6. Future studies comparing these two media systems in well-designed trials should be performed (29).

Problems of Extended Culture and Blastocyst Transfer

Culture media differ in composition, and incubators differ in their O_2 and CO_2 tension and prolonged culture may create genetic and epigenetic changes in the embryo. Recent data showed that transfer on blastocyst stage could be associated with higher pregnancy and neonatal risks.

Extended embryo culture to the blastocyst stage provides some theoretical advantages and disadvantages, while it promotes embryo self-selection, it also exposes those embryos to possible harm due to the *in vitro* environment (30). Table 11.2 summarizes complications of blastocyst transfers.

Premature Birth after Blastocyst Transfer

After adjusting for confounding factors, the risk of preterm birth was significantly greater after blastocyst-stage than after cleaved-stage transfer (31). IVF pregnancies after blastocyst transfer were associated with a higher incidence of premature births (RR 1.27, 95% CI 1.22–1.31) and very preterm births (RR 1.22, 95% CI 1.10–1.35) as compared to cleaved-stage embryos (32). The preterm birth rate was higher with blastocyst transfer versus day 3 transfer (17.2 versus 14.1% = <0.001) (33).

In a systematic review and meta-analysis including six observational studies, there was a significantly higher risk of premature labor (OR 1.32, 95% CI 1.19–1.46) in the blastocyst arm as compared to cleaved embryo transfer (33). In another systematic review and meta-analysis, it was found that blastocyst transfer was associated with premature births (less than 37 weeks) and very preterm births (less than 32 weeks) (30).

In a retrospective, population-based study including 5078 infants after ART, among singletons, there was no significant difference in the odds of preterm birth between blastocyst- and cleavage-stage embryo transfer. Among twins, the crude rates of preterm birth were similar after blastocyst and cleavage-stage embryo transfer. The authors stated that in contrast with the findings from a number of other studies, blastocyst culture in Australia and New Zealand is not associated with increased risk of preterm, low birth weight, or small for gestational age infants. They suggested future studies to assess the long-term outcome of cultures and possible adverse outcomes (34).

In a population-based registry study including IVF singleton deliveries after blastocyst transfer from 2002 through 2013 and cross-linked with the Swedish Medical Birth Registry, deliveries after blastocyst transfer were compared with deliveries after cleaved-stage transfer and deliveries after spontaneous conception. There were 4819 singleton deliveries after blastocyst transfer; 25,747 after cleaved-stage transfer; and 1,196,394 after spontaneous conception. Blastocyst transfer was associated with a higher

TABLE 11.2

Complications of Blastocyst Transfer

Complication	Significance	Reference
Higher preterm labor	RR 1.27, 95% CI (1.22–1.31)	Ginström et al. (35) Källen et al. (31)
Higher very preterm birth	RR 1.22 95% CI (1.10–1.35)	Ginström et al. (35)
Increased monozygotic twinning	2.5% versus 1.71%	Franasiak et al. (37) Kanter et al. (36)
Increased weight of baby	Questionable possibility	Martins et al. (20,30) Kaartinen et al. (41)
Increased perinatal morbidity	OR 1.61; 95% CI (1.14–2.29)	Ginström et al. (35)
Increased incidence of placenta previa	OR 2.08; 95% CI (1.7–2.55)	Ginström et al. (35)
Increased incidence of placental abruption	OR 1.62; 95% CI (1.15–2.29)	Ginström et al. (35)

Abbreviations: CI, confidence interval; OR, odds ratio; RR, relative risk.

Note: There is a higher cancellation rate of embryo transfer in blastocyst culture due to a failure of reaching blastocyst stage, but the incidence is not calculated in the literature.

risk of premature births (OR, 1.17; 95% CI 1.05–1.31) as compared to the spontaneous pregnancy group but not to the cleaved embryo transfer group (35).

Monozygotic Twinning

The incidence of monozygotic twinning after single embryo transfer was lower for day 2–3 transfer (1.71%, 95% CI 1.45–1.98, $n = 162$) than for day 5–6 transfer (2.5%, 95% CI 2.28–2.74; $n = 472$) (36). Franasiak et al. (37) reported 99 monozygotic twins in the cleaved stage (1.9%) and 135 monozygotic twins in the blastocyst transfer group (2.4%). The difference was significant. Mateize et al. (38) reported that the blastocyst transfer was associated with a significant increase in monozygotic twins (OR 2.70; 95% CI 1.36–5.34).

A meta-analysis has shown that monozygotic twin is increased after transfer at the blastocyst stage (39).

Weight of the Baby

There is a controversy concerning the weight of the baby at birth after blastocyst and cleaved embryo transfer. There is a questionable possibility of increased large-for-gestational-age babies (40). Martins et al. (20) in a meta-analysis showed that blastocyst transfer results in a higher rate of large-for-gestational age births. The birth weight after fresh blastocyst transfer was significantly higher than that after transfer at the cleavage stage (41). Ginström (35) showed that blastocyst transfer had a lower birth weight as compared to cleavage transfer (OR 0.83; 95% CI 0.71–0.97).

Perinatal Mortalities

In a large population-based study, perinatal mortality was significantly higher after blastocyst transfer as compared to cleaved embryo transfer (OR 1.61; 95% CI, 1.14–2.29) (35). Similar results were obtained in several studies (30,42).

Congenital Malformation

Källen et al. (31) reported that blastocyst transfer resulted in a higher risk of congenital malformation after adjusting for confounding factors. A meta-analysis of two studies of 22,068 cleaved-stage and 4517 blastocyst-stage births (OR 1.29 95% CI 1.03–1.62) showed increased incidence of malformation (42). However, in a large population-based Swedish study, there was no increased risk of congenital malformation after blastocyst transfer (35).

Epigenetic Disturbances in *In Vitro* Cultured Gametes and Embryos: Implications for Human-Assisted Reproduction

The phenotypic consequences of any observed epigenetic differences between ART and non-ART groups remain largely unclear. The periconceptional period is critical not only for embryonal, placental, and fetal development, but also the outcome at birth; suboptimal *in vitro* culture conditions may also lead to persistent changes in the epigenome influencing disease susceptibilities later in life. Therefore, when considering the safety of human ART from an epigenetic point of view, our main concern should not be whether or not a few rare imprinting disorders are increased, but rather we must be aware of a functional link between interference with epigenetic reprogramming in very early development and adult disease.

Maternal Complications

The risks of placenta previa and placental abruption were higher after blastocyst transfers as compared to cleavage-stage transfer (OR, 2.08; 95% CI, 1.7–2.55) and (OR 1.62; 95% CI 1.15–2.29), respectively (35).

Conclusion

The live birth rate after fresh single embryo transfer was significantly higher in the blastocyst transfer as compared to cleaved embryos; however, the evidence is controversial and was considered to be low quality.

The higher-quality randomized studies and the meta-analysis comparing the live birth rate after blastocyst and cleaved embryos showed no significant difference in the cumulative pregnancy rate per one started cycle.

The question is, why do we continue extended culture to blastocyst? The key answer is the higher pregnancy rate in the fresh transfer; however, the cumulative pregnancy rate per one stimulated cycle is often ignored. By extending the culture of the embryos to the blastocyst stage, there is a risk of arrest of the embryos at any stage before reaching the blastocyst stage, and embryo transfer will be canceled. It is possible that if embryos were transferred at the cleavage stage, they may have survived *in vivo*. Finally, neonatal complications of the baby and maternal possible complications are often ignored. A possible explanation for the adverse perinatal outcome could be that extended culture may trigger genetic and epigenetic changes in the trophoectodermal cells that can lead to abnormal placentation (43).

REFERENCES

1. Steptoe PC, Edwards RG. Birth after the reimplantation of a human embryo. *Lancet.* 1978;2(8085):366.
2. Droesch K, Muasher SJ, Brzyski RG, Jones GS, Simonetti S, Liu HC, Rosenwaks Z. Value of suppression with a gonadotropin-releasing hormone agonist prior to gonadotropin stimulation for *in vitro* fertilization. *Fertil Steril.* 1989;51(2):292–7.
3. Devroey P, Aboulghar M, Garcia-Velasco J, Griesinger G, Humaidan P, Kolibianakis E, Ledger W, Tomás C, Fauser BC. Improving the patient's experience of IVF/ICSI: A proposal for an ovarian stimulation protocol with GnRH antagonist co-treatment. *Hum Reprod.* 2009;24(4):764–74.
4. Abou-Setta AM, Al-Inany HG, Mansour RT, Serour GI, Aboulghar MA. Soft versus firm embryo transfer catheters for assisted reproduction: A systematic review and meta-analysis. *Hum Reprod.* 2005;20:3114–21.
5. Swain JE, Carrell D, Cobo A, Meseguer M, Rubio C, Smith GD. Optimizing the culture environment and embryo manipulation to help maintain embryo developmental potential. *Fertil Steril.* 2016;105(3):571–87.
6. Gardner DK, Vella P, Lane M, Wagley L, Schlenker T, Schoolcraft WB. Culture and transfer of human blastocyts increases implantation rates and reduces the need for multiple embryo transfers. *Fertil Steril.* 1998;69:84–8.
7. Sfontouris IA, Martins WP, Nastri CO, Viana IG, Navarro PA, Raine-Fenning N, van der Poel S, Rienzi L, Racowsky C. Blastocyst culture using single versus sequential media in clinical IVF: A systematic review and meta-analysis of randomized controlled trials. *J Assist Reprod Genet.* 2016;33(10):1261–72.
8. Maheshwari A, Hamilton M, Bhattacharya S. Should we be promoting embryo transfer at blastocyst stage? *Reprod Biomed Online.* 2016;32:142–6.
9. Aziminekoo E, Mohseni Salehi MS, Kalantari V, Shahrokh Tehraninejad E, Haghollahi F, Hossein Rashidi B, Zandieh Z. Pregnancy outcome after blastocyst stage transfer comparing to early cleavage stage embryo transfer. *Gynecol Endocrinol.* 2015;31(11):880–4.
10. Brison DR. Challenges imposed by scientific development in ART. *Hum Fertil.* 2005;8(2):93–6.
11. Crawford S, Boulet SL, Mneimneh AS, Perkins KM, Jamieson DJ, Zhang Y, Kissin DM. Costs of achieving live birth from assisted reproductive technology: A comparison of sequential single and double embryo transfer approaches. *Fertil Steril.* 2016;105(2):444–50.
12. Papanikolaou EG, Camus M, Kolibianakis EM, Van Landuyt L, Van Steirteghem A, Devroey P. *In vitro* fertilization with single blastocyst-stage versus single cleavage-stage embryos. *N Engl J Med.* 2006;354(11):1139–46.
13. Kolibianakis E, Bourgain C, Albano C, Osmanagaoglu K, Smitz J, Van Steirteghem A, Devroey P. Effect of ovarian stimulation with recombinant follicle-stimulating hormone, gonadotropin releasing hormone antagonists, and human chorionic gonadotropin on endometrial maturation on the day of oocyte pickup. *Fertil Steril.* 2002;78:1025–9.

14. Harton GL, Munne S, Surrey M, Grifo J, Kaplan B, McCulloch DH, Griffin DK, Wells D, PGD practitioners. Diminished effect of maternal age on implantation after pre-implantation genetic diagnosis with array comparative genomic hybridization. *Fertil Steril.* 2013;100:1695–703.

15. Utsunomiya T, Ito H, Nagaki M, Sato J. A prospective, randomized study: Day 3 versus hatching blastocyst stage. *Hum Reprod.* 2004;19(7):1598–603.

16. Blake DA, Farquhar CM, Johnson N, Proctor M. Cleavage stage versus blastocyst stage embryo transfer in assisted conception. *Cochrane Database Syst Rev.* 2007;17:CD002118.

17. Glujovsky D, Blake D, Farquhar C, Bardach A. Cleavage stage versus blastocyst stage embryo transfer in assisted reproductive technology. *Cochrane Database Syst Rev.* 2012;11(7):CD002118.

18. De Vos A, Van Landuyt L, Santos-Ribeiro S, Camus M, Van de Velde H, Tournaye H, Verheyen G. Cumulative live birth rates after fresh and vitrified cleavage stage versus blastocyst-stage embryo transfer in the first treatment cycle. *Hum Reprod.* 2016;31:2442–9.

19. Glujovsky D, Farquhar C, Quinteiro Retamar AM, Alvarez Sedo CR, Blake D. Cleavage stage versus blastocyst stage embryo transfer in assisted reproductive technology. *Cochrane Database Syst Rev.* 2016;30(6):CD002118.

20. Martins WP, Nastri CO, Rienzi L, van der Poel SZ, Gracia C, Racowsky C. Blastocyst versus cleavage stage embryo transfer: A systematic review and meta-analysis of the reproductive outcomes. *Ultrasound Obstet Gynecol.* 2017;49(5):583–91.

21. Levi-Setti PE, Cirillo F, Smeraldi A, Morenghi E, Mulazzani GEG, Albani E. No advantage of fresh blastocyst versus cleavage stage embryo transfer in women under the age of 39: A randomized controlled study. *J Assist Reprod Genet.* 2018;35(3):457–65.

22. Vajta G, Rienzi L, Cobo A, Yovich J. Embryo culture: Can we perform better than nature? *Reprod Biomed Online.* 2010;20:453–69.

23. Cimadomo D, Scarica C, Maggiulli R, Orlando G, Soscia D, Albricci L, Romano S, Sanges F, Ubaldi FM, Rienzi L. Continuous embryo culture elicits higher blastulation but similar cumulative delivery rates than sequential: A large prospective study. *J Assist Reprod Genet.* 2018;35(7):1329–38.

24. Youssef MM, Mantikou E, van Wely M, Van der Veen F, Al-Inany HG, Repping S, Mastenbroek S. Culture media for human pre-implantation embryos in assisted reproductive technology cycles. *Cochrane Database Syst Rev.* 2015;24(11):CD007876.

25. Dieamant F, Petersen CG, Mauri AL et al. Single versus sequential culture medium: Which is better at improving ongoing pregnancy rates? A systematic review and meta-analysis. *JBRA Assist Reprod.* 2017;21(3):240–6.

26. Kaser DJ, Bogale B, Sarda V, Farland LV, Williams PL, Racowsky C. Randomized controlled trial of low (5%) versus ultralow (2%) oxygen for extended culture using bipronucleate and tripronucleate human preimplantation embryos. *Fertil Steril.* 2018;109(6):1030–7.

27. Hardarson T, Bungum M, Conaghan J, Meintjes M, Chantilis SJ, Molnar L, Gunnarsson K, Wikland M. Noninferiority, randomized, controlled trial comparing embryo development using media developed for sequential or undisturbed culture in a time-lapse setup. *Fertil Steril.* 2015;104(6):1452–9.

28. Ceschin II, Ribas MH, Ceschin AP, Nishikawa L, Rocha CC, Pic-Taylor A, Baroneza JE. A prospective randomized study comparing two commercially available types of human embryo culture media: G1-PLUS™/G2-PLUS™ sequential medium (Vitrolife) and the GL BLAST™ sole medium (Ingamed). *JBRA Assist Reprod.* 2016;20(1):23–6.

29. Sfontouris IA, Martins WP, Nastri CO, Viana IG, Navarro PA, Raine-Fenning N, van der Poel S, Rienzi L, Racowsky C. Blastocyst culture using single versus sequential media in clinical IVF: A systematic review and meta-analysis of randomized controlled trials. *J Assist Reprod Genet.* 2016;33(10):1261–72.

30. Martins WP, Nastri CO, Rienzi L, van der Poel SZ, Gracia C, Racowsky C. Obstetrical and perinatal outcomes following blastocyst transfer compared to cleavage transfer: A systematic review and meta-analysis. *Hum Reprod.* 2016;31:2561–9.

31. Källen B, Finnstrom O, Lindam A, Nilsson E, Nygren KG, Olausson PO. Blastocyst versus cleavage stage transfer in *in vitro* fertilization: Differences in neonatal outcome? *Fertil Steril.* 2010;94:1680–3.

32. Maheshwari A, Kalampokas T, Davidson J, Bhattacharya S. Obstetric and perinatal outcomes in singleton pregnancies resulting from the transfer of blastocyst-stage versus cleavage-stage embryos generated through *in vitro* fertilization treatment: A systematic review and meta-analysis. *Fertil Steril.* 2013;100(6):1615–21.

33. Dar S, Librach CL, Gunby J et al. Increased risk of preterm birth in singleton pregnancies after blastocyst versus day 3 embryo transfer: Canadian ART register (CARTR) analysis. *Hum Reprod.* 2013;28:924–8.
34. Chambers GM, Chughtai AA, Farquhar CM, Wang YA. Risk of preterm birth after blastocyst embryo transfer: A large population study using contemporary registry data from Australia and New Zealand. *Fertil Steril.* 2015 Oct;104(4):997–1003.
35. Ginström Ernstad E, Bergh C, Khatibi A et al. Neonatal and maternal outcome after blastocyst transfer: A population-based registry study. *Am J Obstet Gynecol.* 2016;214:378.
36. Kanter JR, Boulet SL, Kawwass JF, Jamieson DJ, Kissin DM. Trends and correlates of monozygotic twinning after single embryo transfer. *Obstet Gynecol.* 2015;125:111–7.
37. Franasiak JM, Dondik Y, Molinaro TA et al. Blastocyst transfers is not associated with increased rates of monozygotic twins when controlling for embryo cohort quality. *Fertil Steril.* 2015;103:95–100.
38. Mateize I, Santos-Ribeiro S, Done E, Van Landuyt L, Van de Velde H, Tournaye H, Verheyen G. Do ARTs affect the incidence of monozygotic twinning? *Hum Reprod.* 2016;31(11):2435–41.
39. Hviid KVR, Malchau SS, Pinborg A, Nielsen HS. Determinants of monozygotic twinning in ART: A systematic review and a meta-analysis. *Hum Reprod Update.* 2018;24(4):468–83.
40. Zhu J, Lin S, Li M, Chen L, Lian Y, Liu P, Qiao J. Effect of *in vitro* culture period on birthweight of singleton newborns. *Hum Reprod.* 2014;29:448–54.
41. Kaartinen NM, Kananen KM, Rodriguez-Wallberg KA, Tomas CM, Huhtala HS, Tinkanen HI. Male gender explains increased birthweight in children born after transfer of blastocysts. *Hum Reprod.* 2015;30:2312–20.
42. Dar S, Lazer T, Shah PS, Librach CL. Neonatal outcomes among singleton births after blastocyst versus cleavage stage embryo transfer: A systematic review and meta-analysis. *Hum Reprod Update.* 2014;20:439–48.
43. Rizos D, Lonergan P, Boland MP, Arroyo-García R, Pintado B, de la Fuente J, Gutiérrez-Adán A. Analysis of differential messenger RNA expression between bovine blastocysts produced in different culture systems: Implications for blastocyst quality. *Biol Reprod.* 2002;66:589–95.

12

Use of Mitochondrial Donation

Andy Greenfield

Introduction

In February 2015, both houses of the UK Parliament voted to make lawful two assisted reproductive technologies (ARTs). Collectively known as mitochondrial donation (MD) or mitochondrial replacement, these techniques aim to prevent the transmission of a group of devastating, life-threatening diseases caused by abnormal DNA in the power-generating organelles of most cells, the mitochondria. This was a landmark legislative decision that attracted attention worldwide, not least due to the fact that the success of MD relies on alteration to the inheritable (germ line) components of an individual, i.e., eggs or embryos. Proponents pointed out that for *some* women blighted by mitochondrial disease, who wished to have a genetically related child free from the disease, there was no realistic alternative to MD. Moreover, preclinical data, scrutinized by an independent panel on three separate occasions, indicated that MD was not intrinsically unsafe, notwithstanding the interpretative limitations of preclinical data. Opponents responded in a number of ways, indicating that the desire for genetically related offspring was not in itself a "medical condition," and while being an important consideration, did not outweigh safety concerns associated with a first-in-human intervention. In addition, such alteration to the germ line might, they said, pave the way (or lower the activation barrier) to similar interventions with less worthy aims, i.e., a can of germ line worms might well be opened. Then, in 2017, during the ongoing establishment of a regulatory pathway for MD in the United Kingdom, a report appeared describing the birth of a baby boy in Mexico following MD to prevent mitochondrial disease transmission. The ramifications of this clinical use of MD—scientifically, ethically, legally, and politically—are not yet clear.

Here, the role of mitochondrial DNA (mtDNA) in normal and abnormal physiology and some of the unique characteristics of mtDNA inheritance are briefly introduced. Then, the science behind MD techniques is surveyed, and some of the concerns that have been raised in respect to safety and efficacy by preclinical experimentation in a number of contexts are discussed, followed by discussion of how these have been, or might be, resolved or negotiated in moving from the bench to the clinic. Finally, ethical concerns about MD and their relationship to broader concerns about germ line interventions in medicine are considered. Emphasis is placed on the importance of continued research and regulation in the ART sector, with an emphasis on the regulatory framework developed in the United Kingdom.

Mitochondrial DNA (mtDNA) and Mitochondrial Diseases

Oxidative phosphorylation, the process by which ATP is generated in the cell for use in energy-demanding reactions, occurs in mitochondria (1). It exploits a proton gradient across the inner mitochondrial membrane, generated by electron transport, and is an ancient way of utilizing oxygen for respiration. In this sense, the familiar metaphor of the mitochondrion as a cellular "battery" is incorrect, since batteries only store energy and do not generate it. The ancient origin of the mitochondrion as a free-living microorganism turned endosymbiont is revealed by the retention of an independent mitochondrial genome: mitochondrial DNA (mtDNA). This 16.5 kb circular DNA molecule encodes 37 genes (including 13 coding for polypeptides) required for oxidative phosphorylation, but apparently not for other cellular processes regulated by mitochondria, such as thermogenesis, programmed cell death (apoptosis), and steroid hormone biosynthesis. The vast majority of the approximately 1500 proteins comprising the mitochondrial proteome, which facilitate this wide range of mitochondrial functions, are encoded by nuclear genes (2).

Mutations in both nuclear DNA (nDNA) and mtDNA can result in defective mitochondria, incapable of normal oxidative phosphorylation; these can cause a range of heterogeneous, devastating diseases that mainly, but not exclusively, affect tissues with high energy requirements through aerobic metabolism, such as neural and muscle tissues (3). The prevalence of mitochondrial diseases caused by mutations in nDNA is estimated at 2.9 cases per 100,000 individuals, while that of mitochondrial diseases caused by mutations in mtDNA is 9.6 cases per 100,000 (4). These figures indicate an overall prevalence for mitochondrial disease of around 12–13 cases per 100,000. Elevated mutation rates of mtDNA are thought to arise from oxidative damage to DNA caused by reactive oxidative species produced in mitochondria. Mitochondrial diseases can occur at any age and manifest with a wide range of symptoms. The clinical features, including severity, of mtDNA-dependent mitochondrial diseases (see Table 12.1 for examples of these) are highly variable and depend on a number of factors, including the nature of the mtDNA mutation, the proportion of the mtDNA that is pathogenic versus normal—often called the degree of heteroplasmy—and the particular tissue distribution of the abnormal mtDNA. Polymorphisms in mtDNA also allow it to be classified into distinct haplotypes and, at a population level, into haplogroups. There have been reports that distinct haplogroups might impact on the occurrence and severity of mtDNA-dependent mitochondrial disease (5,6).

The inheritance of mtDNA-based mitochondrial diseases differs from the familiar Mendelian pattern of those caused by mutations in nDNA. mtDNA transmission can be unpredictable, partly due to factors already mentioned, but also due to the nature of mtDNA's exclusive matrilineal inheritance. Sperm-borne mitochondria are eliminated following fertilization by mitophagy (7). Thus, mitochondrial DNA molecules

TABLE 12.1

Some Mitochondrial Diseases Caused by Point Mutations in Mitochondrial DNA

Condition Name	Abbreviation	Gene Mutation Examples	Comment
Leber hereditary optic neuropathy	LHON	*MT-ND1,4,4L, 6* m.3460G>A m.14484T>C m.11778G>A m.10663T>C	Male sex is associated with an increased risk of developing LHON
Mitochondrial encephalopathy with lactic acidosis and stroke-like episodes	MELAS	*MT-TL1* m.3243A>G	*MT-TL1* (m.3243A>G) can also cause CPEO (chronic progressive external ophthalmoplegia), LS, and MIDD
Leigh syndrome	LS	*MT-TV* m.1644G>T	Most common syndrome associated with childhood-onset mitochondrial diseases; can be caused by mutations in 75 different genes, including in nDNA
Myoclonic epilepsy with ragged red fibers	MERRF	*MT-TK* m.8344A>G	Other pathogenic variants in *MT-TF*, *MT-TL1*, *MT-TI*, and *MT-TP*
Maternally inherited diabetes and deafness	MIDD	*MT-TL1* m.3243A>G	Affects up to 1% of patients with diabetes
Neurogenic muscle weakness, ataxia, and retinitis pigmentosa	NARP	*MT-ATP6* m.8993T>G m.8993T>C	Often presents in early childhood; same mutations reported in Leigh syndrome, reflecting clinical continuity

Note: Mutations are described by reference to their position in the mtDNA molecule and the nature of the base change, e.g., m.3243A>G is an A to G transition at position 3243. Particular gene symbols are also sometimes given, e.g., *MT-TL1* refers to the mtDNA-encoded transfer RNA (leucine) 1. Further information on these diseases and associated mutations can be found in Gorman et al., 2016 (3) and at MITOMAP.org.

transmitted to the embryo are derived only from the oocyte, and numbers of these have been estimated to be as high as 500,000–1,000,000 (8,9). However, in human primordial germ cells (embryonic precursors of mature gametes), the amount of mtDNA is around 1000-fold less, and this is known as the *mitochondrial bottleneck* (8). The consequence of the bottleneck is an unpredictability of mitochondrial inheritance, akin to the skewing of ratios associated with multiple sampling of small numbers from a much larger population of variable objects. Thus, in the case of a woman with mtDNA heteroplasmy in her germ line, it is possible for the number of abnormal mitochondria to vary significantly from one oocyte to the next (10), a phenomenon known as *segregation*. This can result in children with highly variable symptoms within a single family.

Mitochondrial Donation: The Basics

There is no effective treatment for mitochondrial diseases, and so the focus has been on the prevention of transmission of pathogenic mtDNA. Women at risk of transmitting mitochondrial disease to their offspring have a number of options: (a) they can remain childless or (b) adopt; (c) they can opt for assisted reproduction using an egg donor (free of mitochondrial disease); or (d) they can choose assisted reproduction and use preimplantation genetic diagnosis (PGD) in an attempt to identify embryos with an acceptably low level of pathogenic mtDNA (11). This last option is suitable for a woman who wants to be genetically related to her offspring (in the standard way that biological mothers are related to their children). However, while PGD can identify the level of heteroplasmy in an embryo, it cannot ensure that embryos with acceptably low levels will be detected. If such embryos are identified, PGD may constitute an effective risk reduction strategy. However, for some women with high levels of heteroplasmy or homoplasmy (100% pathogenic mtDNA) in their germ line, PGD is not a viable strategy.

For the latter class of women, mitochondrial donation (MD) is now a lawful clinical option in the United Kingdom. The principle of MD is the transfer of nuclear genetic material from an oocyte or embryo (zygote) containing abnormal mitochondria to a corresponding oocyte or embryo containing normal mitochondria. In the United Kingdom, there are currently two techniques that can be lawfully performed in the clinic: maternal spindle transfer (MST, Figure 12.1) and pronuclear transfer (PNT, Figure 12.2). MST involves the transfer of the prospective mother's chromosomes, which are attached to the spindle

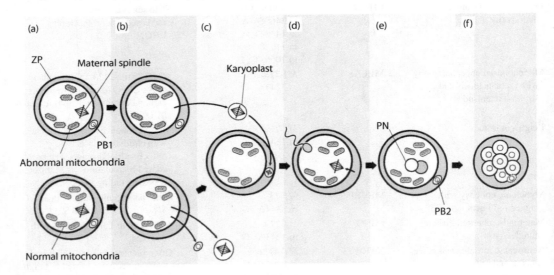

FIGURE 12.1   Methodology for maternal spindle transfer (MST). (a) The affected egg, surrounded by the zona pellucida (ZP), contains the maternal chromosomes on the spindle, and abnormal mitochondria. (b) The maternal spindle is transferred, within a karyoplast, from the affected egg to a donor egg containing normal mitochondria (c), from which the spindle (and the first polar body [PB1]) have been removed. (d) The reconstructed oocyte, containing mostly normal mitochondria, is fertilized, and pronuclei (PN) and the second polar body (PB2) are then produced (e). (f) Embryonic development proceeds (cleavage stage shown).

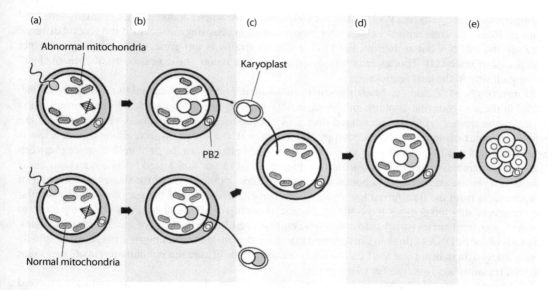

FIGURE 12.2 Methodology for pronuclear transfer (PNT). (a) The affected egg and donor egg are fertilized, generating pronuclei and a second polar body (PB2). (b) The pronuclei from the affected zygote are transferred, within a karyoplast, to the donor embryo (c), from which the pronuclei have been removed. (d) The reconstituted embryo now contains mostly normal mitochondria. (e) Development proceeds as normal.

of the metaphase II (MII)-arrested oocyte (egg), into a donor egg from which the maternal spindle has been removed. This requires transfer of the maternal spindle within a small piece of membrane-bound cytoplasm—the karyoplast. Thus, MST is a form of MII-arrested oocyte reconstruction, actually involving donation of all the constituents of the egg cytoplasm (ooplasm), including mitochondria, but excluding the donor's chromosomes. The reconstructed egg can then be fertilized and used to establish a pregnancy. Some have expressed a preference for MST over PNT because the former, unlike the latter, does not involve the intentional destruction of a fertilized human egg.

In the case of PNT, both the prospective mother's egg and that from a donor are fertilized by sperm from the intended biological father (see Figure 12.2). Once formed, the pronuclei of the fertilized donor egg are removed and discarded; these are then replaced by the pronuclei from the prospective mother's fertilized egg. As with MST, this process ensures that the nDNA of any embryo generated using PNT is genetically related to both the prospective mother and sperm provider in the standard manner of sexual reproduction. However, in the case of MST and PNT, the embryo in question will contain mitochondria predominantly derived from the donor oocyte, that is, normal mitochondria. The contribution of mtDNA from the oocyte donor has led to MD sometimes being known as "three-person IVF," or even "three-parent IVF," in the popular media. The former is a plausible description, since biological material from a third person, containing DNA, is employed by this IVF technique; the latter term, however, is at best misleading since it implies that the donated mtDNA automatically confers on the donor the status of a parent. But this is not a compulsory inference, at least not in any conventional sense of "parent." Of course, "parent" is somewhat polysemous, so caution is required here.

Mitochondrial Donation: Preclinical Assessments of Safety and Efficacy in Model Organisms

Mouse models have been an important tool in establishing the safety and efficacy of MD. PNT has been performed in mice since the mid-1980s, when it was first established that viable offspring were obtained following the transfer of fertilized egg pronuclei into enucleated parthenogenetic eggs (12). One set of experiments directly assessed whether PNT could be used to rescue respiration defects caused by a mtDNA deletion in offspring of the "mitomouse": the data indicated successful rescue (13). Most experimentation suggests that PNT is efficient and reproducible when conducted with normally fertilized zygotes. However, some reports indicate that abnormalities in offspring can occur if the genetic distance between the mtDNA donor and nuclear DNA recipient strains is too great, such as between distinct subspecies of mice (14). This topic is revisited during a discussion of the possibility of "mitonuclear" incompatibility in the next section.

More recently, MST has been investigated in the nonhuman primate *Macaca mulatta* (Rhesus macaque) (15). Unlike a zygote that contains pronuclei, a MII-arrested egg has no nucleus; thus, visualization of its chromosomes requires specialized optics. A successful protocol involved visualization of the spindle complex using polarized microscopy and its removal; the karyoplast containing the spindle was briefly exposed to a fusogen (Sendai virus extract) and then placed into the perivitelline space (between the oocyte membrane and zona pellucida [see Figure 12.1]) of an "enucleated" donor oocyte to allow fusion. Karyoplast and ooplasm donors were chosen to allow examination of the degree of carryover of mitochondria from the transferred karyoplast. Fertilization, cleavage, and blastocyst rates were similar between reconstructed oocytes and controls. Blastocyst quality of MST embryos was also comparable to controls, and pregnancies established using these embryos resulted in the birth of four healthy macaques. Analysis of the mtDNA of three infants showed that there was no detectable contribution from the spindle donor. These data indicate that MST can be safely and successfully used in a nonhuman primate to prevent mtDNA transmission from mother to offspring.

In summary, protocols for MD in animals have been developed over many years and have involved continual refinement to reduce the amount of carryover of mitochondria from the nuclear DNA donor (karyoplast-derived), to prevent premature activation of oocytes or abnormally fertilized oocytes and to optimize the micromanipulations to minimize harm to the reconstructed oocytes or zygotes—all factors that are important in the development of human MD for the clinic. It is also worth noting here that two other meiotic genome sources have also been tested in MD protocols in mice (and humans): the first and second polar bodies (16,17). There are advantages to the use of polar body transfer (PBT) techniques for MD over MST and PNT: polar bodies are "ready-made" karyoplasts for transfer of nuclear DNA and have comparatively low numbers of mitochondria associated with them (17,18). However, unlike MST and PNT, PBT techniques were not made lawful in the United Kingdom by the introduction of the mitochondrial donation regulations in 2016. Such techniques may, however, be the subject of future legislative changes in the United Kingdom, or other jurisdictions.

Mitochondrial Donation: Preclinical Assessments of Safety and Efficacy in Human Research Embryos

While data from mammalian model organisms are reassuring, suggesting that MD *can* be used safely and effectively, given the appropriate experimental design and micromanipulation skills, it is important to generate similar data in human model systems. Moreover, use of human material allows certain questions to be addressed in the context of the human mitochondrial and nuclear genomes and the genetic variation that is commonly found in these.

Initial studies using MST in human oocytes, followed either by fertilization (19) or parthenogenetic activation (20), suggested that MST was, following careful optimization to minimize risks of abnormal fertilization and aneuploidy, able to produce reconstructed eggs that were compatible with preimplantation embryo development to the blastocyst stage and, significantly, with low levels (below 1%) of mtDNA carryover from the transferred karyoplast. Similar data were generated by earlier use of PNT in abnormally fertilized human zygotes (9). More recently, there have been reports of further optimization of both MST and PNT in contexts that more closely resemble the likely clinical context in which they may be used (10,21,22). MST can be performed such that fertilization rates, aneuploidy rates, and blastocyst quality are comparable to controls (10,21). Careful optimization of the timing of PNT also generated blastocysts of comparable quality to controls, as evidenced by single-cell expression profiles (22). In each study, mtDNA carryover was low in cells sampled from the blastocyst, albeit that PNT appears to result in slightly higher levels, perhaps due to the volume of cytoplasm transferred with the pronuclei being larger than with MST.

In all three reports, there were also descriptions of additional experiments that were performed in an attempt to model the behavior of carried-over mtDNA in the context of postimplantation development, a reflection of the practical and legal limits on the length of time for which human research embryos can currently be cultured *in vitro*. These studies involved the derivation and culture of human embryonic stem (hES) cells derived from control and experimental embryos, with, in most cases, extensive passaging in order to determine whether initially low levels of carried-over mtDNA were maintained after multiple rounds of cell division, when mtDNA replication was likely to be a significant factor in determining overall levels. Each study reported a phenomenon that has come to be known as "reversion," in which a minority of the stem cell lines examined (approximately 15%–20%) exhibited an increase in the proportion (commonly to 100%) of carried-over mtDNA. Occasionally, the carried-over mtDNA behaved in an unstable fashion, returning to much lower levels after continued passaging. There is no consensus on the mechanism(s) accounting for reversion: the starting level of carried-over mtDNA was uniformly low in all reports, and there was no clear relationship between the occurrence of reversion and the extent of genetic diversity between the karyoplast- and donor-derived mtDNA haplogroups. As reported, reversion is an unexplained phenomenon affecting some stem cell lines *in vitro*: the most important unknown is whether it is an artefact of cell culture conditions or the unusual biology of human embryonic stem cells, or whether it might indicate the possibility of reversion *in utero* following clinical use of MD, characterized by the elevation of the levels of any carried-over pathogenic mtDNA in postimplantation embryos and fetuses. For this reason, the UK panel that assessed the safety and efficacy of MD in 2016, and reported to the Human Fertilisation and Embryology Authority (HFEA), recommended that all patients should be offered prenatal testing if they become pregnant following MST or PNT and that clinics offering MD should strongly encourage patients and their offspring to take part in long-term follow-up (23).

A number of publications have expressed concern that MD might disrupt functional interactions between mtDNA and the nuclear genome, which are required for normal mitochondrial function and homeostasis (24,25). The logic behind these concerns is essentially an evolutionary one: that mtDNA and nuclear genomes have coevolved to permit mitochondrial-nuclear (mitonuclear) interactions and that MD might place together mtDNA and nuclear gene combinations that have not previously been subject to negative selection and thus may have deleterious consequences. However, others think these concerns are unfounded and that abnormal mitonuclear interactions are unlikely to be any more prevalent in those born following MD than in those born following conventional reproduction (26,27). Some of the aforementioned reports of MD in human oocytes and zygotes describe attempts to assess whether any metabolic abnormalities could be detected in experimental embryos or cells derived from these: no such abnormalities were detected, and they all concluded that the outbred human genome can robustly interact with a variety of common mtDNA haplogroups, presumably reflecting the evolutionary success of such haplogroups. Nevertheless, the possibility of matching nuclear and mitochondrial donor mtDNA haplotypes/haplogroups when MD is used clinically has been suggested in order to mitigate or eliminate the risk of mitonuclear incompatibilities (23,28). It is worth noting, however, that making matching a requirement is likely to limit the availability of egg donors, especially in the case of rare haplogroups.

Regulating Mitochondrial Donation: The UK Journey

The UK regulatory journey, from the first application for an HFEA research license in 2004 by the Newcastle Fertility Centre at Life team, requesting permission to experiment with human embryos to assess the feasibility of PNT, through to the variation of that clinic's license to permit the use of MD in patients in March 2017, took 13 years. And there was extensive debate about the potential for MD for several years prior to 2004. The regulatory pathway was complex, involving four scientific reviews, by independent expert scientific panels, of MD safety and efficacy; the regular licensing of projects by the HFEA to permit ongoing research; consultations concerning public attitudes toward MD, organized by the HFEA and Sciencewise; and much discussion on ethics, policy, and design of a robust mechanism to allow HFEA regulation of MD (29). This mechanism involves two stages: (a) any clinic wishing to perform MD must demonstrate its competence in the relevant technique—these are very difficult embryological techniques to perform and are unlikely to ever be commonplace—and this demonstration would result in a variation to the clinic license, permitting MD to be performed; (b) patients must be approved on a *case-by-case* basis—only those for whom PGD is unlikely to be successful should be permitted at this stage. In addition, patients should be offered prenatal testing to assess levels of pathogenic mtDNA in the fetus. Finally, follow-up of children born following MD is strongly encouraged. In February 2018, applications by Newcastle to perform PNT on named patients with MERFF syndrome (Table 12.1) were approved by the HFEA.

Attitudes toward the ways in which MD regulation—from research to clinic—established in the United Kingdom are typically varied, with some applauding the meticulous nature of the regulatory pathway, others complaining about how long it took, and some making the accusation that the process was rushed or defective in some other way. Notwithstanding this diverse opinion, it is perhaps instructive to look at an alternative approach to introducing MD into the clinic before assessing the UK's approach. There have been two recent peer-reviewed reports of the use of MD to establish pregnancies. The first involved the use of PNT in the case of a 30-year-old nulligravid woman with unexplained infertility (30). The rationale of the intervention relies on the speculative hypothesis that mitochondrial deficiencies in the oocyte may cause infertility in some older women (31). The woman became pregnant following transfer of five embryos; a triplet pregnancy ensued that was surgically reduced to twins. But neither fetus survived beyond midgestation, probably due to obstetric complications of the multiple pregnancy. The fetuses lacked detectable mtDNA from the intended mother (i.e., pronuclei-associated mtDNA). Following this report, the use of MST was described in the case of a woman with Leigh syndrome (32). In this case, a live birth occurred following transfer of a single XY euploid embryo. The neonate had detectable pathogenic mtDNA in its tissues, ranging from 2.36% to 9.23%, but was reported to be healthy at 7 months. This case has been the subject of much discussion and criticism (33–35). It transpired that the embryo had been generated in the United States but the pregnancy had been established in Mexico, allegedly in an attempt to circumvent regulatory prohibitions on establishing the pregnancy in the United States—although its legality in the Mexican context has also been questioned (34). The UK regulation of MD, and IVF more generally, through the HFEA, appears to be a bastion of clarity and patient-centered wisdom when compared to these cases. The HFEA insists on clinics reducing their multiple pregnancy rate, aiming for 10%, and inspects clinics against this metric; it also does not permit MD as a speculative treatment for infertility. Moreover, the code of practice concerning MD prohibits any UK clinic from importing eggs or embryos that have undergone MD overseas. This means that any embryos generated by use of MD in the United Kingdom must be created in ways that are compliant with the HFEA Code of Practice, even if these are for subsequent export.

Finally, it is hoped that future uses of MD will first be reported in peer-reviewed journals. There have been instances of reports of the clinical use of MD in newspaper articles in advance of any peer-reviewed publication. This form of publicity is not especially helpful, since it results in a tendency to offer instantaneous assessment of the intervention, and an associated narrative concerning its significance, in the absence of the data that actually allow genuine assessment. This can lead to unrealistic expectations on behalf of prospective patients. MD publications should include full details of protocols used, and comprehensive clinical data, so that expert opinion can be formed on the basis of a complete evidence base. This sort of transparency, including provision of follow-up data, is vital.

Mitochondrial Donation: Ethical Considerations

Scrutiny of MD has not been limited to scientific and clinical assessments. While safety and efficacy have ethical dimensions, even a safe and efficacious MD technology is opposed by some. Here, are some of the ethical concerns about MD that have been expressed.

Safety and Efficacy

Offering an intervention that is neither safe nor efficacious would itself be unethical, so establishing the safety and efficacy of MD is undoubtedly important. In the United Kingdom, there were four independent panel reviews of MD safety between 2011 and 2016. At each stage, there was a direction of travel toward increasing satisfaction of the likely safety and efficacy of the methods. Of course, in such an exercise of using scientific evidence to inform policy, there will come a stage at which the question is: *safe enough*? This is to acknowledge the fact that a possible gap will always exist between the best inferences from preclinical data and actual outcomes of first-in-human clinical applications. It has been observed by some that no other innovation in ART has received the sort of scrutiny that MD has. But that observation is perhaps best interpreted as an implicit suggestion that other ART methodologies (including those now considered to be routine, in addition to more innovative and speculative "add-ons") could benefit from more, and better, scientific scrutiny through research.

The most contentious elements of MD from the perspective of safety and efficacy appear to be the risks that (a) carried-over pathogenic mtDNA might persist in the child at dangerous levels—perhaps due to a phenomenon analogous to the reversion seen *in vitro*; or that (b) mitonuclear interactions may be disrupted (see the section "Mitochondrial Donation: Preclinical Assessments of Safety and Efficacy in Human Research Embryos"). The expert panel reporting to the HFEA recommended that prenatal testing be offered to women who become pregnant following MD, as an acknowledgment of the risk of (a) and recommended that haplogroup/haplotype matching be considered due to (b). Moreover, given the additional risks associated with any first-in-human intervention, it is also recommended that MD be offered only to women for whom PGD is not a viable option, that is, for women who have consistently high levels of abnormal mtDNA in their oocytes. Like PGD, MD should currently be viewed as a risk-reduction strategy in these women, rather than a guaranteed way of preventing transmission of mitochondrial disease. These techniques require further refinements as they unfold in the clinic, the most significant of which would be to find a way to completely eliminate carryover of pathogenic mtDNA (36). This would eliminate any possibility of reversion and also avoid establishing significant heteroplasmy in MD offspring, which some reports, mostly based on experiments in mouse inbred strains, suggest should be avoided (21,37,38). But, given the strength of their desire to have genetically related children free of mitochondrial disease, and the possibility that some might simply risk the lottery of continued "natural" reproduction, the existing risks of MD were considered likely to be acceptable to some women.

Family Resemblances

This latter comment leads to another point of contention: are these potential harms, which in any case would not accrue to the consenting woman but to the future child, *justified* given the existence of safe alternatives? The use of an egg donor, for example, would result in a child free of disease. But in this case, such as in the case of adoption, the mother would not be genetically related to the child (although she would bear it). *Now* the question is whether the desire for genetic relatedness should be respected to the extent that the above risks are deemed acceptable. If the history of MD, in terms of the time and expense spent on preclinical research and associated administrative and policy-related work, comes down to respecting the insistence on genetic relatedness, does this constitute a good investment? Is this not a use of a risky ART for social purposes, as some have argued? But the desire that humans have to reproduce, in ways that usually result in biological connections and resemblances between parents and children, is one that runs deep, culturally and historically (see the following section on "Identity Crisis"). It is one of the major drivers of IVF itself. Because of this, it must be viewed as a serious factor when considering the merits of an innovative but potentially risky ART.

Identity Crisis?

The notion of personal identity is relevant to a number of questions raised by MD (39). For example, who precisely is the individual treated by MD? How does MD affect the identity of the child born following its use? This latter question is difficult and potentially ambiguous because it depends on our understanding of the term *identity*. Philosophers have wrestled with the concept of identity and offered distinct interpretations, such as the distinction between numerical and narrative identity. It is a reasonable question to ask, for example, what distinct sorts of narrative might develop around individuals born following MD, and whether these might be positive or negative (40)? Famously, the moral philosopher Derek Parfit discussed the issue (or problem) of "nonidentity": any child born following a particular intervention in planned human reproduction, such as an intentional delay in reproducing or the use of an ART, will be a different child to the one who would have been born had there been no intervention (41–43). From this perspective, the prospective parents engaged in MD are best viewed as attempting to ensure that a certain *type* of child is born, i.e., a child free of mitochondrial disease. The "problem" arising is that it is not then possible to claim that any *individual* is actually harmed by, or benefits from, the intervention in question, which seems counterintuitive (and problematic if one thinks all clinical interventions must aim at benefit and the avoidance of harm). Neither is MD a therapy or treatment in one other conventional sense, since the prospective mother will not herself be treated for her symptoms (although she would benefit from the satisfaction of her desire, i.e., the birth of a related child free from mitochondrial disease), and the entity that could arguably be said to be treated, namely, the embryo, must first be *created* as a condition of that treatment. These are deep waters. One thing seems clear: the hoped-for absence of mitochondrial disease is a significant aspect of the identity of any individual born following MD, and a *good* one.

Following on from this, one other expression of concern related to identity is whether mtDNA itself conveys any specific "traits." For this concern to make sense, we must assume that mitochondrial disease is not *itself* included in any list of specific traits influenced by mtDNA (since it clearly is a trait and its avoidance is at the center of MD's rationale). Rather, the concern here might be clarified by imagining the following scenario (borrowed from another context [44]): imagine you are in a maternity hospital and you hear exclamations of joy and wonder as relatives examine newborns on the ward. "Look, she has her mum's eyes and grandpa's nose..!" and other similar expressions of excitement at recognizing newly formed family resemblances, are heard. Perhaps the concern *here* is that a child born following MD might have her mother's eyes, her grandpa's nose, and her *mitochondrial donor's ears*, for example. (This is, perhaps, the anxiety implicit in the term "three-parent IVF," sometimes used to refer to MD.) Of course, since there is no legal entitlement to know the identity of the mitochondrial donor used in MD in the United Kingdom, such a scenario is unlikely to eventuate, but as a thought experiment, it nevertheless makes the point. It seems to me that such an eventuality is also very unlikely in a biological sense, since we are here concerned only with *differences* (polymorphisms) between the biological mother's (pathogenic) mtDNA (hopefully replaced) and the donor's mtDNA, such as might exist between two distinct mtDNA haplotypes. I know of no evidence that such sequence differences could significantly influence a complex trait such as ear or nose shape or similar: the contribution made by such mtDNA variation would likely be swamped by contributions made by the thousands of (also varying) maternally and paternally derived nuclear genes that play a role in the regulation of mitochondrial activity. (This is not to say, of course, that differences between even closely related mtDNA haplotypes do not influence some [perhaps dispositional] aspects of human biology.) But even if there is an extremely small, theoretical risk of such familiar "trait" transmission specifically from the mtDNA donor, the overwhelming consideration for all those involved is, surely, that any child be free of mitochondrial disease and otherwise healthy.

"Framing" Mitochondrial Donation

It is commonplace to see evaluations of the language and distinctive metaphors that are used to describe technological innovations like MD. For example, is MD a straightforward example of "donation?" The egg donor effectively supplies all the constituents of the donated ooplasm, including mitochondria, plus a whole host of other biomolecules. Presumably, the term *donation* refers to the *intention* with which the technique is used, i.e., to offer functional *mitochondria*, rather than other ooplasm constituents, which are not central to that explanation. Some take such critiques further, suggesting that MD consists of nuclear transfer, and that, therefore, there is an unhappy similarity between MD and somatic cell nuclear transfer, or "cloning." Again, these are relatively superficial criticisms. It is true that nDNA is transferred between eggs/embryos, but the nuclear genomes in question are meiotic, not somatic, and so there is no possibility of generating "clones" through such methods. Moreover, the *intention* with which the technique is performed is again central to its justification. Superficially, there is much in common between the technique of pouring oil into a car engine and pouring in concentrated nitric acid: but these two acts would be entirely distinct in terms of their ethical evaluation. Such issues are related to how MD is framed in terms of the problem that it aims to alleviate, its potential harms and benefits, its relationship to other interventions in human futures, and the metaphors or tropes used to convey these; but ultimately evaluating the ethical acceptability of MD will require more than simply a framing analysis.

Mitochondrial Donation as a Gateway-Assisted Reproductive Technology

One pervasive objection to MD is the idea that legislation to permit interventions in the human germ line increases the likelihood, and the acceptability, of other such interventions, including alteration to the sequence of embryonic nDNA for reproductive purposes. This is a form of slippery slope argument: the path to nuclear genome modification will be traveled more easily, potentially unintentionally, due to the introduction (and possible social normalization) of MD. The first point to make about this argument is that it assumes that modification of nuclear genes would be ethically unacceptable. But it is by no means clear that this would be the case in *all* circumstances. For example, the use of a technology like genome editing (45), *if safe and efficacious*, to prevent the birth of a child with cystic fibrosis, in the case of at-risk parents, is not *obviously* any more ethically contentious than the use of lawful PGD to effect the same end, *in the same context* (44). This suggests that the anxiety expressed by the slippery slope argument is more likely to concern the imagined prospect of uncontrolled usage of germ line interventions in an attempt to gain mastery over all aspects of human biology and human futures, and even to intentionally inflict harm. But this inference is not compulsory: we can regulate technologies to limit their legitimate domains of application, i.e., flatten the slope or make it less slippery. For example, in the United Kingdom, PGD can be used to prevent the birth of individuals at risk of serious inheritable disorders, such as cystic fibrosis and mitochondrial diseases; but it cannot be used lawfully to select the sex of a child merely to accommodate parental preferences. In addition, MD in the United Kingdom can be used *only* to prevent the transmission of serious mitochondrial diseases; it cannot be used as a (speculative) treatment for infertility. Such restrictions are upheld by robust regulatory frameworks and associated oversight, and these will continue to be important as MD evolves as a clinical intervention.

Summary and Conclusion

After years of preclinical experimentation and multifaceted assessment, MD has entered the clinic in the United Kingdom, and other countries may follow suit in introducing legislative and administrative frameworks to permit its regulation. Such regulation is *vital*: there is still much to learn about MD, and clinical data, appropriately generated, will provide crucial clues as to how it might be refined in years to come. Good regulation should be viewed not as *stifling* to medical and scientific progress, but as *facilitating*. Continued preclinical research is also extremely important. New techniques, such as polar body transfer or genome editing, may in the future assist in establishing robust safety and efficacy.

As a first-in-human germ line intervention, MD will continue to be an exemplar of biotechnological innovation in the ART sector, and thus rightly attract attention from scientists, clinicians, bioethicists, and policymakers. We must continue to remember the particularities of MD, i.e., how it operates and what it aims to achieve. It cannot be compared in any *simple* way with, for example, the use of genome editing to correct a pathogenic mutation in a nuclear gene of a human zygote (46), although clear similarities exist in the rationales for both (47). As made clear earlier, nuclear gene mutations can also cause mitochondrial disease, and thus it is a good question whether the ethical justification for MD might be employed, without significant alteration to its shape, to make the case for using nuclear genome editing as an ART to prevent mitochondrial disease (29). Of course, MST and PNT involve no alteration of DNA sequences and therefore raise overlapping but distinct safety concerns—but in terms of the *intentions* with which MD or nuclear genome editing might be used, there are ethical similarities to be had. Ethical and scientific debate concerning MD is likely to be ongoing. It is hoped that its clinical use, with strict regulation (48), will be a success.

Acknowledgments

I wish to thank a number of colleagues for helpful discussions concerning mitochondrial donation over recent years. First, I thank Peter Braude, Frances Flinter, Robin Lovell-Badge, Caroline Ogilvie, and Tony Perry for their wise counsel; and colleagues at the HFEA, especially Peter Thompson, Juliet Tizzard,

David Archard, Lee Rayfield, and Sally Cheshire for help and advice on this topic, and ARTs more generally. I also wish to thank Tim Lewens and Mary Herbert for making useful comments on a draft of this review. I thank Gareth Clarke for assistance with the production of the figures. Finally, thoughts expressed here are mine and do not necessarily represent those of my colleagues or any organizations with which I am associated.

REFERENCES

1. Smeitink J, van den Heuvel L, DiMauro S. The genetics and pathology of oxidative phosphorylation. *Nat Rev Genet.* 2001;2:342–52.
2. Calvo SE, Mootha VK. The mitochondrial proteome and human disease. *Annu Rev Genomics Hum Genet.* 2010;11:25–44.
3. Gorman GS, Chinnery PF, DiMauro S, Hirano M, Koga Y, McFarland R, Suomalainen A, Thorburn DR, Zeviani M, Turnbull DM. Mitochondrial diseases. *Nat Rev Dis Primers.* 2016;2:16080.
4. Gorman GS, Schaefer AM, Ng Y. et al. Prevalence of nuclear and mitochondrial DNA mutations related to adult mitochondrial disease. *Ann Neurol.* 2015;77:753–9.
5. Wei W, Gomez-Duran A, Hudson G, Chinnery PF. Background sequence characteristics influence the occurrence and severity of disease-causing mtDNA mutations. *PLOS Genet.* 2017;13:e1007126.
6. Wallace DC. The mitochondrial genome in human adaptive radiation and disease: On the road to therapeutics and performance enhancement. *Gene.* 2005;354:169–80.
7. Song WH, Yi YJ, Sutovsky M, Meyers S, Sutovsky P. Autophagy and ubiquitin-proteasome system contribute to sperm mitophagy after mammalian fertilization. *Proc Natl Acad Sci USA.* 2016;113:E5261–70.
8. Floros VI, Pyle A, Dietmann S. et al. Segregation of mitochondrial DNA heteroplasmy through a developmental genetic bottleneck in human embryos. *Nat Cell Biol.* 2018;20:144–51.
9. Craven L, Tuppen HA, Greggains GD. et al. Pronuclear transfer in human embryos to prevent transmission of mitochondrial DNA disease. *Nature.* 2010;465:82–5.
10. Kang E, Wu J, Gutierrez NM. et al. Mitochondrial replacement in human oocytes carrying pathogenic mitochondrial DNA mutations. *Nature.* 2016;540:270–5.
11. Smeets HJ, Sallevelt SC, Dreesen JC, de Die-Smulders CE, de Coo IF. Preventing the transmission of mitochondrial DNA disorders using prenatal or preimplantation genetic diagnosis. *Ann N Y Acad Sci.* 2015;1350:29–36.
12. Mann JR, Lovell-Badge RH. Inviability of parthenogenotes is determined by pronuclei, not egg cytoplasm. *Nature.* 1984;310:66–7.
13. Sato A, Kono T, Nakada K, Ishikawa K, Inoue S, Yonekawa H, Hayashi J. Gene therapy for progeny of mito-mice carrying pathogenic mtDNA by nuclear transplantation. *Proc Natl Acad Sci USA.* 2005;102:16765–70.
14. Ma H, Marti Gutierrez N, Morey R. et al. Incompatibility between nuclear and mitochondrial genomes contributes to an interspecies reproductive barrier. *Cell Metab.* 2016;24:283–94.
15. Tachibana M, Sparman M, Sritanaudomchai H. et al. Mitochondrial gene replacement in primate offspring and embryonic stem cells. *Nature.* 2009;461:367–72.
16. Ma H, O'Neil RC, Marti Gutierrez N. et al. Functional human oocytes generated by transfer of polar body genomes. *Cell Stem Cell.* 2017;20:112–9.
17. Wang T, Sha H, Ji D, Zhang HL, Chen D, Cao Y, Zhu J. Polar body genome transfer for preventing the transmission of inherited mitochondrial diseases. *Cell.* 2014;157:1591–604.
18. Supplementary report to the HFEA 2014. Review of the Safety and Efficacy of Polar Body Transfer to Avoid Mitochondrial Disease. Available at: https://www.hfea.gov.uk/media/2610/2014-10-07_-_polar_body_transfer_review_-_final.pdf
19. Tachibana M, Amato P, Sparman M. et al. Towards germline gene therapy of inherited mitochondrial diseases. *Nature.* 2013;493:627–31.
20. Paull D, Emmanuele V, Weiss KA. et al. Nuclear genome transfer in human oocytes eliminates mitochondrial DNA variants. *Nature.* 2013;493:632–7.
21. Yamada M, Emmanuele V, Sanchez-Quintero MJ. et al. Genetic drift can compromise mitochondrial replacement by nuclear transfer in human oocytes. *Cell Stem Cell.* 2016;18:749–54.
22. Hyslop LA, Blakeley P, Craven L. et al. Towards clinical application of pronuclear transfer to prevent mitochondrial DNA disease. *Nature.* 2016;534:383–6.

23. Report to the HFEA 2016. Scientific review of the safety and efficacy of methods to avoid mitochondrial disease through assisted conception: 2016 update. Available at: https://www.hfea.gov.uk/media/2611/fourth_scientific_review_mitochondria_2016.pdf

24. Reinhardt K, Dowling DK, Morrow EH. Medicine. Mitochondrial replacement, evolution, and the clinic. *Science*. 2013;341:1345–6.

25. Morrow EH, Reinhardt K, Wolff JN, Dowling DK. Risks inherent to mitochondrial replacement. *EMBO Rep*. 2015;16:541–4.

26. Chinnery PF, Craven L, Mitalipov S, Stewart JB, Herbert M, Turnbull DM. The challenges of mitochondrial replacement. *PLOS Genet*. 2014;10:e1004315.

27. Eyre-Walker A. Mitochondrial replacement therapy: Are mito-nuclear interactions likely to be a problem? *Genetics*. 2017;205:1365–72.

28. Dobler R, Dowling DK, Morrow EH, Reinhardt K. 2018. A systematic review and meta-analysis reveals pervasive effects of germline mitochondrial replacement on components of health. *Hum Reprod Update*. 2018;24:519–34.

29. Nuffield Council on Bioethics *Novel Techniques for the Prevention of Mitochondrial DNA Disorders: An Ethical Review*. London: Nuffield Council on Bioethics; 2012.

30. Zhang J, Zhuang G, Zeng Y, Grifo J, Acosta C, Shu Y, Liu H. Pregnancy derived from human zygote pronuclear transfer in a patient who had arrested embryos after IVF. *Reprod Biomed Online*. 2016;33:529–33.

31. Kristensen SG, Pors SE, Andersen CY. Improving oocyte quality by transfer of autologous mitochondria from fully grown oocytes. *Hum Reprod*. 2017;32:725–32.

32. Zhang J, Liu H, Luo S. et al. Live birth derived from oocyte spindle transfer to prevent mitochondrial disease. *Reprod Biomed Online*. 2017;34:361–8.

33. Gleicher N, Kushnir VA, Albertini DA, Barad DH. First birth following spindle transfer. *Reprod Biomed Online*. 2017;35:542–3.

34. Palacios-Gonzalez C, Medina-Arellano MJ. Mitochondrial replacement techniques and Mexico's rule of law: On the legality of the first maternal spindle transfer case. *J Law Biosci*. 2017;4:50–69.

35. Chan S, Palacios-Gonzalez C, De Jesus Medina Arellano M. Mitochondrial replacement techniques, scientific tourism, and the global politics of science. *Hastings Cent Rep*. 2017;47:7–9.

36. Greenfield A, Braude P, Flinter F, Lovell-Badge R, Ogilvie C, Perry ACF. Assisted reproductive technologies to prevent human mitochondrial disease transmission. *Nat Biotechnol*. 2017;35:1059–68.

37. Sharpley MS, Marciniak C, Eckel-Mahan K. et al. Heteroplasmy of mouse mtDNA is genetically unstable and results in altered behavior and cognition. *Cell*. 2012;151:333–43.

38. Burgstaller JP, Johnston IG, Jones NS. et al. MtDNA segregation in heteroplasmic tissues is common in vivo and modulated by haplotype differences and developmental stage. *Cell Rep*. 2014;7:2031–41.

39. Liao SM. Do mitochondrial replacement techniques affect qualitative or numerical identity? *Bioethics*. 2017;31:20–6.

40. Scully JL. A mitochondrial story: Mitochondrial replacement, identity and narrative. *Bioethics*. 2017;31:37–45.

41. Parfit D. *Reasons and Persons*. Oxford University Press, Oxford: Clarendon Press; 1987.

42. Newson AJ, Wrigley A. Is mitochondrial donation germ-line gene therapy? Classifications and ethical implications. *Bioethics*. 2017;31:55–67.

43. Wrigley A, Wilkinson S, Appleby J. Mitochondrial replacement: Ethics and identity. *Bioethics*. 2015;29:631–8.

44. Greenfield A. Carry on Editing. *British Medical Bulletin* 2018;127:23–31.

45. Nuffield Council on Bioethics *Genome Editing: An Ethical Review*. London, UK: Nuffield Council on Bioethics; 2016.

46. Ma H, Marti-Gutierrez N, Park SW. et al. Correction of a pathogenic gene mutation in human embryos. *Nature*. 2017;548:413–9.

47. Scott R, Wilkinson S. Germline genetic modification and identity: The mitochondrial and nuclear genomes. *Oxf J Leg Stud*. 2017;37:886–915.

48. Bredenoord AL, Appleby JB. Mitochondrial replacement techniques: Remaining ethical challenges. *Cell Stem Cell*. 2017;21:301–4.

13

Controversies in Recurrent Implantation Failure: From Theory to Practice

Efstratios Kolibianakis, Pavlidi Olga, and Christos A. Venetis

Introduction

Although assisted reproductive technologies (ARTs) have helped numerous couples to achieve live birth, this is not feasible in a significant proportion of cases, despite several attempts. Repeated implantation failure (RIF) remains a difficult problem both for clinicians, struggling to help patients, as well as for patients, anxiously seeking solutions.

Controversies in the Definition of Repeated Implantation Failure

It is without saying that if the definition of a condition varies, it becomes very difficult to estimate its real incidence as well as to draw conclusions on the efficacy of the proposed treatments.

Unfortunately, a significant variability in the definition of RIF exists. Many variables have been used for this purpose, including the number of embryos transferred, the number of previous *in vitro* fertilization (IVF) attempts, embryo quality, and maternal age (1). Using different combinations of these variables, several definitions of RIF have been proposed (2). Currently, no universally accepted definition of RIF is available.

RIF was initially defined as a cumulative transfer of eight cleavage stage embryos or four blastocysts not leading to a positive pregnancy test 14 days after oocyte pickup (3). According to the European Society of Human Reproduction and Embryology, Preimplantation Genetic Diagnosis Consortium, RIF is considered as a failure to achieve clinical pregnancy after three or more unsuccessful transfers of high-quality embryos or after the cumulative transfer of 10 or more embryos in multiple transfers (4). More recently, RIF has been defined as the failure of pregnancy achievement after the transfer of at least four good-quality embryos in a minimum of three fresh or frozen cycles in women under the age of 40 years (5).

In a relevant systematic review, 119 studies using arbitrary definitions for RIF were evaluated (2). The most common single variable used for definition of RIF was the number of failed/unsuccessful cycles, which was more than three. Using the number of embryos transferred cumulatively in combination with the number of unsuccessful cycles, the most common definition was "cumulative transfer of 10 or more embryos during three or more unsuccessful or failed cycles."

It becomes evident that research on the causes of RIF, as well as on its management, might lead to diverging conclusions and controversies, not only because of potential problems associated with study design, but also due to the use of different definitions of RIF.

Controversies in the Management of RIF

RIF and Preimplantation Genetic Testing for Aneuploidy

Preimplantation genetic testing for aneuploidy (PGT-A) has been used in patients with RIF to identify and transfer chromosomally normal embryos, with the aim increase the probability of pregnancy. In a retrospective study, significantly higher pregnancy rates were present following array comparative genomic hybridization (array CGH) ($n = 43$) as compared to embryo transfer without PGT-A ($n = 33$) (68.3% versus 21.2%, $p = 0.609$, respectively) (6). However, the therapeutic value of this strategy needs to be confirmed in relevant randomized controlled trials (RCTs).

Embryo Manipulation and RIF

Although assisted hatching has been shown to increase the probability of live birth in women with RIF (relative risk [RR]: 2.51, 95% confidence interval [CI]: 1.06–5.96), this was based on a pooled analysis of only two small RCTs including 250 patients (7). Evidently, conclusions based on a small number of patients analyzed, although supporting the need for further research, cannot be used to shape routine clinical practice.

Intracytoplasmic Morphologically Selected Sperm Injection versus Intracytoplasmic Sperm Injection in Patients with RIF

Intracytoplasmic morphologically selected sperm injection (IMSI) has been proposed as a treatment in couples with RIF. This, however, is currently based on a subgroup analysis of an RCT in patients younger than 35 years of age, with two or more failed attempts ($n = 139$), and oligoasthenoteratozoospermia, who were treated by IMSI or intracytoplasmic sperm injection (ICSI) (clinical pregnancy rate: 29.8% versus 12.9%, respectively; $p = .017$). Prior to introducing IMSI in routine clinical practice, however, this finding should be confirmed by appropriate RCTs.

RIF and Acquired Uterine Conditions

It is generally accepted that submucosal fibroids of any type negatively affect IVF outcome and implantation. On the contrary, subserosal fibroids have no impact on implantation and IVF outcome. Although intramural fibroids have been suggested to exert a negative impact on the probability of pregnancy, it is still not clear whether this effect is associated with their number (8) and diameter (9). The exact pathophysiologic mechanism supporting a negative effect of intramural fibroids on endometrial receptivity is not clear. Gene expression profiling of leiomyomas has shown that only few alterations are present in genes related to the window of implantation (10–12). Not unexpectedly, a beneficial effect of intramural fibroids excision has not been shown in a meta-analysis by Pritts et al. (13), while a Cochrane systematic review suggested that the effect of myomectomy on fertility could not be evaluated due to insufficient published evidence. Apparently, the knowledge gap that exists in routine clinical practice regarding the effect and optimal management of uterine fibroids extends to patients with RIF.

A similar situation is present regarding adenomyosis. Although published meta-analyses suggest that its presence is associated with significantly lower clinical pregnancy rates ([RR 0.72; 95% CI 0.55–0.95] [14], [OR 0.73; 95% CI 0.60–0.90] [15]), significant heterogeneity in the included studies limits the value of the conclusions drawn. In addition, the basis for the impaired implantation associated with the adenomyosis is not clear (16–20). Not surprisingly, it is still not known which is the best treatment approach for women with adenomyosis seeking fertility. No comparative studies exist between conservative (14) and surgical treatment (15,21) in women with adenomyosis. Moreover, the consequences of surgical treatment for a future pregnancy have not been evaluated (22,23).

RIF and Endometrial Polyps

The role of endometrial polyps in RIF is indirectly shown by their higher incidence in these patients (up to 45%) (24) as compared to patients undergoing their first ART attempt (11%–22%) (25). Due to the lack of high-quality prospective studies in women with endometrial polyps undergoing IVF, their proposed unfavorable effect on implantation is based on indirect evidence from studies comparing IVF outcome in patients with and without polyps. These studies, however, have also produced controversial results supporting (26) or negating a beneficial effect of polypectomy (27,28), which complicates the overall assessment of the contribution of endometrial polyps in RIF.

Chronic Endometritis in Patients with RIF

The association between chronic endometritis and RIF is based on its higher incidence in patients with RIF (range: 15%–60%) (29–32) as compared to asymptomatic infertile patients before their first IVF attempt (range: 3%–15%) (31,33). However, scarce data exist regarding the value of antibiotics for treating women with chronic endometritis and RIF. In a retrospective study, similar ongoing pregnancy rates were observed between women with histologically confirmed chronic endometritis who were either treated ($n = 68$) or not ($n = 20$) by antibiotics (29.4% versus 25.0%, respectively, $p = .701$) (34). In addition, alternative treatments such as hysteroscopic removal of bacterial biofilms have been proposed (35), although they are still not supported by relevant RCTs.

Manipulating Endometrium in Patients with RIF

Endometrial injury has been proposed as a method to increase the probability of pregnancy both in the overall population as well as in patients with RIF. However, currently published relevant studies are of moderate quality and apply different methods of endometrial injury in different types of patients. More importantly, a biological mechanism supporting endometrial injury is still lacking.

A systematic and meta-analysis by the Cochrane group in women who had more than two failed embryo transfers, that included 474 women in four RCTs, a significant increase of probability of live birth was observed after endometrial scratching (RR: 1.96, 95% CL: 1.21–3.16) (36). However, the quality of evidence was considered low.

Endocrine Causes in RIF

Endocrine disorders may play a role in RIF, affecting implantation through the interaction of various hormones with their corresponding receptors in endometrium. Vitamin D deficiency, polycystic ovary syndrome (PCOS), and thyroid disease have been implicated in RIF; however, their exact role is not yet fully understood.

LT4 Supplementation

Conflicting evidence exists regarding the value of LT4 supplementation for increasing the probability of delivery and lowering the probability of miscarriage rate in women with subclinical hypothyroidism or euthyroid women with TSH concentration above 2.5 mIU/mL, while such information is not currently available in women with RIF (37,38). The probability of live birth in women with thyroid autoimmunity (TAI) is significantly lower compared to women without TAI (odds ratio [OR] 0.73; 95% CI 0.54–0.99, $p = .04$; $I^2 = 41\%$), while the presence of TAI has been associated with an increased risk of spontaneous miscarriage (39). However, it appears that treatment of these women is not beneficial regarding the probability of pregnancy (40), while no data exist in women who in addition suffer from RIF.

Vitamin D Supplementation

In a meta-analysis by Chu et al. (41) in women undergoing ART, the probability of live birth was significantly higher in women replete in vitamin D as compared to women with deficient or insufficient vitamin D status (OR 1.33, 95%CI: 1.08–1.65). However, it is not yet clear whether vitamin D supplementation in the latter group is beneficial either in the general population or in women with RIF.

Metformin

Although it has been shown that early pregnancy loss (EPL) is significantly decreased (0.19 95% CI: 0.12–0.28, $p < .001$) in women with PCOS treated with metformin, it is not yet known whether such treatment is beneficial for pregnancy achievement in women with RIF (42).

Intrauterine Administration of Immune Cells in Patients with RIF

The endometrium plays a key role in the process of implantation, which is thought to be affected by the immune system. Intrauterine administration of autologous peripheral blood mononuclear cells (PBMCs) has been investigated in this respect as an inflammation inducer (43). A nonrandomized trial showed that intrauterine administration of autologous PBMC (35 women/35 cycles) increased live birth rates in women who had more than two failed embryo transfers (PBMC treated group, $n = 17$: 55.6%— nontreated group, $n = 18$: 7.6%, $p = .013$) (44). However, this intervention has not been evaluated in relevant RCTs.

Administration of Human Chorionic Gonadotropin in Patients with RIF

Intrauterine administration of synthetic or natural hCG around the time of ET has been suggested to improve the outcomes of assisted reproduction treatment based on the fundamental role of hCG in embryo implantation and early stages of pregnancy (45). hCG may promote peritrophoblastic immune tolerance, which facilitates trophoblast invasion by inducing an increase in endometrial T-cell apoptosis (46). However, its administration as a priming agent prior to embryo transfer has not yet been studied in patients with RIF.

Administration of Atosiban in Patients with RIF

The concept of atosiban administration is based on its interference with the oxytocin/prostaglandin F2a system minimizing uterine contractility after embryo transfer. A recently published meta-analysis evaluated the impact of atosiban administration on live birth rate in women who had experienced two or more consecutive IVF-ET attempts in which at least one to two high-quality embryos were transferred. Atosiban was associated with an increased probability of live birth rate (OR: 2.89, 95% CI: 1.78–4.67) (47). However, this outcome was based on pooling the results from only two RCTs including 390 patients. Thus, further trials are required prior to utilization of atosiban routinely in patients with RIF.

Administration of Growth Hormone in Patients with RIF

Administration of growth hormone (GH) during ovarian stimulation has been shown to improve success rates of IVF in poor responders, probably by exerting a beneficial effect on oocyte quality (48). Regarding RIF, in patients with at least two failed IVF cycles, a higher probability of live birth has been observed in an RCT comparing cotreatment with GH (OR:6,4, 51.4%, 95% CI: 35.6–67.0 $p = .002$) versus no cotreatment (17.1%, 95% CI: 8.1–32.7) (49). However, this study has not yet been repeated, and its conclusion was based on the analysis of only 70 patients producing wide confidence intervals in the estimates obtained.

Immunotherapy in Patients with RIF

It has recently been suggested that immune-inflammatory factors, such as antiphospholipid antibodies, antinuclear antibodies, and dysregulated T- and natural killer (NK)-cell-mediated immune responses play a role in RIF. Several immunotherapeutic modalities, such as prednisone or intravenous immunoglobulin G (IVIG) administration have been suggested to increase the probability of pregnancy.

Intravenous Immunoglobulin G

In a meta-analysis on the use of IVIG in patients with RIF, Clark et al. (50) suggested that administration of IVIG increases the probability of live birth. However, the validity of its conclusions, which was based on pooling data from three relevant RCTs (51–53), is questionable. One of the studies included, the study by Sher et al. (52), was not an RCT and reported live birth rates in patients with two IVF failures who, besides IVIG, received heparin/aspirin treatment. No independent control group was present in that study, and thus the reasoning behind its inclusion in the meta-analysis by Clark et al. (50) is unclear. The second study by De Placido et al. (51) was an RCT which, however, included patients who cannot be strictly classified as RIF, since according to that study's inclusion criteria, besides three or more failed attempts of embryo transfer after IVF replacing at least three embryos, they had also two or more very early abortions (less than 8 weeks) or biochemical pregnancies. The third study by Stephenson et al. (53) was a double-blind, placebo-controlled RCT evaluating the addition of IVIG in 54 women with repeated unexplained IVF failure, defined as at least two previous fresh or frozen embryo transfers, each of which resulted in failure of implantation, a biochemical pregnancy, or a spontaneous abortion at 8 or less weeks of gestation. In each prior cycle, at least two good-quality embryos had been replaced in the presence of an endometrial thickness of 7 mm or more on the day of hCG injection. Similar live birth rates were present in the IVIG and the placebo group, respectively (15% versus 12%, respectively; $p = .52$). Thus, currently published evidence does not appear to support the use of IVIG in patients with RIF.

Tacrolimus

Tacrolimus inhibits T-cell activation by binding to the intracytoplasmic FK-binding protein and has been used for immunosuppression after transplantation (54). Although it has been evaluated in patients with RIF (55) with promising results, currently no RCTs exist to support its use.

Hydroxychloroquine

Hydroxychloroquine is an antimalarial drug often used as treatment in various autoimmune diseases, particularly systemic lupus erythematosus. Its immunomodulatory effect has led to its administration in patients with RIF (56). However, currently, there is a lack of RCTs supporting its clinical effectiveness.

Granulocyte Colony-Stimulating Factor

Granulocyte colony-stimulating factor (G-CSF) is involved in a granulocytic and myelocytic proliferation and has been used in patients with RIF. The meta-analysis by Zhang et al. (57) showed that the probability of clinical pregnancy was increased in patients with RIF after G-CSF administration (RR: 2.07, 95% CI: 1.64–2.61, $p < 0.001$). This result was based on pooling data from five abstracts and three fully published papers (960 patients, 8 RCTs).

Male Factor

Multiple studies have reported the negative effect of high sperm DNA fragmentation (DF) on clinical pregnancy following IVF and/or ICSI treatment (58). However, the hypothesis that sperm DF is an important cause of RIF is not supported by the currently published literature. No obvious differences in sperm DNA fragmentation were present between patients with RIF ($n = 35$) defined as the failure to achieve a clinical pregnancy following the transfer of four good-quality embryos in a minimum of three fresh and frozen embryo cycles in women aged younger than 40 years and fertile controls ($n = 7$) (34.7%, versus 35.5%, $p = .930$) (59).

Lifestyle Factors

Maternal obesity has been negatively associated with implantation, clinical pregnancy, and live birth rate (60), and in this respect, it might be perceived as a contributing factor to RIF. However, there are no data to support a direct association. The same is true for smoking, which although there is no doubt regarding its negative association with implantation (61,62), no data exist to support a direct association with RIF.

Progesterone

Considering the importance of late follicular serum progesterone for the achievement of pregnancy after a fresh ET (63), it seems likely that it might contribute to RIF in a proportion of patients. If this is true, the incidence of progesterone elevation on the day of hCG administration would be expected to be higher in patients with increased numbers of failed IVF cycles. Data to support this hypothesis stem from a study in which women with two or more previous failed IVF/ETs had a significantly higher prevalence of progesterone elevation compared with women with one failed IVF/ET or no failed IVF/ETs (64). Thus, it might be possible that a proportion of patients with an elevated progesterone level on the day of triggering final oocyte maturation might experience repeated implantation failure, due to its known negative association with the probability of pregnancy. This is especially true given the fact that women with a history of progesterone elevation have approximately six times higher odds of exhibiting progesterone elevation in their next cycle (65). Therefore, it is interesting to evaluate whether appropriate management of elevated progesterone, when present in patients with RIF, could improve the probability of pregnancy. In this respect, Magdi et al. in a prospective cohort study, compared the freeze-all policy ($n = 81$) with fresh embryo transfer ($n = 90$) in women who had at least three previous failed embryo transfers with four or more high-quality embryos transferred in total (66). A significantly higher probability of ongoing pregnancy was present in women with RIF treated by the freeze-all approach (40.7%) as compared to women treated by a fresh transfer (21.1%) (OR: 2.57 CI: 1.31–5.04, $p = .005$). Thus, based on a single study, the application of a freeze-all policy in patients with elevated progesterone appears to be beneficial in patients with RIF (66).

Cytoplasmic Transfer

Cytoplasmic transfer between oocytes was initially developed in order to treat infertile patients exhibiting persistent poor embryonic development and recurrent implantation failure after IVF. This is performed by microinjection of 5%–15% of the ooplasm from a young fertile donor oocyte into a defective recipient oocyte (67), resulting in the birth of several children worldwide (68). However, besides the fact that the effectiveness of the method has not been tested in relevant RCTs, the long-term health effects of induced mitochondrial heteroplasmy in the children born is yet unknown, and thus the method is strictly experimental.

Coculture and Hyaluronic Acid–Enriched Transfer Medium in Patients with RIF

Use of coculture and of hyaluronic acid–enriched medium have been claimed to increase the probability of pregnancy in patients with RIF. However, regarding coculture, this is based on data from retrospective studies (69), while for hyaluronan, higher clinical pregnancy (35.2% versus 10.0%, $p = .004$) and ongoing pregnancy/delivery rates (31.3% versus 4.0%, $p = .0005$) have been reported in an RCT (70).

Freeze-All and RIF

The "freeze-all" strategy during which all created embryos are frozen for later transfer needs to be explored in RIF patients. Apparently, transfer of embryos in the normal endometrium of a natural or of an artificially prepared cycle (71) bypasses whatever effect ovarian stimulation has on endometrial receptivity, on the expense of introducing an additional intervention such as embryo freezing. This strategy has been shown to increase the probability of pregnancy in high-responder patients (72); however, data for patients with RIF are still not available.

TABLE 13.1

Interventions from Randomized Controlled Trials or Meta-Analyses That Appear to Offer a Benefit in Patients with Repeated Implantation Failure

Intervention	Author	Number of RCTs	Number of Patients	Live Birth RR 95% CI
GH	Altmae et al. (49)	1	70	3.00 1.35–6.65
Hyaluronan	Friedler et al. (70)	1	101	3.52 9.76–40.82
Assisted hatching	Martins et al. (7)	2	250	2.51 1.06–5.96
Atosiban	Huang et al. (47)	2	390	RR: 2.16 1.51–3.10
Endometrial scratching	Nastri et al. (36)	4	474	RR: 1.96 1.21–3.16
G-CSF	Zhang et al. (57)	8	960	RR: 2.07 1.64–2.61

Abbreviations: CI, confidence interval; G-CSF, granulocyte colony-stimulating factor; GH, growth hormone; LBR, live birth rate; OR, odds ratio; RCT, randomized controlled trial; RR: relative risk.

Conclusion

The current absence of a consensus in the definition of RIF leads to significant methodologic and interpretational problems of available research. Currently, management of RIF consists of either non-evidence-based interventions or interventions evaluated in a small number of patients and RCTs (Table 13.1). Table 13.1 summarizes interventions used in RIF patients for which there is some evidence (originating from RCTs or meta-analyses) of benefit in terms of the probability of pregnancy. Apparently, the statistical power of these studies to produce solid conclusions that can confidently guide clinical practice is very limited. The need to produce a consensus definition of RIF that can in turn be used in future well-designed RCTs is more than obvious.

REFERENCES

1. Laufer N, Simon A. Recurrent implantation failure: Current update and clinical approach to an ongoing challenge. *Fertil Steril.* 2012;97:1019–20.
2. Polanski LT, Baumgarten MN, Quenby S et al. What exactly do we mean by "recurrent implantation failure?" A systematic review and opinion. *Reprod Biomed Online.* 2014;28:409–23.
3. Coulam CB. Implantation failure and immunotherapy. *Hum Reprod.* 1995;10:1338–40.
4. Thornhill AR, deDie-Smulders CE, Geraedts JP et al. ESHRE PGD Consortium "Best practice guidelines for clinical preimplantation genetic diagnosis (PGD) and preimplantation genetic screening (PGS)." *Hum Reprod.* 2005;20:35–48.
5. Coughlan C, Ledger W, Wang Q et al. Recurrent implantation failure: Definition and management. *Reprod Biomed Online.* 2014;28:14–38.
6. Greco E, Bono S, Ruberti A et al. Comparative genomic hybridization selection of blastocysts for repeated implantation failure treatment: A pilot study. *Biomed Res Int.* 2014;2014:457913.
7. Martins WP, Rocha IA, Ferriani RA et al. Assisted hatching of human embryos: A systematic review and meta-analysis of randomized controlled trials. *Hum Reprod Update.* 2011;17:438–53.
8. Oliveira FG, Abdelmassih VG, Diamond MP et al. Impact of subserosal and intramural uterine fibroids that do not distort the endometrial cavity on the outcome of in vitro fertilization-intracytoplasmic sperm injection. *Fertil Steril.* 2004;81:582–7.

9. Christopoulos G, Vlismas A, Salim R et al. Fibroids that do not distort the uterine cavity and IVF success rates: An observational study using extensive matching criteria. *BJOG.* 2017;124:615–21.

10. Luo X, Xu J, Chegini N. The expression of Smads in human endometrium and regulation and induction in endometrial epithelial and stromal cells by transforming growth factor-β. *J Clin Endocrinol Metab.* 2003;88:4967–76.

11. Horcajadas JA, Pellicer A, Simon C. Wide genomic analysis of human endometrial receptivity: New times, new opportunities. *Hum Reprod Update.* 2007;13:77–86.

12. Horcajadas JA, Goyri E, Higon MA et al. Endometrial receptivity and implantation are not affected by the presence of uterine intramural leiomyomas: A clinical and functional genomics analysis. *J Clin Endocrinol Metab.* 2008;93:3490–8.

13. Pritts EA, Parker WH, Olive DL. Fibroids and infertility: An updated systematic review of the evidence. *Fertil Steril.* 2009;91:1215–23.

14. Vercellini P, Consonni D, Dridi D et al. Uterine adenomyosis and in vitro fertilization outcome: A systematic review and meta-analysis. *Hum Reprod.* 2014;29:964–77.

15. Younes G, Tulandi T. Effects of adenomyosis on *in vitro* fertilization treatment outcomes: A meta-analysis. *Fertil Steril.* 2017;108:483–90.e3.

16. Agarwal A, Gupta S, Sharma RK. Role of oxidative stress in female reproduction. *Reprod Biol Endocrinol.* 2005;3:28.

17. Tremellen K, Russell P. Adenomyosis is a potential cause of recurrent implantation failure during IVF treatment. *Aust N Z J Obstet Gynaecol.* 2011;51:280–3.

18. Benagiano G, Habiba M, Brosens I. The pathophysiology of uterine adenomyosis: An update. *Fertil Steril.* 2012;98:572–9.

19. Brosens J, Verhoeven H, Campo R et al. High endometrial aromatase P450 mRNA expression is associated with poor IVF outcome. *Hum Reprod.* 2004;19:352–6.

20. Kissler S, Hamscho N, Zangos S et al. Uterotubal transport disorder in adenomyosis and endometriosis—A cause for infertility. *BJOG.* 2006;113:902–8.

21. Rocha TP, Andres MP, Borrelli GM et al. Fertility-sparing treatment of adenomyosis in patients with infertility: A systematic review of current options. *Reprod Sci.* 2018;25:480–6.

22. Grimbizis GF, Mikos T, Tarlatzis B. Uterus-sparing operative treatment for adenomyosis. *Fertil Steril.* 2014;101:472–87.

23. Osada H. Uterine adenomyosis and adenomyoma: The surgical approach. *Fertil Steril.* 2018;109:406–17.

24. Pinheiro A, Antunes A, Jr., Andrade L et al. Expression of hormone receptors, Bcl2, Cox2 and Ki67 in benign endometrial polyps and their association with obesity. *Mol Med Rep.* 2014;9:2335–41.

25. Fatemi HM, Kasius JC, Timmermans A et al. Prevalence of unsuspected uterine cavity abnormalities diagnosed by office hysteroscopy prior to *in vitro* fertilization. *Hum Reprod.* 2010;25:1959–65.

26. Tiras B, Korucuoglu U, Polat M et al. Management of endometrial polyps diagnosed before or during ICSI cycles. *Reprod Biomed Online.* 2012;24:123–8.

27. Yang JH, Yang PK, Chen MJ et al. Management of endometrial polyps incidentally diagnosed during IVF: A case-control study. *Reprod Biomed Online.* 2017;34:285–90.

28. Kilic Y, Bastu E, Ergun B. Validity and efficacy of office hysteroscopy before in vitro fertilization treatment. *Arch Gynecol Obstet.* 2013;287:577–81.

29. Bouet PE, El Hachem H, Monceau E et al. Chronic endometritis in women with recurrent pregnancy loss and recurrent implantation failure: Prevalence and role of office hysteroscopy and immunohistochemistry in diagnosis. *Fertil Steril.* 2016;105:106–10.

30. Johnston-MacAnanny EB, Hartnett J, Engmann LL et al. Chronic endometritis is a frequent finding in women with recurrent implantation failure after in vitro fertilization. *Fertil Steril.* 2010;93:437–41.

31. Romero R, Espinoza J, Mazor M. Can endometrial infection/inflammation explain implantation failure, spontaneous abortion, and preterm birth after in vitro fertilization? *Fertil Steril.* 2004;82:799–804.

32. Conway D, Ketefian A, Shamonki M. Chronic endometritis: A common finding in good prognosis patients with failed implantation following IVF. *Fertil Steril.* 2010;94:S175.

33. Kasius JC, Fatemi HM, Bourgain C et al. The impact of chronic endometritis on reproductive outcome. *Fertil Steril.* 2011;96:1451–6.

34. Yang R, Du X, Wang Y et al. The hysteroscopy and histological diagnosis and treatment value of chronic endometritis in recurrent implantation failure patients. *Arch Gynecol Obstet.* 2014;289:1363–9.

35. Park HJ, Kim YS, Yoon TK et al. Chronic endometritis and infertility. *Clin Exp Reprod Med.* 2016;43:185–92.
36. Nastri CO, Lensen SF, Gibreel A et al. Endometrial injury in women undergoing assisted reproductive techniques. *Cochrane Database Syst Rev.* 2015;(3):CD009517.
37. Cai Y, Zhong L, Guan J et al. Outcome of *in vitro* fertilization in women with subclinical hypothyroidism. *Reprod Biol Endocrinol.* 2017;15:39.
38. Jatzko B, Vytiska-Bistorfer E, Pawlik A et al. The impact of thyroid function on intrauterine insemination outcome—A retrospective analysis. *Reprod Biol Endocrinol.* 2014;12:28.
39. Toulis KA, Goulis DG, Venetis CA et al. Risk of spontaneous miscarriage in euthyroid women with thyroid autoimmunity undergoing IVF: A meta-analysis. *Eur J Endocrinol.* 2010;162:643–52.
40. Dhillon-Smith RK, Middleton LJ, Sunner KK et al. Levothyroxine in women with thyroid peroxidase antibodies before conception. *N Engl J Med.* 2019;380:1316–25.
41. Chu J, Gallos I, Tobias A et al. Vitamin D and assisted reproductive treatment outcome: A systematic review and meta-analysis. *Hum Reprod.* 2018;33:65–80.
42. Lautatzis ME, Goulis DG, Vrontakis M. Efficacy and safety of metformin during pregnancy in women with gestational diabetes mellitus or polycystic ovary syndrome: A systematic review. *Metabolism.* 2013;62:1522–34.
43. Makrigiannakis A, BenKhalifa M, Vrekoussis T et al. Repeated implantation failure: A new potential treatment option. *Eur J Clin Invest.* 2015;45:380–4.
44. Yoshioka S, Fujiwara H, Nakayama T et al. Intrauterine administration of autologous peripheral blood mononuclear cells promotes implantation rates in patients with repeated failure of IVF-embryo transfer. *Hum Reprod.* 2006;21:3290–4.
45. Cole LA. Biological functions of hCG and hCG-related molecules. *Reprod Biol Endocrinol.* 2010;8:102.
46. Kayisli UA, Selam B, Guzeloglu-Kayisli O et al. Human chorionic gonadotropin contributes to maternal immunotolerance and endometrial apoptosis by regulating Fas-Fas ligand system. *J Immunol.* 2003;171:2305–13.
47. Huang QY, Rong MH, Lan AH et al. The impact of atosiban on pregnancy outcomes in women undergoing *in vitro* fertilization-embryo transfer: A meta-analysis. *PLOS ONE.* 2017;12:e0175501.
48. Kolibianakis EM, Venetis CA, Diedrich K et al. Addition of growth hormone to gonadotrophins in ovarian stimulation of poor responders treated by in-vitro fertilization: A systematic review and meta-analysis. *Hum Reprod Update.* 2009;15:613–22.
49. Altmae S, Mendoza-Tesarik R, Mendoza C et al. Effect of growth hormone on uterine receptivity in women with repeated implantation failure in an oocyte donation program: A randomized controlled trial. *J Endocr Soc.* 2018;2:96–105.
50. Clark DA, Coulam CB, Stricker RB. Is intravenous immunoglobulins (IVIG) efficacious in early pregnancy failure? A critical review and meta-analysis for patients who fail *in vitro* fertilization and embryo transfer (IVF). *J Assist Reprod Genet.* 2006;23:1–13.
51. Placido G D, Zullo F, Mollo A et al. Intravenous immunoglobulin (IVIG) in the prevention of implantation failures. *Ann N Y Acad Sci.* 1994;734:232–4.
52. Sher G, Matzner W, Feinman M et al. The selective use of heparin/aspirin therapy, alone or in combination with intravenous immunoglobulin G, in the management of antiphospholipid antibody-positive women undergoing *in vitro* fertilization. *Am J Reprod Immunol.* 1998;40:74–82.
53. Stephenson MD, Fluker MR. Treatment of repeated unexplained *in vitro* fertilization failure with intravenous immunoglobulin: A randomized, placebo-controlled Canadian trial. *Fertil Steril.* 2000;74:1108–13.
54. Shrestha BM. Two decades of tacrolimus in renal transplant: Basic science and clinical evidences. *Exp Clin Transplant.* 2017;15:1–9.
55. Nakagawa K, Kwak-Kim J, Ota K et al. Immunosuppression with tacrolimus improved reproductive outcome of women with repeated implantation failure and elevated peripheral blood TH1/TH2 cell ratios. *Am J Reprod Immunol.* 2015;73:353–61.
56. Ghasemnejad-Berenji H, Ghaffari Novin M, Hajshafiha M et al. Immunomodulatory effects of hydroxychloroquine on Th1/Th2 balance in women with repeated implantation failure. *Biomed Pharmacother.* 2018;107:1277–85.

57. Zhang L, Xu WH, Fu XH et al. Therapeutic role of granulocyte colony-stimulating factor (G-CSF) for infertile women under *in vitro* fertilization and embryo transfer (IVF-ET) treatment: A meta-analysis. *Arch Gynecol Obstet*. 2018;298:861–71.

58. Simon L, Zini A, Dyachenko A et al. A systematic review and meta-analysis to determine the effect of sperm DNA damage on *in vitro* fertilization and intracytoplasmic sperm injection outcome. *Asian J Androl*. 2017;19:80–90.

59. Coughlan C, Clarke H, Cutting R et al. Sperm DNA fragmentation, recurrent implantation failure and recurrent miscarriage. *Asian J Androl*. 2015;17:681–5.

60. Bellver J, Pellicer A, Garcia-Velasco JA et al. Obesity reduces uterine receptivity: Clinical experience from 9,587 first cycles of ovum donation with normal weight donors. *Fertil Steril*. 2013;100:1050–8.

61. Benedict MD, Missmer SA, Vahratian A et al. Secondhand tobacco smoke exposure is associated with increased risk of failed implantation and reduced IVF success. *Hum Reprod*. 2011;26:2525–31.

62. Soares SR, Simon C, Remohi J et al. Cigarette smoking affects uterine receptiveness. *Hum Reprod*. 2007;22:543–7.

63. Venetis CA, Kolibianakis EM, Bosdou JK et al. Progesterone elevation and probability of pregnancy after IVF: A systematic review and meta-analysis of over 60 000 cycles. *Hum Reprod Update*. 2013;19:433–57.

64. Liu L, Zhou F, Lin X et al. Recurrent IVF failure is associated with elevated progesterone on the day of hCG administration. *Eur J Obstet Gynecol Reprod Biol*. 2013;171:78–83.

65. Venetis CA, Kolibianakis EM, Bosdou JK et al. Basal serum progesterone and history of elevated progesterone on the day of hCG administration are significant predictors of late follicular progesterone elevation in GnRH antagonist IVF cycles. *Hum Reprod*. 2016;31:1859–65.

66. Magdi Y, El-Damen A, Fathi AM et al. Revisiting the management of recurrent implantation failure through freeze-all policy. *Fertil Steril*. 2017;108:72–7.

67. Cohen J, Scott R, Alikani M et al. Ooplasmic transfer in mature human oocytes. *Mol Hum Reprod*. 1998;4:269–80.

68. Barritt JA, Brenner CA, Malter HE et al. Mitochondria in human offspring derived from ooplasmic transplantation. *Hum Reprod*. 2001;16:513–6.

69. Zeyneloglu HB, Kahraman S. The use of coculture in assisted reproductive technology: Does it have any impact? *Curr Opin Obstet Gynecol*. 2009;21:253–9.

70. Friedler S, Schachter M, Strassburger D et al. A randomized clinical trial comparing recombinant hyaluronan/recombinant albumin versus human tubal fluid for cleavage stage embryo transfer in patients with multiple IVF-embryo transfer failure. *Hum Reprod*. 2007;22:2444–8.

71. Arefi S, Hoseini A, Farifteh F et al. Modified natural cycle frozen-thawed embryo transfer in patients with repeated implantation failure: An observational study. *Int J Reprod Biomed (Yazd)*. 2016;14:465–70.

72. Bosdou JK, Venetis CA, Tarlatzis BC et al. Higher probability of live-birth in high, but not normal, responders after first frozen-embryo transfer in a freeze-only cycle strategy compared to fresh-embryo transfer: A meta-analysis. *Hum Reprod*. 2019;34:491–505.

14

Fibroids: To Remove or Not

Abdel-Maguid Ramzy

Introduction

Uterine myomas (leiomyomata, fibroids) are the most common tumor of the reproductive tract, with a cumulative incidence of 70% in women of reproductive age (1). These benign monoclonal tumors are more common and are associated with the most severe symptoms in women of African descent. Compared with Caucasian women with symptomatic myomas, women of African descent typically present to their provider at a younger age and with a significantly worse myoma burden as in larger size and number (2). Fibroids vary greatly in their size, number, and location within the uterus—all factors that could negatively impact a woman's fertility. Regardless of their location, size, or number, uterine fibroids are found in about 5%–10% of women with infertility (3). For approximately 1.0%–2.4% of women with infertility, fibroids are the only abnormal findings (4,5). The adverse effects include both a reduction in fertility and an association with early pregnancy complications (6,7). Uterine myomas are associated with a variety of clinical problems including menorrhagia, pelvic pressure, as well as pregnancy complications, and adverse obstetric outcomes such as preterm labor and delivery, placenta previa, intrauterine growth retardation, increased rate of cesarean section, and postpartum hemorrhage (8–10).

Risk Factors for the Development of Uterine Myomas

Early menarche, nulliparity, caffeine and alcohol consumption, obesity, and high blood pressure have all been found to increase the risk of developing uterine myomata (11). Epidemiological evidence indicates that the prevalence of uterine fibroids increases as a woman gets older. At the same time, assisted reproductive technology (ART) statistics suggest that women are delaying childbearing, which increases their risk of both age-related and fibroid-related impacts on fertility.

Pathophysiology in Relation to Impact of Location of Uterine Myomas and *In Vitro* Fertilization Outcome

Various systems have been proposed so far to describe myomas. Still, none takes into account all the parameters that determine the heterogeneity of these tumors. Traditionally, based on their location in relationship to the endometrial cavity, myomas are classified as submucosal, intramural, or subserosal (12). It is essential that the criteria for differentiating intramural from subserosal myomas be clearly stated. The operational definition for a subserosal location was that all fibroids for that patient had 50% of their volume projecting beyond the outer uterine contour. If one or more of the uterine fibroids were projecting 50% or were clearly intramural, they were defined as "intramural" (IM) (13). Somigliana et al. have argued that because the thickness of a normal uterine wall is 15–20 mm, all fibroids that do not distort the uterine cavity and with a mean diameter of more than 30 mm may be classified as subserosal, even if the lesion takes up the entire uterine wall (14). The International Federation of Gynecology and Obstetrics (FIGO) classification, introduced by Munro and colleagues in 2011, is based on the relationship of the fibroid with the uterine wall for causes of abnormal uterine bleeding in nongravid women of reproductive age. According to this classification, nine types of myomas have been described, from type 0 (pedunculated intracavitary fibroids) to type 7 (pedunculated subserosal fibroids). Type 8, the last one representing fibroids, cannot otherwise be classified (viz. cervical, parasitic, etc.) (15).

The current existing evidence indicates that these effects are directly dependent on the proximity of the fibroid to the endometrium (16). The glandular atrophy in the endometrium overlying the fibroid is one of the most commonly observed histological alterations associated with fibroids (17,18). More recently, experiments of Rackow and Taylor have demonstrated that the presence of submucosal and intramural fibroids results in a global reduction in endometrial HOX gene expression, which is not limited to the focal area overlying the fibroid(s). The authors suggested the observed impaired endometrial receptivity might be mediated by a diffusible signaling molecule(s) that is secreted from the fibroid but exerts its effects across the entire endometrium (19).

As for the effect of uterine fibroids on the chance of a woman to get pregnant and keep her pregnancy to term, it is prudent to refer back to spontaneous pregnancies to have a broad idea of the pathophysiology of the problem. Pritts et al. carried out a systematic literature review and meta-analysis of existing controlled studies looking into the clinical pregnancy rate, spontaneous abortion rate, ongoing pregnancy, live birth rate, implantation rate, and preterm delivery rate in women with and without fibroids, and in women who underwent myomectomy. They mapped clearly the location/effect relationship of uterine fibroids versus pregnancy outcome. They stated that fertility outcomes are decreased in women with submucosal fibroids, and removal seems to confer benefit. Subserosal fibroids do not affect fertility outcomes, and removal does not confer benefit. Women with intramural fibroids appeared to have decreased fertility but the results of therapy are unclear (20).

Arguments against the Removal of Myomas

In 1992, Seoud et al. found in a retrospective cohort study of 58 women undergoing ART with a history of prior myomectomy ($n = 47$) or myomas *in situ* ($n = 11$) that there were similar clinical pregnancy rates between the groups, and in comparison to the overall IVF population (21). However in this study, it is noted that 10 of the 11 subjects with myomas *in situ* had subserosal myomas, and 50.7% of the myomectomy group had subserosal myomas removed. The groups were similar in age and duration of infertility, but the myomectomy group had a significantly higher incidence of primary infertility compared with the myoma group (74.5% versus 45.5%, $P < .001$). An additional limiting factor includes the fact that overall pregnancy rates were much lower when this study was performed during the early days of ART.

By a retrospective study by our group from Egypt, Ramzy et al. raised this issue back in 1998, when we were encouraged to go ahead with IVF and not surgery first for those patients having myomas less than 7 cm, as we have shown that they do not affect the implantation or miscarriage rates in IVF or ICSI. In our study among 406 patients, 51 (12.6%) were found to have uterine corporeal myomata. The study concluded that uterine corporeal myomata, not encroaching on the cavity and less than 7 cm in mean diameter, do not affect the implantation or miscarriage rates in IVF or ICSI (22).

In another study from our group, Aboulghar et al. in 2004 in a cohort study compared 63 infertile women with intramural myomas to 100 age-matched controls without myomas undergoing the same stimulation protocol for IVF. Of the 63 women with myomas, 19 underwent myomectomy prior to IVF, and the authors concluded that clinical pregnancy rates were not statistically different between groups (36% myomectomy versus 29% intramural myoma with no myomectomy versus 36% controls) (23). In 2004 as well, Oliveira et al. from Brazil in a retrospective, matched-control study included 245 women with subserosal and/or intramural fibroids that did not compress the uterine cavity (fibroid group) and 245 women with no evidence of fibroids anywhere in the uterus (control group). They concluded that patients having subserosal or intramural leiomyomas of less than 4 cm not encroaching on the uterine cavity have IVF-ICSI outcomes comparable to those of patients without such leiomyomas. Therefore, they might not require myomectomy before being scheduled for assisted reproduction cycles. However, they recommended caution for patients with fibroids greater than 4 cm and that such patients may need to be submitted to treatment before they are enrolled in IVF-ICSI cycles. Whether or not women with fibroids greater than 4 cm would benefit from fibroid treatment remains to be determined (24). The same limitations came from Bari, Italy, where Vimercati et al. in a retrospective single-center assessment of clinical outcomes of IVF/ICSI cycles in 224 cycles from patients with fibroids or who had undergone myomectomy, versus 215 cycles with no fibroids, concurred that myomas less than 4 cm do not need interference. Because they are intramural and not encroaching on the cavity, they pose no threat on the pregnancy and live birth rates of the pregnancy cycle following IVF. They went even further to withhold myomectomy in larger myomas (greater than 4 cm), and offer them more cycles to increase their chances of getting pregnant (25).

Another prospective, randomized, multicenter clinical trial study, though not including IVF/ICSI cycles, investigated the association of non-cavity-distorting uterine fibroids and pregnancy outcomes after ovarian stimulation-intrauterine insemination in 900 couples with unexplained infertility, of which 102 had one or more uterine fibroids among African and non-African American women. They concluded that there are no differences in conception and live birth rates in women with non-cavity-distorting fibroids and those without fibroids (26).

Arguments for the Removal of Myomas

On a different note, starting in 1995, Farhi et al. found a different effect of uterine myomata on the outcome of ART cycles. They concluded that implantation rate and pregnancy outcome are impaired in women with uterine leiomyomata only when they cause deformation of the uterine cavity. They advised that in patients with leiomyomata associated with an abnormal uterine cavity, surgical treatment should be considered prior to IVF because of the reduced implantation rate (27).

In 1998 as well, Eldar-Geva et al., in a retrospective comparative study, including 106 ART cycles in 88 patients with uterine fibroids (33 subserosal, 46 intramural without cavity distortion, and 9 submucosal) was compared with that of 318 ART cycles in age-matched patients without fibroids (28), concluded that pregnancy and implantation rates were significantly lower in the groups of patients with intramural and submucosal fibroids, even when there was no deformation of the uterine cavity. Pregnancy and implantation rates were not influenced by the presence of subserosal fibroids. They recommended surgical or medical treatment should be considered in infertile patients who have intramural and/or submucosal fibroids before resorting to ART treatment.

Concerning intramural fibroids, Bulletti and colleagues reported significant improvement in spontaneous pregnancy rate in a cohort of 106 women with fibroids of various types (submucosal, intramural, and subserosal) who underwent myomectomy, compared to 106 women with fibroids who did not undergo myomectomy (42% versus 11%) (29). The same group reported a significant improvement in pregnancy and delivery rate in IVF/ICSI cycles following myomectomy for intramural and subserosal fibroids in women with normal uterine cavity but with at least one intramural fibroid larger than 5 cm (pregnancy rate 34% in the myomectomy group versus 15% in the group with fibroids *in situ* and delivery rate 25% versus 12%, respectively) (30).

On the same note to these findings, Bulletti et al. in 2004, in a trial of 168 women with non-cavity-distorting myomas (one to five myomas; at least one greater than 5 cm and no submucosal component) compared outcomes among those who underwent laparoscopy before IVF versus women with myomas and no surgery prior to IVF. Investigators reported a superior cumulative pregnancy rate (34% [28/84] versus 15% [13/84], $P < .05$) and live birth delivery rate (25% [21/84] versus 12% [10/84], $P < .05$) in the group undergoing laparoscopy compared with the nonsurgical group. The benefit of myomectomy was observed in the surgical group of women who had at least one fibroid with a diameter greater than 5 cm and a normal uterine cavity, but age differences between groups were not reported or taken into consideration in the analysis. Additional limitations include lack of comparison of fibroid size and number between groups and potential selection bias as the subjects choose which intervention they received (surgery versus no surgery). Thus, while these trials suggest that myomectomy may improve pregnancy rates, concerns about selection bias and confounding by age make it difficult to recommend myomectomy to improve pregnancy and live birth rates (31).

Khalaf et al. in 2006 thought that it was unwise to adopt the conservative approach in cases having uterine myomas and enrolled patients for IVF treatment cycles. They have shown, through their study in 2006 including 322 women without fibroids (control group) and 112 women with fibroids (study group), that these cases underwent 606 IVF/ICSI cycles (32). They concluded that regarding the cumulative pregnancy rates after three IVF cycles, even the small myomas, significantly reduce the ongoing pregnancy rate at each cycle of IVF/ICSI by 40% and the live birth rate at each cycle by 45%. The same group carried out a systematic review and meta-analysis in 2010, including 19 observational studies comprising 6087 IVF cycles, on myomas that do not distort the cavity. They reached the conclusion that the presence of non-cavity-distorting intramural fibroids is associated with adverse pregnancy outcomes in women undergoing IVF treatment (33).

In a recent retrospective, matched, single-center, cohort study in 2016, including 163 women with fibroids and matched with 326 controls in a 1:2 ratio, Christopoulos et al. from London, United Kingdom, concluded that the presence of non-cavity-distorting fibroids appears to negatively affect clinical pregnancy in patients undergoing their first IVF/ICSI cycle, when matched with controls of the same age (34). They further observed that the deleterious effect of fibroids was significant in women with two or more fibroids and in women with fibroids 30 mm in diameter or larger.

In a retrospective cohort study, including 51 cases with type 3 fibroid uterus (type 3 myomas are totally extracavitary but abut the endometrium, FIGO classification) versus 453 cases control, Lei Yan et al. concluded that type 3 myomas have a significant negative effect on the main IVF-ICSI outcomes, including implantation rate, clinical pregnancy rate, and live birth rate, but do not significantly increase the clinical miscarriage rate. The deleterious impact was remarkable in women with type 3 fibroids with diameter greater than 2.0 cm (35).

Whether For or Against: Check the Uterine Cavity First

The two most commonly used modalities to evaluate the effects of fibroids on the uterine are discussed. The sensitivity and specificity of HSG for detection of intrauterine lesions may be as low as 50% and 20%, respectively (36). Transvaginal ultrasound was initially considered to have a sensitivity of as high as 90%–100% and a specificity of 87%–98% (37). However, subsequent studies failed to reproduce the initial reports and showed sensitivities of as low as 69% (38) and specificity of 11% for accurate identification of submucosal fibroids (39). More recently, saline infusion sonography or sonohysterography (SHG), particularly the three-dimensional (3D) mode, has gained popularity as an accurate imaging modality for the evaluation of uterine cavity (40). The expertise to use this office modality and the proper settings, including the availability of the needed disposables as well as asepsis, is an obvious limitation. Hysteroscopy is considered the gold standard for evaluation of the uterine cavity. Compared to hysteroscopy, 2D and 3D SHG have sensitivities of 98% and 100%, respectively. More importantly, 2D and 3D SHG are reported to have specificities of 100%. In contrast, the specificity of transvaginal ultrasound can be as low as 11% when compared to hysteroscopy or 3D sonohysterogram (41). In addition to hysteroscopy, magnetic resonance imaging (MRI) is another reliable diagnostic modality that may accurately identify and localize the fibroids, especially in complicated cases. Because it is expensive, MRI is usually performed as an ancillary imaging method (42).

Counseling Patients

The decision to do a myomectomy before an IVF cycle is not an easy one. You will always be faced with the question: "Do you think it is essential, doctor?" To answer this question, you have to have clear-cut evidence that this woman will more likely face less of a chance to get pregnant following an IVF cycle unless she has a myomectomy. Or if she gets pregnant, she will probably lose her baby. We have to bear in mind that these patients are desperate. They consider IVF as the salvage for their long-standing misery as they believe it is a "once and for all" means for them to fulfill their dream of having a baby. Suggesting myomectomy before IVF may not be welcomed by these patients, as other than being "a surgery" with all its risks and fears, it is a setback or at the very least a delay in their "time-to-pregnancy" path. Remember that a good number of these patients are in their late 30s. In the back of their minds, they know that they do not have the luxury of waiting, as their fertile days will soon perish (43).

What about the Effect of Previous Myomectomy on the Success of the IVF Cycles?

What effects do the presence of uterine fibroids have on the success of ART cycles? Some studies advise against myomectomy before enrolling a patient for IVF, while other studies show evidence that myomectomy will promote the possibility of positive outcome of these cycles. Another angle we should take into consideration is the fact that myomectomy is considered a major surgery. As with any major surgical procedure, myomectomy carries risks, such as bleeding, infection, and damage to other organs. Furthermore, myomectomy is associated with adhesion formation, although this may be argued that it is not a concern for women who are planning to pursue ART (44,45). However, the adhesions around the fimbrial ends of the tubes, whether partial or complete occlusion of the ostia of the tube, will inevitably lead to fimbrial phimosis or in more grave cases, hydrosalpinx. The latter is proven to cause failure of the outcome of IVF/ICSI cycles. This will entitle another surgical procedure before enrolling the patient to a new cycle to excise or occlude the tube. It is to be considered that intestinal adhesions are not to be ignored. At the very least, they may cause some localized discomfort or colicky pain in some cases.

In general, when considering the effects of myomectomy on IVF outcomes in particular, there are few studies available. Two recent studies have attempted to underscore the fact that previous myomectomy does not adversely affect IVF outcomes. Narayan et al. investigated the effect of myomectomy in 27 patients who had undergone hysteroscopic myomectomy for submucosal fibroids (46). Their delivery rate was not significantly different from a group of control patients without fibroids (37% versus 22%; $p = .13$). Surrey et al. also described IVF outcomes in 101 patients after myomectomy for submucosal fibroids compared with 1448 controls. The pregnancy rates were 68% and 62%, respectively ($p = .24$) (47). Thus, previous myomectomy does not appear to negatively affect pregnancy rates in IVF cycles.

While surgical myomectomy has been the traditional treatment for fibroids, over the last several years, nonsurgical approaches have begun to increase in popularity. Several alternative approaches, such as uterine artery embolization and laparoscopic cryomyolysis, have recently been investigated. However, due to safety concerns, women who desire to retain fertility have generally been excluded from studies on these treatments (48). Thus, the data on pregnancy outcomes for these procedures are scarce and, furthermore, the safety of the procedures needs to be evaluated before reproductive outcomes can be discussed (49).

Conclusion

Cases with uterine myomata who are seeking fertility through ART should be handled on an individualized basis. Since pregnancy-related concerns depend on the location and size of the leiomyoma, the importance of an in-depth discussion of a management plan between patients and physicians cannot be overemphasized. In counseling the patient with your final decision, the age of the patient and her ovarian reserve should be taken into consideration given the time lapse that will have to be imposed before pursuing another ART cycle (Figure 14.1). From several studies, it is concluded that subserosal myomas less than 7 cm in size and intramural myomas less than 4–5 cm in diameter that do not encroach upon the endometrium appear to have little effect on IVF outcomes. Larger intramural and subserosal myomas present a clinical dilemma, and more studies are needed to clarify a definitive plan for management. Myomectomy should be considered in women affected with submucosal and/or intramural fibroids, encroaching on the cavity, who are pursuing fertility treatments, particularly in cases of previously failed IVF/ICSI cycles. High-resolution 2D transvaginal sonography may serve as an initial screening tool for the assessment of uterine

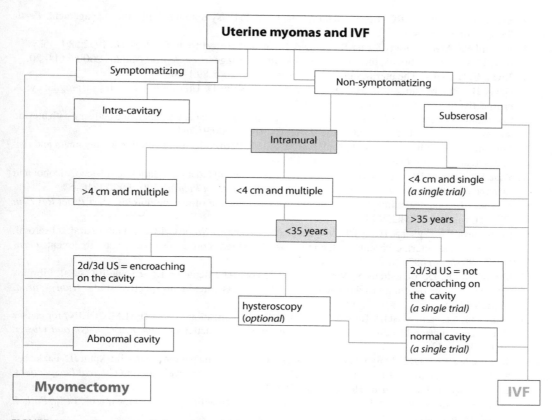

FIGURE 14.1   A flowchart outlining a suggested line of management for cases with uterine myomas who are counseled to enroll in assisted reproductive technology cycles.

myomas in this respect. In cases with deep implanted intramural myomas and submucous myomas, 3D SHG is an essential, more accurate diagnostic tool. In addition, hysteroscopy should be considered an invaluable additional tool in the proper assessment of the uterine cavity of IVF patients with fibroids. This tool is valuable in studying the endometrium overlying those myomas that compromise the uterine cavity such as submucous myomas, or in cases with intramural myomas impacted deep enough to encroach on the uterine cavity. In addition, evaluate the endometrium and uterine cavity before enrolling the patient in a new or repeat ART cycle. Hysteroscopic myomectomy should be considered the gold standard for the treatment of submucous myomas. On a different but significant note, myomectomy has long been regarded as the standard treatment for the various symptoms associated with fibroids, such as pelvic pressure, pain, or menorrhagia. Alternative treatment modalities, such as uterine artery embolization, laparoscopic myolysis, or MRI-guided focused ultrasound should not be routinely employed until their safety and efficacy have been more fully evaluated. On a final note, further research is needed to resolve the argument forward.

REFERENCES

1. Baird DD, Dunson DB, Hill MC, Cousins D, Schectman JM. High cumulative incidence of uterine leiomyoma in black and white women: Ultrasound evidence. *Am J Obstet Gynecol.* 2003;188:100–7.
2. Peddada SD, Laughlin SK, Miner K, Guyon JP, Haneke K, Vahdat HL et al. Growth of uterine leiomyomata among premenopausal black and white women. *Proc Natl Acad Sci USA.* 2008;105:19887–92.
3. Donnez J, Jadoul P. What are the implications of myomas on fertility? A need for a debate? Hum. *Reprod.* 2002;17:1424–30.

4. Buttram VC J, Reiter RC. Uterine leiomyomata: Etiology, symptomatology, and management. *Fertil Steril.* 1981;36:433–45.
5. Verkauf BS. Myomectomy for fertility enhancement and preservation. *Fertil Steril.* 1992;58:1–15.
6. Bajekal N, Li TC. Fibroids, infertility and pregnancy wastage. *Hum Reprod Update.* 2000;6:614–20.
7. Taylor E, Gomel V. The uterus and fertility. *Fertil Steril.* 2008;89:1–16.
8. Davis JL, Ray-Mazumder S, Hobel CJ, Baley K, Sassoon D. Uterine leiomyomas in pregnancy: A prospective study. *Obstet Gynecol.* 1990;75:41–4.
9. Coronado GD, Marshall LM, Schwartz SM. Complications in pregnancy, labor, and delivery with uterine leiomyomas: A population-based study. *Obstet Gynecol.* 2000;95:764–9.
10. Vergani P, Locatelli A, Ghidini A, Andreani M, Sala F, Pezullo JC. Large uterine leiomyomata and risk of cesarean delivery. *Obstet Gynecol.* 2007;109:410–4.
11. Wise LA, Palmer JR, Harlow BL et al. Risk of uterine leiomyomata in relation to tobacco, alcohol and caffeine consumption in the Black Women's Health Study. *Hum Reprod.* 2004;19(8):1746–54.
12. McLucas B. Diagnosis, imaging and anatomical classification of uterine fibroids. *Best Pract Res Clin Obstet Gynaecol.* 2008;22:627–42.
13. Eldar-Geva T, Meagher S, Healy DL, MacLachlan V, Breheny S, Wood C. Effect of intramural, subserosal, and submucosal uterine fibroids on the outcome of assisted reproductive technology treatment. *Fertil Steril.* 1998;70(4):687–91.
14. Somigliana E, De Benedictis S, Vercellini P, Nicolosi AE, Benaglia L, Scarduelli C et al. Fibroids not encroaching the endometrial cavity and IVF success rate: A prospective study. *Hum Reprod.* 2011;26:834–9.
15. Munro MG, Critchley HOD, Broder MS et al. FIGO classification system (PALM-COEIN) for causes of abnormal uterine bleeding in nongravid women of reproductive age. *Int J of Gynecol and Obstet.* 2011;113(1):3–13.
16. Maguire M, Segars JH. Benign uterine disease: Leiomyomata and benign polyps. In: Aplin JD, Fazleabas AT, Glasser SR, Giudice LC, editors. *The Endometrium: Molecular, Cellular and Clinical Perspectives.* 2nd ed. London, UK: Informa HealthCare; 2008:797–812.
17. Deligdish L, Loewenthal M. Endometrial changes associated with myomata of the uterus. *J Clin Pathol.* 1970;23(8):676–80.
18. Sharma SP, Misra SD, Mittal VP. Endometrial changes—A criterion for the diagnosis of submucous uterine leiomyoma. *Indian J Pathol Microbiol.* 1979;22(1):33–6.
19. Rackow BW, Taylor HS. Submucosal uterine leiomyomas have a global effect on molecular determinants of endometrial receptivity. *Fertil Steril.* 2010;93(6):2027–34.
20. Pritts EA, Parker WH, Olive DL. Fibroids and infertility: An updated systematic review of the evidence. *Fertil Steril.* 2009;91(4):1215–23.
21. Seoud M, Patterson R, Musher S, Coddington C. Effects of myoma or prior myomectomy on *in vitro* fertilization (IVF) performance. *J Assist Reprod Genet.* 1992;9:217–21.
22. Ramzy AM, Sattar M, Amin Y, Mansour RT, Serour GI, Aboulghar MA. Uterine myomata and outcome of assisted reproduction. *Hum Reprod.* 1998;13(1):198–202.
23. Aboulghar MM, Al-Inany HG, Aboulghar MA, Serour GI, Mansour RT. The effect of intramural fibroids on the outcome of IVF. *Mid East Fertil Soc J.* 2004;9:263–7.
24. Oliveira FG, Abdelmassih VG, Diamond MP, Dozortsev D, Melo NR, Abdelmassih R. Impact of subserosal and intramural uterine fibroids that do not distort the endometrial cavity on the outcome of *in vitro* fertilization–intracytoplasmic sperm injection. *Fertil Steril.* 2004;81(3):582–7.
25. Vimercati A, Scioscia M, Lorusso F, Laera AF, Lamanna G, Coluccia A et al. Do uterine fibroids affect IVF outcomes? *Reprod Biomed Online.* 2007;15(6):686–91.
26. Styer AK, Jin S, Liu D et al. Association of uterine fibroids and pregnancy outcomes after ovarian stimulation-intrauterine insemination for unexplained infertility. *Fertil Steril.* 2017;107(3):756–62.e3.
27. Farhi J, Ashkenazi J, Feldberg D, Dicker D, Orvieto R, Ben Rafael Z. Effect of uterine leiomyomata on the results of *in-vitro* fertilization treatment. *Hum Reprod.* 1995;10(10):2576–78.
28. Eldar-Geva T, Meagher S, Healy DL, MacLachlan V, Breheny S, Wood C. Effect of intramural, subserosal, and submucosal uterine fibroids on the outcome of assisted reproductive technology treatment. *Fertil Steril.* 1998;70(4):687–91.
29. Bulletti C, De Ziegler D, Polli V, Flamigni C. The role of leiomyomas in infertility. *J Am Assoc Gynecol Laparosc.* 1999;6(4):441–5.

30. Bulletti C, DE Ziegler D, Levi Setti P, Cicinelli E, Polli V, Stefanetti M. Myomas, pregnancy outcome, and *in vitro* fertilization. *Ann N Y Acad Sci.* 2004;1034:84–92.

31. Bulletti C, De Ziegler D, Levi Setti P, Cicinelli E, Polli V, Stefanetti M. Myomas, pregnancy outcome, and *in vitro* fertilization. *Ann N Y Acad Sci.* 2004;1034:84–92.

32. Khalaf Y, Ross C, El-Toukhy T, Hart R, Seed P, Braude P. The effect of small intramural uterine fibroids on the cumulative outcome of assisted conception. *Hum Reprod.* 2006;21(10):2640–4.

33. Sunkara SK, Khairy M, El-Toukhy T, Khalaf Y, Coomarasamy A. The effect of intramural fibroids without uterine cavity involvement on the outcome of IVF treatment: A systematic review and meta-analysis. *Hum Reprod.* 2010;25(2):418–29.

34. Christopoulos G, Vlismas A, Salim R, Islam R, Trew G, Lavery S. Fibroids that do not distort the uterine cavity and IVF success rates: An observational study using extensive matching criteria. *BJOG.* 2017;124(4):615–21.

35. Yan L, Yu Q, Zhang YN, Guo Z, Li Z, Niu J, Ma J. Effect of type 3 intramural fibroids on in vitro fertilization–intracytoplasmic sperm injection outcomes: A retrospective cohort study. *Fertil Steril.* 2018;109(5):817–22.

36. Soares SR, Barbosa dos Reis MM, Camargos AF. Diagnostic accuracy of sonohysterography, transvaginal sonography, and hysterosalpingography in patients with uterine cavity diseases. *Fertil Steril.* 2000;73(2):406–11.

37. Indman PD. Abnormal uterine bleeding. Accuracy of vaginal probe ultrasound in predicting abnormal hysteroscopic findings. *J Reprod Med.* 1995;40(8):545–8.

38. Cepni I, Ocal P, Erkan S, Saricali FS, Akbas H, Demirkiran F, Idil M, Bese T. Comparison of transvaginal sonography, saline infusion sonography and hysteroscopy in the evaluation of uterine cavity pathologies. *Aust N Z J Obstet Gynaecol.* 2005;45(1):30–5.

39. Sylvestre C, Child TJ, Tulandi T, Tan SL. A prospective study to evaluate the efficacy of two- and three-dimensional sonohysterography in women with intrauterine lesions. *Fertil Steril.* 2003;79(5):1222–5.

40. Makris N, Kalmantis K, Skartados N, Papadimitriou A, Mantzaris G, Antsaklis A. Three-dimensional hysterosonography versus hysteroscopy for the detection of intracavitary uterine abnormalities. *Int J Gynaecol Obstet.* 2007;97(1):6–9.

41. de Kroon CD, Louwé LA, Trimbos JB, Jansen FW. The clinical value of 3-dimensional saline infusion sonography in addition to 2-dimensional saline infusion sonography in women with abnormal uterine bleeding: Work in progress. *J Ultrasound Med.* 2004;23:1433–40.

42. Dueholm M, Lundorf E, Sørensen JS, Ledertoug S, Olesen F, Laursen H. Reproducibility of evaluation of the uterus by transvaginal sonography, hysterosonographic examination, hysteroscopy and magnetic resonance imaging. *Hum Reprod.* 2002;17(1):195–200.

43. Ramzy AM. Myomectomy before IVF: Which fibroids need to be removed? Debate. *Middle East Fertil Soc J.* 2011;(16):38–44.

44. Dubuisson JB, Fauconnier A, Chapron C, Kreiker G, Nörgaard C. Second look after laparoscopic myomectomy. *Hum Reprod.* 1998;13:2102–6.

45. Fauconnier A, Dubuisson JB, Ancel PY, Chapron C. Prognostic factors of reproductive outcome after myomectomy in infertile patients. *Hum Reprod.* 2000;15:1751–7.

46. Narayan R, Rajat R, Goswamy K. Treatment of submucous fibroids, and outcome of assisted conception. *J Am Assoc Gynecol Laparosc.* 1994;1:307–11.

47. Surrey ES, Minjarez DA, Stevens JM, Schoolcraft WB. Effect of myomectomy on the outcome of assisted reproductive technologies. *Fertil Steril.* 2005;83:1473–9.

48. Somigliana E, Vercellini P, Daguati R, Pasin R, De Giorgi O, Crosignani PG. Fibroids and female reproduction: A critical analysis of the evidence. *Hum Reprod Update* 2007;13:465–76.

49. Kolankaya A, Arici A. Myomas and assisted reproductive technologies: When and how to act? *Obstet. Gynecol Clin North Am.* 2006;33:145–52.

15

Limitations of Endometrioma Surgery in In Vitro Fertilization: Possibilities of Early Disease Control

Vasilios Tanos and Elsie Sowah

Introduction

Endometrioma affects 17%–44% of women with endometriosis (1). Approximately 17% of women suffering from infertility are diagnosed with an endometrioma (2). The pathogenesis of endometrioma is characterized by sequential and progressive damage of healthy ovarian tissue. During menses, implantation of regurgitated endometrial cells on the ovarian surface (via tubal lumen) causes a series of biochemical mechanisms including persistent inflammation, bleeding (at implantation site) and invagination of the ovarian cortex, adhesions, cystic formations, tissue alterations, and deformity (3). Invagination of the ovarian cortex secondary to metaplasia of celomic epithelium in the context of cortical inclusion cysts has also been proposed as a possible mechanism of endometrioma formation (4). Hence, the endometrioma pseudocapsule is ovarian epithelium containing the follicular structures and oocytes. Upon opening the endometrioma after irrigation, endoscopic imaging reveals pinkish tissue that is the ovarian epithelium. The ovarian tissue that is identifiable during endoscopic imaging is embedded thus with endometriotic cells that can continue to proliferate and even migrate if not destroyed (5).

In addition, ovarian endometriosis, whether superficial or deep, is a marker of more significant pelvic and intestinal endometriotic lesions (6). Despite the fact that diagnosis of an endometrioma can be done by transvaginal ultrasound examination at a very early stage, the identification of which patients will deteriorate by developing larger endometrioma remains a major challenge.

Although cyclic pelvic pain, dyspareunia, bleeding, dysuria, and infertility are the most common presentations, symptomatology does not indicate the extent or progression of the disease. Endometriosis awareness among general practitioners and the public is still very poor. Misdiagnosis and undertreatment occur frequently. As a result, endometrioma is often diagnosed when the cyst is very large, or the disease has reached an advanced stage. Hence, many infertility patients present with endometrioma and tubal factor problems with an indication for an *in vitro* fertilization (IVF) treatment.

A systematic review of the literature was performed to identify the course of action in treating endometrioma prior to IVF. In addition, nine current guidelines by international gynecological societies were used as a tool to guide identification of the current gaps in research and evidence for clinical practice. Research also focused on the pros and cons as well as outcomes of endometrioma surgical treatment before IVF. Based on the evidence and conclusions of our research, an algorithm for the options in the management of endometrioma prior to IVF is proposed.

Materials and Methods

Materials

A literature review was performed by searching Internet/online databases and former papers and presentations. Internet-based resources included the following: (a) search engines: Google and Google Scholar; (b) research databases: PubMed and Ovid Embase; and (c) library database: St. George's University of London Hunter Database. Numerous scientific journals both print-based and some web-based were accessed through the databases. Main titles included *Fertility and Sterility, American Journal of Obstetrics and Gynecology, European Journal of Obstetrics and Gynecology and Reproductive Biology, Reproductive BioMedicine Online, Human Reproduction,* and *PlosOne.*

Methods

The search terms used were "ovarian endometrioma," "endometrioma + surgery," "endometrioma + surgery + IVF," and "endometrioma + ART." PubMed was used as the primary source of literature due to the highest yield of relevant material.

Results were further filtered by publication date within 10 years. From the final 180 articles, titles and publication dates were used to further distinguish relevant literature and isolate prospective studies. Figure 15.1 outlines the database search process carried out.

Characteristics of Selected Studies

Thirty-three articles matching our search criteria were analyzed and categorized into pros/cons of endometrioma surgery prior to IVF depending on the evidence presented.

Among the 33 articles, 25 were published in the last 10 years, and the remaining were published in the last 15 years.

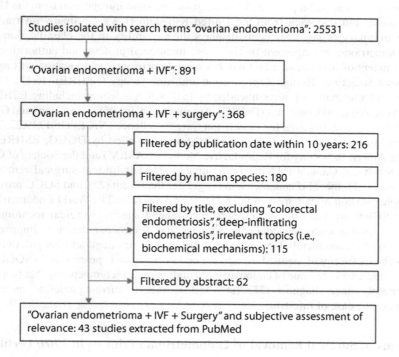

FIGURE 15.1 Methodology used to isolate relevant articles on endometrioma surgery prior to *in vitro* fertilization.

Fourteen articles provided evidence in support of surgical removal prior to ART. There were two retrospective case-control studies, two retrospective cohort studies, and one retrospective analysis. Additionally, there were one committee opinion, one scientific impact paper, one pooled analysis, one literature review, one systematic review, and two meta-analyses. Notably there were only two prospective studies: a prospective cohort study and a prospective randomized study (Table 15.2).

Nineteen articles provided evidence against removal. There were seven retrospective studies and six prospective studies. Additionally, there were two meta-analyses, two literature reviews, one systematic review, and one scientific impact paper (Table 15.3).

Five articles provided evidence for both pro and con removal of endometrioma prior to IVF, a combined total patient population of 6088 (7–11). In seven studies, the research design, number of patients and characteristics, and results extraction were not clear and were excluded from our calculations.

For the analysis of current evidence on implantation and pregnancy rates between surgical removal of endometrioma and no surgery prior to IVF, only four studies matched the selection criteria. The following exclusion criteria were applied to the search: (a) sample population: women with endometrioma, intervention group: women having surgical treatment prior to IVF, and control group: women with unremoved endometrioma going into IVF; (b) primary outcomes: implantation rate and pregnancy rate; (c) interventional studies (no review papers); and (d) publication date within the last 10 years. An exception was made to the fourth criteria in order to include Wong et al. (12) and Garcia-Velasco et al. (13). The publication date criteria resulted in many relevant studies being excluded. Among the four studies selected, two are retrospective case-control studies (13,14) and two are retrospective cohort studies (12,15).

Results

Guidelines

Overall, eight international gynecological societies have published guidelines regarding endometriosis and endometrioma management prior to IVF. One guideline from Europe, two from the United States, two from Canada, and one each from the United Kingdom (UK), Germany/Austria, and France (16–27). The summary of key statements displays the variability in the classification of concerns regarding endometrioma management by the above mentioned professional authorities. Presurgery assessment of extent of disease, size and number of endometrioma, and location was recommended by the European Society of Human Reproduction and Embryology (ESHRE) (16,17). Consideration of ovarian reserve was explicitly recommended by half (4/8) guidelines including ESHRE, German Society for Gynecology and Obstetrics (DGGG), American College of Obstetricians and Gynecologists (ACOG), and the National Institute for Health and Care Excellence (NICE) (16,17,19,22–24). Surgical removal of endometrioma prior to IVF was overtly recommended by DGGG, ESHRE, and NICE (16,19,22). The American Society for Reproductive Medicine (ASRM) and the Society of Obstetricians and Gynaecologists of Canada (SOGC) both support size-conditional surgical removal—ASRM recommends surgical removal if endometrioma is greater than 4 cm (25), and SOGC provides support for laparoscopic excision of endometrioma greater than 3 cm (26). The World Endometriosis Society (WES) and ESHRE are the only societies to recommend specific surgical techniques: ESHRE recommends excision of endometrioma over drainage and electrocoagulation to improve pregnancy rate (17), and WES recommends laparoscopic excision over drainage and coagulation to enhance fertility (18). The inefficacy of medical therapy for endometriomas is prominent in SOGC and DRGG (26,19). SOGC addresses the issue of endometrioma malignancy, recommending that biopsy should be considered for early cancer diagnosis (27). Table 15.1 outlines the current guidelines on the removal of endometrioma in the case of infertility.

Pros and Cons of Surgical Removal of Endometrioma Prior to *In Vitro* Fertilization

The total population across both pros/cons, including control and study patients was 40,724.

TABLE 15.1

Guidelines for the Treatment of Endometrioma in Context of Infertility

Guideline	Key Statements	Reference
ESHRE (Europe)	Presurgery assessment of extent of disease, size and number of endometrioma(s), and location (unilateral, bilateral) is essential. Excision of endometrioma increases postoperative pregnancy rate versus drainage and electrocoagulation. Women must be counseled on risk to ovarian reserve.	Dunselman et al. (16) Saridogan et al., Working Group of ESGE, ESHRE, and WES (17)
WES (Global/Canada)	Laparoscopic excision preferred over laparoscopic ablation to enhance fertility. No clear recommendation for best surgical approach for deep endometriosis in women with infertility. Medical management alongside laparoscopic surgery does not enhance fertility.	Johnson and Hummelsloj et al. for World Endometriosis Society Montpellier Consortium (18)
DGGG (Germany/ Austria)	Surgical removal recommended for improvement of fertility. Consider ovarian reserve in repeat operations.	Ulrich et al. (19)
CNOGF (France)	Surgical removal not recommended to improve chance of fertility. Discovery of endometrioma during IVF treatment should not interrupt treatment. Preservation of fertility must be discussed with patients undergoing surgery for endometriomas.	Chauffour et al. (20) Collinet et al. (21)
NICE (United Kingdom)	When infertility associated, multidisciplinary team and fertility specialist input are essential. Laparoscopic ovarian cystectomy with excision of cyst wall improves spontaneous pregnancy and reduces recurrence. Consider ovarian reserve.	NICE Guideline (22)
ACOG (United States)	No specific recommendation about surgical removal of endometrioma to preserve fertility. Consider ovarian reserve in repeat operations. IVF recommended over repeat surgery after initial unsuccessful surgery, in absence of pain.	ACOG Practice Bulletin (23) Armstrong (24)
ASRM (United States)	Insufficient evidence to recommend resection of endometriomas to improve IVF outcomes. Endometriomas greater than 4 cm should be removed surgically to improve access to follicles and possibly ovarian response.	Practice Committee of the American Society of Reproductive Medicine (25)
SOCG (Canada)	No specific recommendations for surgical removal of endometriomas in infertility Laparoscopic treatment of minimal/mild endometriosis improves pregnancy rates. Laparoscopic excision of endometriomas greater than 3 cm may improve fertility. Medical therapies of endometriomas for infertility are ineffective. Biopsy of endometriosis and ovarian masses recommended (malignancy).	Leyland et al. (26) Le and Giede (27)

Abbreviations: ACOG, American College of Obstetricians and Gynecologists; ASRM, American Society for Reproductive Medicine; CNOGF, Collège National des Gynécologues et Obstétriciens Français; DGGG, German Society for Gynecology and Obstetrics; ESHRE, European Society of Human Reproduction and Embryology; NICE, National Institute for Health and Care Excellence; SOCG, Society of Obstetricians and Gynaecologists of Canada; WES, World Endometriosis Society.

Pros of Surgical Removal of Endometrioma Prior to IVF

The total patient population of articles supporting removal of endometrioma before ART was 30,741. Table 15.2 summarizes the "pros" of surgical removal of endometrioma prior to IVF according to current evidence.

Three articles provided evidence that removal of endometrioma reduces the risk of abscess and infection. The risk of endometrioma rupture with or without pelvic abscess development is supported by five studies within the systematic review carried out by Somigliana et al. (28). The ASRM committee opinion (25)

TABLE 15.2

Pros of Surgical Removal of Endometrioma Prior to Assisted Reproductive Technology

Benefits of Endometrioma Excision Prior to *In Vitro* Fertilization (IVF)	PROS Number of Patients	Type of Study(ies)	References
Avoidance of Abscesses, Infection			
Risks of ruptured endometrioma	–	Systematic review (2006)	Somigliana et al. (28)
Abscesses, infection, further progression of endometriosis, contamination with content of endometrioma	–	Committee opinion	ASRM (25)
Contamination of follicular fluid with endometrioma contents can affect IVF outcome	314	Retrospective case-control study	Benaglia et al. (29)
Improved IVF Outcomes			
Removal of large (5 cm) endometriomas improves follicular production and number of oocytes retrieved during IVF	26	Retrospective analysis study	Ferrero et al. (30)
Removal of large, greater than 4 cm endometriomas can result in improved fertility outcomes	–	Committee opinion	ASRM (25)
Surgical removal of endometrioma greater than 4 cm increases pregnancy rate and decreases recurrence rate	–	Literature review	Rizk et al. (31)
Lower mean oocyte retrieval and higher cycle cancellation rate during IVF/ICSI in women with endometriomas compared to normal	5753 103 64 1039	Meta-analysis Prospective cohort study Retrospective cohort study Meta-analysis	Hamdan et al. (9) Ashrafi et al. (11) Mao et al. (10) Chun et al. (32)
No difference in fertilization, implantation, and pregnancy rates between pre-ICSI endometrioma surgery and control groups	99	Prospective randomized study	Demirol et al. (33)
Higher live birth rate post-IVF among patients without endometrioma versus with endometrioma	61	Retrospective cohort study	Benaglia et al. (62)
Implantation rate lower in women with endometrioma even of 10–25 mm versus women with simple ovarian cyst	168	Retrospective case-control	Kumbak et al. (8)
Diagnosis of Malignancy at an Early Stage			
Surgical removal avoids risk of malignancy associated with endometrioma, i.e., endometrioid-type	– 23,114	Scientific impact paper Pooled analysis of case-control studies	Jayaprakasan et al./ RCOG (7) Pearce et al. (34)

Abbreviations: ASRM, American Society for Reproductive Medicine; RCOG, Royal College of Obstetricians and Gynecologists.

reports that this rupture may result in abscesses, infection, and further progression of endometriosis as well as contamination of the ovary or peritoneum with endometrioma content. Contamination of follicular fluid via accidental aspiration of endometrioma contents, which occurred in 19/314 total patients (6.1%), resulted in lower adjusted clinical pregnancy (0.63; 95% confidence interval [CI]: 0.49–0.87, $p = .005$) and live birth relative risks (RRs) (0.60; 95% CI: 0.51–0.86, $p = .003$) among the exposed group versus the control group, respectively (29).

Ten articles, with a combined total patient population of 7313, provide evidence that removal of endometrioma prior to IVF may improve IVF outcomes as measured by increase in follicular production, oocyte retrieval, fertilization, implantation, and pregnancy rates, and reduced cycle cancellation rate. Three studies found that removal of large endometriomas improves IVF outcomes (25,30,31). One study found that among patients with unilateral endometrioma measuring greater than 5 cm, the differences in IVF outcomes between the ovary with endometrioma and the healthy ovary were as follows: (a) less follicles produced ovary with endometrioma versus healthy ovary (total number of follicles: 2.6 ± 1.3 and 4.8 ± 2.0, respectively; $p < .0001$); (b) less total number of retrieved oocytes (2.0 ± 1.2 and 4.2 ± 1.7, respectively; $p = < .01$); and (c) less number of oocytes retrieved which are suitable for fertilization (0.5 ± 1.1 and 3.3 ± 1.5, respectively; $p = < .01$) (30). Four studies, including a combined total of 6895 patients, demonstrated a lower mean oocyte retrieval during IVF/intracytoplasmic sperm injection (ICSI) in women with endometriomas compared to normal (standardized mean difference [SMD]) $= -0.23$ [95% CI $= -0.37, -0.10$] [9], [6.6 ± 3.74 versus 10.4 ± 5.25; $p < .001$] [11], [5.7 ± 3.1 versus 10.4 ± 4.4; $p < .05$] [10], [MD $= -1.50$; 95% CI, -2.84 to -0.15, $p = .03$] [32]). Among 64 total patients undergoing IVF, comparing 32 endometrioma cases and 32 tubal-associated cases, there was a higher cycle cancellation rate among endometrioma patients (18.3% and 1.7%, respectively; $p < .05$) (10). One study compared IVF outcomes in 85 patients with endometriomas measuring 10–50 mm versus 83 patients with simple ovarian cyst measuring 10–35 mm found lower implantation rate in women with endometrioma compared to the cyst group (13.9 and 16.4, respectively; $p = .03$) (8). A randomized control study of 99 patients with endometrioma, randomized to ovarian endometrioma cystectomy pre-ICSI or no surgery, found no statistically significant difference in fertilization (86% and 88%, respectively), implantation (16.5% and 18.5%, respectively), and pregnancy rates (34% and 38%, respectively) between pre-ICSI surgery and control groups (33).

Two articles, with a combined patient population of 23,114, provided evidence that removal of endometrioma can also help in diagnosis of malignancy at an early stage. The lifetime probability of developing ovarian cancer increases from 1% to 2% in the presence of endometrioma (7). In their pooled analysis of case-control studies, covering a total patient population of 23,114, Pearce et al. (34) found that endometriosis is associated with increased risks of clear-cell (OR: 3.05; $p < .0001$), low-grade serous (OR: 2.11; $p < .0001$), and endometrioid invasive (OR: 2.04; $p < .0001$) ovarian cancers.

Cons of Surgical Removal of Endometrioma

The total patient population of articles providing evidence against the benefit of endometrioma surgery before ART was 9983. Table 15.3 summarizes the "cons" of surgical removal of endometrioma prior to IVF according to current evidence.

Evidence that surgical removal of endometrioma damages ovarian reserve and function—reduced ovarian reserve; increased gonadotropin stimulation; lower embryo transfer, implantation, and pregnancy rates; increased risk of cycle cancellation—was provided by 16 articles, with a total patient population of 9603. Eight studies provided evidence that surgical removal of endometrioma negatively affects ovarian reserve. These eight studies included a mix of retrospective (14,35), prospective (36,37), meta-analysis/systematic review (9,38,39), and the Royal College of Obstetricians and Gynaecologists (RCOG) scientific impact paper (7). Among 1642 women with infertility across three age groups (younger than 30, 31–35, younger than 36), there was a lower anti-Müllerian hormone (AMH) in patients with previous endometrioma cystectomy (1.23 ± 0.15) as compared to patients with greater than 3 cm endometrioma (2.22 ± 0.23) and patients with nonendometrioma causes of infertility (3.08 ± 0.1) ($p < .0001$) (35). In the retrospective case control of 428 women undergoing IVF, of which 142 had *in situ* endometrioma at time of IVF, 112 had laparoscopic endometrioma cystectomy pre-IVF and 174 women with tubal infertility,

TABLE 15.3

Cons of Surgical Removal of Endometrioma Prior to *In Vitro* Fertilization

	CONS		
Disadvantages of Endometrioma Excision Prior to IVF	**Number of Patients**	**Type of Study(ies)**	**References**
Damage to Ovarian Function and Reserves			
Surgical removal can result in reduced ovarian reserve	428	Retrospect case control study	Bongioanni et al. (14)
	–	Scientific impact paper	Jayaprakasan et al./
	63	Prospective case-control study	RCOG (7)
	1642	Retrospective analysis	Turcuoglu and
	60	Prospective cohort study	Melekoglu (37)
	291	Meta-analysis	Hwu et al. (35)
	5753	Meta-analysis	Uncu et al. (36)
	–	Systematic review	Raffi et al. (38)
			Hamdan et al. (9)
			Somigliana et al. (39)
Decreased postsurgery pregnancy rates as compared with other types of endometriosis	359	Retrospective observational cohort study	Maignien et al. (43)
Laparoscopic removal of endometrioma reduces ovarian reserve (low AMH) and increases FSH	193	Prospective study (2014)	Alborzi et al. (40)
Excision of endometrioma may remove healthy ovarian tissue	326	Retrospective cohort study	Perlman and Kjer (42)
	59	Prospective study	Muzii (41)
Lower mean number oocytes retrieved in women with decreased ovarian reserve caused by endometrioma cystectomy versus idiopathic	167	Retrospective case control study	Roustan et al. (61)
Lower embryo quality and implantation rate found to be associated with endometriotic cyst presence during IVF potentially caused by disease itself and not by the cystic mass	168	Retrospective case-control comparison study	Kumbak et al. (8)
Surgical removal may result in requirement of higher doses of gonadotrophins for ovarian stimulation	–	Scientific impact paper	Jayaprakasan et al./
	99	Randomized controlled trial	RCOG (7)
			Demirol et al. (33)
Limited Added Benefit versus No Surgery			
Ovarian responsiveness and oocyte quality did not significantly differ between endometrioma and nonendometrioma in women undergoing IVF	29	Prospective observational study	Filippi et al. (44)
Oocyte quality not improved after surgery	–	Literature review	Ruiz-Flores and Garcia-Velasco (45)
Presence of endometrioma in controlled ovarian hyperstimulation is not associated with reduced number of oocytes retrieved from affected ovary	243	Retrospective case-control study (unilateral endometrioma)	Almog et al. (60)
Endometrial receptivity similar in endometrioma and control groups; no significant impact on implantation, pregnancy rates	103	Prospective cohort study (unilateral/bilateral, less than 3 cm)	Ashrafi et al. (11)

Abbreviations: AMH, anti-Müllerian hormone; FSH, follicle-stimulating hormone; IVF, *in vitro* fertilization.

there were higher cycle cancellation rates in the cystectomy group (7.5% in endometrioma *in situ*, 9.8% in surgery, 2.9% in tubal factor; $p < .02$) (14). Among 237 patients who were treated for endometrioma via cystectomy, there was a statistically significant decrease in AMH after surgery (mean difference: -1.13 ng/mL; 95% CI: -0.37 to -1.88) (38). Another study of 193 patients with endometriomas undergoing laparoscopic cystectomy showed that surgical removal of endometrioma results in reduced ovarian reserve (AMH preoperative was 3.86 ± 3.58; average postoperative by 9 months was 1.83 ± 2.06; $p < .001$) (40).

Two studies with a combined total patient population of 385 women with endometrioma showed that excision of endometrioma may remove healthy ovarian tissue: according to a histological analysis of endometrioma tissue (59 patients), endometriotic tissue can cover up to 98% of the entire cyst wall (median of 60%) and reach up to 2 mm in depth (41); furthermore, proportionally more endometrioma cystectomies disclosed ovarian stroma versus dermoid cystectomies (80.3% and 17.2%, respectively; $p < .001$) (42). Since their study found higher implantation rates (28% and 19%, respectively; $p = .02$) and embryo transfer rates (79.7% and 70.7%, respectively; $p = .03$) in women with simple cyst versus endometrioma, Kumbak et al. (8) propose that poorer IVF outcomes due to presence of endometriotic cyst during IVF may be attributable to the disease itself rather than the cystic mass (8). Higher doses of gonadotrophin may be required for ovarian stimulation in patients with endometrioma surgically removed pre-IVF versus patients with intact endometrioma (7); this is supported by data from the randomized controlled trial (RCT) of 99 patients with endometrioma, which found that those who had endometrioma surgically removed pre-IVF required more days of stimulation (14.0 ± 2.5, $p < .001$) as compared with those who went directly to IVF (10.8 ± 2.6, $p < .001$) (33). A recent retrospective study investigated ART outcomes in endometrioma versus other types of endometriosis and found that previous endometrioma removal surgery was independently associated with lower pregnancy rates with ART (multivariate analysis OR: 0.39 [0.18–0.89; $p = .16$]) (43).

A limited benefit of surgery—based on ovarian responsiveness, oocyte quality, and endometrial receptivity—was reported by four articles with a combined total patient population of 375. A recent prospective study of women with unilateral endometrioma found no difference in (a) ovarian responsiveness (3.7 ± 2.4 and 4.1 ± 1.7; $p = .54$); (b) number of suitable oocytes (3.1 ± 2.6 and 3.5 ± 2.3; $p = .51$); (c) number of "high-quality" embryos (1.8 ± 2.1 and 1.8 ± 1.4; $p = .00$); and (d) fertilization rate (64% and 64%, $p = 0.96$) between the affected versus intact ovary, respectively (44). Additionally, one literature review concluded that despite often lower numbers of oocytes retrieved, oocyte quality remains the same after surgery (45). Finally, one prospective cohort study of 103 patients proposed that endometrial receptivity and accessibility are similar in the presence of endometrioma and without; comparing normal and affected ovaries in patients with unilateral endometrioma, there is no statistical significance in the difference in fertilization rates (72.4% and 69.6%, $p = .644$) (11).

Surgical Removal of Endometrioma and IVF Outcomes

The association between surgical removal of endometrioma and IVF outcomes as represented by implantation and pregnancy rates was investigated in the literature. Across the four selected studies, 326 patients had endometrioma surgically removed prior to IVF, and 307 patients went directly to IVF. In three of the four studies there is a nonsignificant difference in implantation and pregnancy rates, respectively, between the two groups. The only study reporting a statistically significant result found an 8.2% implantation rate for the surgical removal group versus 12% in the direct-to-IVF group and a 14.9% pregnancy rate in the surgical removal group versus 24.9% in the direct-to-IVF group (15) (Table 15.4).

Discussion

Age Seems to Play a Pivotal Role in the Decision-Making on Endometrioma Management

A retrospective cohort study showed that long-term recurrence of endometriosis is higher among younger women as compared to older women (46). Larger cyst size and younger age were reportedly associated with recurrence in a 2014 retrospective study comparing recurrence rates across subgroups of 550 women

TABLE 15.4

Comparison of Implantation and Pregnancy Rates between Surgical Removal of Endometrioma and No Surgery Prior to *In Vitro* Fertilization

| Reference | Study Design | Endometrioma Patients | | IR | | PR | | SS |
		Surgery Prior to IVF	Directly to IVF	Surgery Prior to IVF (%)	Directly to IVF (%)	Surgery Prior to IVF (%)	Directly to IVF (%)	
Bongioanni et al. (14)	Retrospective case control 2004–2009	112	142	24.6	24.2	44.1	48.4	NS
Coccia et al. (15)	Retrospective cohort 2012–2014	67	72	8.2	12.2	14.9	24.6	$p < 0.05$
Garcia-Velasco et al. (13)	Retrospective matched case control 1997–2001	133	56	12.8	14.1	30	29	NS
Wong et al. (12)	Retrospective cohort study 1995–2002	34	37	18	19	49	36	NS

Abbreviations: IR, implantation rate; PR, pregnancy rate per embryo transfer; SS, statistical significance.

with endometrioma (47). Older age was found to be associated with lower AMH for both cystectomy and control groups (35). Moreover, among women who had endometrioma removed surgically pre-IVF, higher pregnancy rates were found among women aged younger than 35 years (34.5%) as compared to women aged older than 35 years (29.5%) (48). Research to investigate surgery for younger patients presenting with endometrioma is minimal, though transvaginal hydrolaparoscopy has been recommended in adolescent patients with ovarian endometrioma measuring less than 3 cm (49).

Size and Type of Endometrioma Can Influence Appropriateness of Surgical Management

Studies have shown that bilateral and larger than 7 cm endometrioma are more associated with damage to ovarian reserve due to surgery, as compared with unilateral and smaller than 7 cm (50). Regarding laparoscopic surgical removal, damage to ovarian tissue may be proportionally related to the size of endometrioma: excision of cysts measuring greater than 4 cm results in more significant damage (51). Recently, Cocci et al. (15) saw that size is perhaps the most significant factor with regard to ovarian retrieval: for each millimeter increase in size, there is a decline in predicted number of oocytes retrieved. Bilateral ovarian endometrioma removal presents a worse outcome as compared to unilateral: the decline in ovarian reserve, independent of age and destruction of the ovarian parenchyma, still predicts a worse outcome versus unilateral and no surgery (15). Ashrafi et al. (11) found in their prospective cohort study that clinical outcomes, such as fertilization, maturation rate, and total formed embryos, were no different between unilateral endometrioma and no endometrioma. This is consistent with findings by Yu et al. (52) that there were no significant associations found among laterality of endometrioma, ovarian reserve, and pregnancy outcome of IVF/ICSI for women with infertility having undergone laparoscopic cystectomy.

Ovarian Reserves

Most studies employ the stripping technique to treat endometrioma in order to reduce recurrence at the expense of significant damage to healthy ovarian tissue. One retrospective, cross-sectional study found that AMH was not reduced in patients with endometrioma independently, but that it is reduced in patients with previous endometrioma removal surgery (53). In a recent prospective case-control that compared women without endometrioma, women with endometrioma, and women who had surgical removal of endometrioma, it was found that damage to ovarian reserve increases, respectively, across the three groups (37). This presents the possibility that ovarian reserve damage may be proportional to the extent and frequency of surgery; again, with all employing stripping technique. In many of these studies, it is suggested therefore to assess ovarian reserve before undertaking surgical removal of endometrioma, and that this factor may be significant enough to recommend against surgical removal. This recommendation is also consistent with many of the guidelines (Table 15.1). Proper preoperative evaluation, and adequate training and experience of the laparoscopist, are crucial parameters and determine the long-term success of the endoscopic approach (54,55).

Surgery as a Means of Preserving Ovarian Tissue

Surgical removal of endometrioma can enable cryopreservation of ovarian tissue. During surgical removal of endometrioma, healthy fragments of ovarian cortex can be isolated and subsequently cryopreserved, reported to be a highly effective technique for fertility preservation (56). Furthermore, Carrillo et al. (56) recommend that ovarian tissue preservation through cryotherapy is individualized based on factors that overlap with those we have identified as priorities for surgical management of endometrioma: patients' age, ovarian reserve status, presence of bilateral lesions, and repeated surgery.

Since endometrioma progressively damages ovarian reserves, it seems logical that surgical treatment of an endometrioma at smaller size, preferably less than 3 cm, would enormously save healthy ovarian tissue. The problem is that we lack the scientific knowledge to identify those patients who will rapidly deteriorate and develop larger lesions. Gynecologists who perform transvaginal hydrolaparoscopy can operate on small endometrioma less than 3 cm with precision and safety using the 5Fr instruments (57).

Proposal for Individualization of Management by Case Identification

The guidelines display a current lack of standards with regard to clinical decision-making on surgical removal of endometrioma prior to IVF. This is due to a lack of RCTs and consequent inability to create evidence-based guidance to which the global community can align practices. Based on the published literature, clinical assessment of endometrioma should direct to endoscopic establishment of diagnosis. High-risk adolescents in addition to older women seeking fertility treatment can benefit from early diagnosis of endometrioma. It is therefore essential that early identification of eligible patients is improved and standardized through stepwise clinical reasoning and diagnostic testing as presented in Figure 15.2.

New ultrasound scanning machines enable accurate diagnosis of endometrioma as small as 1.5 cm, depending on the knowledge of the operator and the body mass index of the patient. In addition to endometrioma diagnosis, the myometrial and the subendometrial areas should be meticulously examined, as adenomyosis and adenomyotic cysts may be found. Magnetic resonance imaging (MRI) can offer more information regarding the exact position of the lesion and multiple pathologies. Subsequently, hysteroscopic surgery can treat the subendometrial adenomyotic cysts. Proceed to transvaginal hydrolaparoscopy (TVHL) when endometrioma measuring less than 3 cm is identified. Bigger endometrioma can be directed straight to IVF or treated with laparoscopic surgery. Figure 15.2 outlines all options regarding endometrioma management.

Performing standard laparoscopic surgery using 5 mm bipolar instruments on small endometrioma less than 5 cm minimizes the probability of preserving the healthy ovarian tissue. Rather, smaller endometrioma size enables an "easier" operation to be performed that results in less damage to healthy ovarian tissue: for example, surgery with 5F bipolar ball or Argon/Plasma jet laser (57). This reflects the change to transvaginal surgery as a preferable technique over standard laparoscopy in the case of small endometrioma prior to IVF (57). Carrillo et al. (56) summarized various factors influencing postsurgery ovarian reserve, one of which was the competence of the surgeon as measured by the ability of the surgeon to minimize removal of healthy tissue, identify the extent of endometriotic infiltration and the borders of the lesion, and minimize coagulation during the procedure.

Recently, Roman et al. proposed plasma energy ablation as an alternative to cystectomy, finding first in their pilot study (58) of eight women that this technique may spare 90% of healthy ovarian parenchyma that would be removed during cystectomy. In a subsequent study (30 women with unilateral endometrioma and no previous surgery), they found a statistically significant reduction in ovarian volume and AFC ($p < .001$) among women who were operated on by cystectomy as compared to those operated on by plasma energy ablation; this association was independent of age, previous pregnancy, and endometrioma size (59).

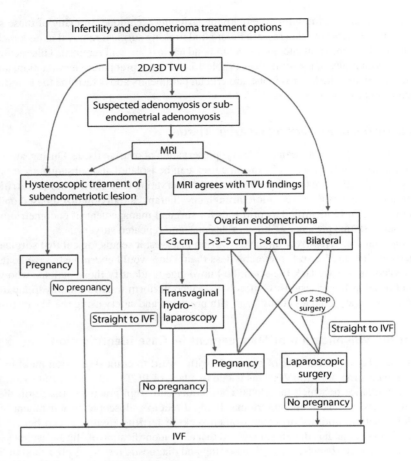

FIGURE 15.2   Infertility and endometrioma treatment options.

Prevention and Early Diagnosis

The scarcity of research and guidelines presents an opportunity for expertise-driven decision-making, but also reveals the urgent need to institute prevention measures. The three areas for prevention are (a) public health, education, and epidemiology; (b) training; and (c) research. Suggested measures for prevention and early treatment of endometrioma are presented in Table 15.5.

TABLE 15.5

Suggested Measures for Prevention and Early Treatment of Endometrioma

Public Health, Education, Epidemiology	Training	Research
Raise awareness among the public	In ultrasound techniques	Initiate randomized controlled trials, prospective studies
Health promotion (nutrition, exercise)	In microsurgery and create specialized centers	Focus on endometrioma surgery techniques
Preventive measures:	In improving early diagnosis and management	Clarify the pathogenesis
Identify high-risk patients based on age, family history, endometriosis markers		Classify possible subtypes
Regular ultrasound monitoring		Consider the possibility of vaccination in high-risk adolescents
Refer patients to endo-clinics		

Preventative medicine interventions focusing on public health, education, and epidemiology will enable a more informed and empowered patient population. This change may result in patients seeking care earlier or trying to reduce their risk factors—both of which can improve outcomes.

Training is a core area of improvement when it comes to improving service delivery to optimize fertility outcomes for these patients. Training in ultrasound techniques is essential in early diagnosis of endometrioma. Training gynecologists to recognize high-risk cases based on risk factors is an additional skill that would be required for effective prevention at the service delivery level.

Finally, as evidenced by the scope of current data, there is an urgent need for research, namely, RCTs and prospective studies. Only with RCTs will evidence-based guidelines be possible.

Limitations of Review

There are important limitations with both quality and quantity of available evidence. The lack of RCTs investigating surgical management of endometrioma and IVF significantly impacts the quality of evidence. Lack of RCTs results in (a) the inability to have internationally consistent guidelines and (b) a high level of inconsistency and contradiction in the pro/con analysis results. Overall, despite endometriosis and endometrioma being two relatively high-yield research areas, endometrioma in IVF is a contemporary issue that is reflected in the limited existing data; available data often refer to endometriosis as whole, which resulted in exclusion from our analysis, and among studies specific to endometrioma, there is very limited material evaluating surgical treatment in the IVF context. This is evidenced by the minimal number of recent studies matching our search criteria on surgical removal of endometrioma versus nonsurgical as pre-IVF treatments (four studies). Despite making exceptions to the exclusion criteria in order to include more studies, the analysis is extremely limited.

There are specific limitations to acknowledge with regard to the literature. The articles cited in the pro/con analysis in which there was insufficient information on study size and patient characteristics may have provided biased or skewed data based on unknown factors relating to population characteristics. Regarding diagnosis of malignancy following surgical removal of endometrioma, for which two articles were cited in Table 15.2, the majority of available data is limited to theoretical deduction or speculation, rather than statistically significant conclusions, due to lack of (prospective studies or RCTs) studies investigating this specific association.

We were limited by default (inclusion criteria) to both implantation and pregnancy rates as indicators of IVF success (Table 15.4); this resulted in excluding numerous studies that appropriately investigated surgical removal of endometrioma prior to IVF but used one, not both, or completely different outcome measures, i.e., embryo transfer, live birth rate, and fertilization rate. Finally, it should be acknowledged that in the study by Wong et al. (12), incorporated in Table 15.4 because it met our criteria, among endometrioma patients who went directly to IVF (37), 23% had undergone a previous excision (12).

Conclusive Remarks

Reputable international gynecological societies published guidelines on diagnosis and treatment of endometriosis and endometrioma in patients with infertility and pain; however, all acknowledge the lack of strong evidence regarding endometrioma management.

Surgery for endometriosis/endometriomas provides good chances for spontaneous pregnancy and increases ART pregnancy rate. Surgery outcomes depend significantly on the patient's age, size of endometrioma, interest in fertility preservation, and the surgeon's skills and experience. Endometriosis is a very aggressive disease that severely compromises the quality of life and fertility of women, and TVHL can provide the best way for early diagnosis and treatment of high-risk patients.

Minimal invasive surgery of the endometriomas offers safe and effective management. Several reports demonstrated that recurrent operations of endometriomas, operating on bilateral endometriomas and big endometriomas larger than 7 cm are associated with diminished pregnancy rates; this evidence must guide the laparoscopist gynecologist in his or her adjustment and modification of surgery protocols and especially the timing of operation. An individualized approach to decision-making on surgical removal of endometrioma and a well-trained laparoscopic surgeon are essential to guiding management and improving fertility outcomes.

REFERENCES

1. Jenkins S, Olive DL, Haney AF. Endometriosis: Pathogenetic implications of the anatomic distribution. *Obstet Gynecol.* 1986;67(3):335–8.
2. Carnahan M, Fedor J, Agarwal A et al. Ovarian endometrioma: Guidelines for selection of cases for surgical treatment or expectant management. *Expert Rev Obstet Gynecol.* 2013;8(1):29–55.
3. Hughesdon P. The structure of endometrial cysts of the ovary. *Br J Obstet Gynecol.* 1957;64(4):481–7.
4. Donnez J, Nisolle M, Smets M et al. Large ovarian endometriomas. *Hum Reprod.* 1996;11(3):641–6.
5. Tanos V, El Akhras S. The effect of hemostatic method on ovarian reserve following endometrioma excision. *Global J Reprod Med.* 2017;1(3):555564.
6. Redwine D. Ovarian endometriosis: A marker for more extensive pelvic and intestinal disease. *Fertil Steril.* 1999;72(2):310–5.
7. Jayaprakasan K, Becker C, Mittal M et al. on behalf of the Royal College of Obstetricians and Gynaecologists. The Effect of Surgery for Endometriomas on Fertility. Scientific Impact Paper No. 55. *Br J Obstet Gynaecol.* 2017;125:e19–28.
8. Kumbak B, Kahraman S, Karlikaya G et al. *In vitro* fertilization in normoresponder patients with endometriomas: Comparison with basal simple ovarian cysts. *Gynecol Obstet Invest.* 2008;65:212–6.
9. Hamdan M, Dunselman G, Li T et al. The impact of endometrioma on IVF/ICSI outcomes: A systematic review and meta-analysis. *Hum Reprod Update.* 2015;21(6):809–25.
10. Mao Y-H, Zhou C, Zaccabri A. Outcome of the IVF for the patients with endometrioma associated infertility. *J Reprod Contracept.* 2009;20(1):19–26.
11. Ashrafi M, Fakheri T, Kiani K et al. Impact of the endometrioma on ovarian response and pregnancy rate in *in vitro* fertilization cycles. *Int J Fertil Steril.* 2014;8(1):29–34.
12. Wong B, Gillman N, Oehninger S et al. Results of *in vitro* fertilization in patients with endometriomas: Is surgical removal beneficial? *Am J Obstet Gynecol.* 2004;191(2):597–605.
13. Garcia-Velasco J, Mahutte N, Corona J et al. Removal of endometriomas before *in vitro* fertilization does not improve fertility outcomes: A matched, case–control study. *Fertil Steril.* 2004;81(5):1194–7.
14. Bongioanni F, Revelli A, Gennarelli G et al. Ovarian endometriomas and IVF: A retrospective case-control study. *Reprod Biol Endocrin.* 2011;9(81).
15. Coccia M, Rizzello F, Capezzuoli T et al. Bilateral endometrioma excision: Surgery-related damage to ovarian reserve. *Reprod Sci.* 2018;20(10):1–8.
16. Dunselman GA, Vermeulen N, Becker C et al. ESHRE guideline: Management of women with endometriosis. *Hum Reprod.* 2014;29(3):400–12.
17. Saridogan E, Becker C, Feki A et al. Recommendations for the surgical treatment of endometriosis—Part 1: Ovarian endometrioma. *Gynecol Surg.* 2017;14:27.
18. Johnson N, Hummelshoj L for World Endometriosis Society Montpellier Consortium. Reply: Consensus on current management of endometriosis. *Hum Reprod.* 2013;28(11):3163–4.
19. Ulrich U, Buchweitz O, Greb R et al. National German Guideline (S2k): Guideline for the diagnosis and treatment of endometriosis: Long version—AWMF Registry No 015-045. *Geburtshilfe Frauenheilkd.* 2014;74:1104–18.
20. Chauffour C, Pouly J, Gremeau A. Endométriome et prise en charge en FIV, RPC Endométriose CNGOF-HAS. *Gynécol Obstét Fertil Sénologie.* 2018;46(3):349–56.
21. Collinet P, Fritel X, Revel-Delhom C et al. Management of endometriosis. *J Gynecol Obstet Hum Reprod.* 2018;47(7):265–74.
22. Endometriosis: diagnosis and management [Internet]. National Institute for Health and Care Guidelines. 2017. Available from: https://www.nice.org.uk/guidance/ng73 (accessed July 6, 2018).
23. American College of Obstetricians and Gynecologists, Falcone T, Lue J. Practice bulletin: Management of endometriosis. *Obstet Gynecol.* 2010;116(1):223–36.
24. Armstrong C. ACOG updates guideline on diagnosis and treatment of endometriosis. *Am Fam Physician.* 2011;83(1):84–5.
25. The Practice Committee of the American Society of Reproductive Medicine. Endometriosis and infertility: A committee opinion. *Fertil Steril.* 2012;98(3):591–8.
26. Leyland D, Casper R, Laberge P et al. SOGC Clinical Practice Guideline. Endometriosis: Diagnosis and management. *Journal of Obstetrics and Gynaecology Canada.* 2010;32(7, Supplement 2):S1–S3.
27. Le T, Giede C, Salem S. Initial evaluation and referral guidelines for management of pelvic/ovarian masses. *J Obstet Gynaecol Can.* 2009;31(7):668–73.

28. Somigliana E, Vercellini P, Vigano P et al. Should endometriomas be treated before IVF-ICSI cycles? *Hum Reprod Update.* 2006;12(1):57–64.

29. Benaglia L, Cardellicchio L, Guarneri C et al. IVF outcome in women with accidental contamination of follicular fluid with endometrioma content. *Eur J Obstet Gynecol Reprod Biol.* 2014; 181:130–4.

30. Ferrero S, Scala C, Tafi E et al. Impact of large ovarian endometriomas on the response to superovulation for *in vitro* fertilization: A retrospective study. *Eur J Obstet Gynecol Reprod Biol.* 2017;213:17–21.

31. Rizk B, Turki R, Lofty H et al. Surgery for endometriosis-associated infertility: Do we exaggerate the magnitude of effect? *Facts Views Vis ObGyn.* 2015;7(2):109–18.

32. Chun Y, Geng Y, Li Y, Chen C, Gao Y. Impact of ovarian endometrioma on ovarian responsiveness and IVF: A systematic review and meta-analysis. *Reprod Biomed Online.* 2015;31(1):9–19. Available from: https://doi.org/10.1016/j.rbmo.2015.03.005

33. Demirol A, Guven S, Baykal C et al. Effect of endometrioma cystectomy on IVF outcome: A prospective randomized study. *Reprod Biomed Online.* 2006;12(5):639–43. Available from: www.rbmonline.com/Article/2182

34. Pearce CL, Templeman C, Rossing MA et al. on behalf of the Ovarian Cancer Association Consortium. Association between endometriosis and risk of histological subtypes of ovarian cancer: A pooled analysis of case-control studies. *Lancet Oncol.* 2012;13(4):385–94.

35. Hwu Y-M, Wu F S-Y, Li S-H et al. The impact of endometrioma and laparoscopic cystectomy on serum anti-Müllerian hormone levels. *Reprod Biol Endocrinol.* 2011;9:80.

36. Uncu G, Kasapoglu I, Ozerkan K et al. Prospective assessment of the impact of endometriomas and their removal on ovarian reserve and determinants of the rate of decline in ovarian reserve. *Hum Reprod.* 2013;28(1):2140–5.

37. Turkcuoglu I, Melekoglu R. The long-term effects of endometrioma surgery on ovarian reserve: A prospective case-control study. *Gynecol Endocrinol.* 2018;34(7):612–5.

38. Raffi F, Metwally M, Amer S. The impact of excision of ovarian endometrioma on ovarian reserve: A systematic review and meta-analysis. *J Clin Endocrinol Metab.* 2012;97(9):3146–54.

39. Somigliana E, Berlanda N, Benaglia L et al. Surgical excision of endometriomas and ovarian reserve: A systematic review on serum anti-Müllerian hormone level modifications. *Fertil Steril.* 2012;98(6): 1531–8.

40. Alborzi S, Keramati P, Younesi M et al. The impact of laparoscopic cystectomy on ovarian reserve in patients with unilateral and bilateral endometriomas. *Fertil Steril.* 2014;101(2):427–34.

41. Muzii L, Bianchi A, Bellati F et al. Histologic analysis of endometriomas: What the surgeon needs to know. *Fertil Steril.* 2007;87(2):362–6.

42. Perlman S, Kjer JJ. Ovarian damage due to cyst removal: A comparison of endometriomas and dermoid cysts. *Acta Obstet Gynecol Scand.* 2016; 95:285–90.

43. Maignien C, Santulli P, Gayet V et al. Prognostic factors for assisted reproductive technology in women with endometriosis-related infertility. *Am J Obstet Gynecol.* 2017;216(3):280. e1-280.e9

44. Filippi F, Benaglia L, Paffoni A et al. Ovarian endometriomas and oocyte quality: Insights from *in vitro* fertilization cycles. *Fertil Steril.* 2014;101(4):988–93.e1

45. Ruiz-Flores F, Garcia-Velasco JA. Is there a benefit for surgery in endometrioma-associated infertility? *Curr Opin Obstet Gynecol.* 2012;24(3):136–40.

46. Tandoi I, Somigliana E, Riparini J et al. High rate of endometriosis recurrence in young women. *J Pediatr Adolesc Gynecol.* 2011;24(6):376–9.

47. Maul LV, Morrison JE, Schollmeyer T et al. Surgical therapy of ovarian endometrioma: Recurrence and pregnancy rates. *JSLS.* 2014;18(3):1–8.

48. Barri PN, Coroleu B, Tur R et al. Endometriosis-associated infertility: Surgery and IVF, a comprehensive therapeutic approach. *Reprod Biomed Online.* 2010;21(2):179–85. Available from: https://doi.org/10.1016/j.rbmo.2010.04.026

49. Gordts St, Puttemans P, Gordts Sy et al. Ovarian endometrioma in the adolescent: A plea for early-stage diagnosis and full surgical treatment. *Gynecol Surg.* 2015;12(1):21–30.

50. Chen Y, Pei H, Chang Y et al. The impact of endometrioma and laparoscopic cystectomy on ovarian reserve and the exploration of related factors assessed by serum anti-Müllerian hormone: A prospective cohort study. *J Ovarian Res.* 2014;7:108. Available from: https://doi.org/10.1186/s13048-014-0108-0

51. Tang Y, Chen SL, Chen X et al. Ovarian damage after laparoscopic endometrioma excision might be related to the size of cyst. *Fertil Steril.* 2013;100(2):464–9.

52. Yu HT, Huang HY, Lee CL et al. Side of ovarian endometrioma does not affect the outcome of *in vitro* fertilization/intracytoplasmic sperm injection in infertile women after laparoscopic cystectomy. *J Obstet Gynaecol Res*. 2015;41(5):717–21.

53. Streuli I, de Ziegler D, Gayet V et al. In women with endometriosis anti-Müllerian hormone levels are decreased only in those with previous endometrioma surgery. *Hum Reprod*. 2012;27(11):3294–303.

54. Pados G, Tsolakidis D, Bontis J. Laparoscopic management of the adnexal mass. *Ann N Y Acad Sci*. 2006;1092:211–28.

55. Jones KD, Sutton CJG. Recurrence of chocolate cysts after laparoscopic ablation. *J Minim Invasive Gynecol*. 2002;9(3):315–20.

56. Carrillo L, Seidman DS, Cittadini E et al. The role of fertility preservation in patients with endometriosis. *J Assist Reprod Genet*. 2016;33(3):317–23.

57. Gordts St, Puttemans P, Gordts Sy et al. Transvaginal endoscopy and small ovarian endometriomas: Unravelling the missing link. *Gynecol Surg*. 2014;11(1):3–7.

58. Roman H, Pura I, Tarta O et al. Vaporization of ovarian endometrioma using plasma energy: Histologic findings of a pilot study. *Fertil Steril*. 2011;95(5):1853–6.e4.

59. Roman H, Auber M, Mokdad C et al. Ovarian endometrioma ablation using plasma energy versus cystectomy: A step toward better preservation of the ovarian parenchyma in women wishing to conceive. *Fertil Steril*. 2011;96(6):1396–400.

60. Almog B, Shehata F, Sheizaf B et al. Effects of ovarian endometrioma on the number of oocytes retrieved for *in vitro* fertilization. *Fertil Steril*. 2011;95(2):525–7.

61. Roustan A, Perrin J, Debals-Gonthier M et al. Surgical diminished ovarian reserve after endometrioma cystectomy versus idiopathic DOR: Comparison of *in vitro* fertilization outcome. *Hum Reprod*. 2015;30(4):840–7.

62. Benaglia L, Bermejo A, Somigliana E et al. Pregnancy outcome in women with endometriomas achieving pregnancy through IVF. *Hum Reprod*. 2012;27(6):1663–7.

Index

A

Accreditation, 87
ACOG, *see* American College of Obstetricians and Gynecologists
Active conception cycle, 21
AFC, *see* Antral follicle count
American College of Obstetricians and Gynecologists (ACOG), 148
American Society for Reproductive Medicine (ASRM), 148
AMH, *see* Anti-Müllerian hormone
Anti-Müllerian hormone (AMH), 1, 4, 104, 151; *see also* Ovarian markers
Antral follicle count (AFC), 6–7; *see also* Ovarian markers
Area under the curve (AUC), 2, 34
Array CGH, 57
ARTs, *see* Assisted reproductive technologies
ASRM, *see* American Society for Reproductive Medicine
Assisted reproductive technologies (ARTs), 4, 33, 86, 104, 107, 116, 128; *see also* Embryo cryopreservation
    live birth rate in autologous cycles, 44
    segmentation concept, 42
AUC, *see* Area under the curve

B

Biopsy, 56
    cleavage-stage embryo, 59
    polar biopsy, 58–59
    trophectoderm biopsy, 59
Blastocyst culture, 107, 113
    baby weight, 112
    congenital malformation, 112
    epigenetic disturbances, 112
    extended culture, 107
    in vitro fertilization outcome, 108–109
    maternal complications, 112
    monozygotic twinning, 112
    perinatal mortalities, 112
    pregnancy rate and live birth rate, 108
    type of media and extended culture, 109–110
Blastocyst transfer, 107
    complications, 111
    premature birth after, 111–112
    problems of extended culture and, 111
BMI, *see* Body mass index
Body mass index (BMI), 49

C

cc2, *see* Second-cell cycle
CCCT, *see* Clomiphene citrate challenge test
CCS, *see* Comprehensive chromosome screening

CGH, *see* Comparative genomic hybridization
Chemokines, 16
Chromosomal mosaicism, 60; *see also* Preimplantation genetic screening
CI, *see* Confidence interval; Corpus luteum
Cleavage-stage embryo, 59
CLIA, *see* Clinical Laboratory Improvement Amendments
Clinical Laboratory Improvement Amendments (CLIA), 19
Clinical pregnancy rate (CPR), 27
Clomiphene citrate challenge test (CCCT), 1, 5; *see also* Ovarian reserve tests
Comparative genomic hybridization (CGH), 56
    array, 57
Comprehensive chromosome screening (CCS), 58
Conception and live births, 12
Confidence interval (CI), 6, 108
Control charts, 92
Controlled ovarian stimulation (COS), 14
Corpus luteum (CL), 71
COS, *see* Controlled ovarian stimulation
CPR, *see* Clinical pregnancy rate
Cryopreservation, 60; *see also* Preimplantation genetic screening
Cytokines, 16

D

DC, *see* Direct cleavage
Decidualization biomarker, 13
Degree of heteroplasmy, 117
DET, *see* Double embryo transfer
DF, *see* DNA fragmentation
DGGG, *see* German Society for Gynecology and Obstetrics
Diagnostic Systems Laboratories Inc. (DSL), 5
Diminished ovarian reserve (DOR), 3
Direct cleavage (DC), 34
DNA fragmentation (DF), 132
Donation, 124
DOR, *see* Diminished ovarian reserve
Double embryo transfer (DET), 63; *see also* Single embryo transfer
DSL, *see* Diagnostic Systems Laboratories Inc.
Dynamic ovarian reserve tests, 5; *see also* Ovarian reserve tests

E

E2, *see* Estradiol
Early pregnancy loss (EPL), 27, 131
ECM, *see* Extracellular matrix
Eeva (Early Embryo Viability Assessment) System, 34
EF, *see* Endometrial fluid

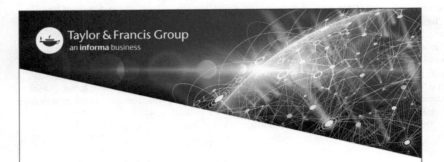